Sterilization of People with Mental Disabilities

STERILIZATION OF PEOPLE WITH MENTAL DISABILITIES

Issues, Perspectives, and Cases

Ellen Brantlinger

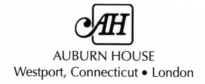

AUBURN HOUSE
Westport, Connecticut • London

Library of Congress Cataloging-in-Publication Data

Brantlinger, Ellen A.
    Sterilization of people with mental disabilities : issues,
perspectives, and cases   /   Ellen Brantlinger.
        p.   cm.
    Includes bibliographical references and index.
    ISBN 0–86569–225–4 (alk. paper)
    1. Sterilization, Eugenic.   2. Mentally handicapped.   I. Title.
    HQ751.B7   1995
    363.9′7—dc20   94–38499

British Library Cataloguing in Publication Data is available.

Library of Congress Catalog Card Number: 94–38499
ISBN: 0–86569–225–4

First published in 1995

Auburn House, 88 Post Road West, Westport, CT 06881
An imprint of Greenwood Publishing Group, Inc.

Printed in the United States of America

The paper used in this book complies with the
Permanent Paper Standard issued by the National
Information Standards Organization (Z39.48–1984).

10 9 8 7 6 5 4 3 2 1

To Readers and Thinkers:

Wilda

Rose

Pam

Mamie

Contents

Preface

This book is focused on a controversial issue about which opinions are ambivalent and volatile. Sterilization of people with mental retardation qualifies as controversial on at least four fronts. First, it is integrally related to sexuality, one of the foremost unmentionable topics about which controversy abounds. Second, it is one of a number of touchy and disputed issues related to fertility and fertility control. Third, the idea of disability makes people uncomfortable; consequently, disability concerns are often denied and ignored. Fourth, it is an area of discrimination in that people with disabilities are treated differently than people without disabilities.

People generally avoid controversial issues, so, as a result, the various problems that cluster around them are ignored and evaded rather than dealt with and resolved. Circumstances embedded in controversy typically involve high stakes and serious risks—in this case, pregnancy, infertility, loss of personal control over the body, and sexually transmitted disease. Therefore, rather than avoiding controversy, it is crucial that our discomforts be confronted and the issues be addressed.

Before getting on with the content of this book, a brief personal history might clarify my incentives for "jumping out of the frying pan into the fire." For whatever reason, my nurturing instincts have always been strong. I "mothered" dolls at an early age, attended to younger neighborhood children, and worried about every problematic social situation I observed. When I was 11, friends who square danced with my parents took on a foster child with Down syndrome. I felt lucky to care for her while they danced. Because of the dire need for foster care for children with disabilities, they soon had acquired many more children. I got my first acquaintance with microcephaly, hydrocephaly, and many forms of cerebral palsy. It is not really surprising, then, that I became a special education teacher. I worked with students with hearing impairments, mental retardation, physical disabilities, and emotional handicaps. During more than 30 years in the field, I experienced the growing pains and external and internal conflicts of special education.

My launch into sexuality issues was different. Perhaps like many of my generation, I experienced the anxieties of limited and distorted information about sex. While teaching—particularly the years teaching adolescents—I could not escape observing the impact of sexual feelings and drives. In one position, after I had been married six years and wanted very much to become pregnant, I witnessed four of my 14- to 19-year-old "educable mentally retarded" girls get pregnant in one year. Although I made attempts at sexuality education, I did it discreetly—school regulations forbade materials with information about sex, and discussions even in response to student questions were forbidden.

While pursuing my doctorate, I needed a course in sociology. My oldest child was born just before the semester started, and I wanted a night course so that my husband could take care of the baby when he was home from work. A course nebulously called "The Family" was listed, but required faculty authorization. The instructor told me that I would have to come in for an interview. It turned out to be the first course taught at the Kinsey Sex Institute. I was 1 of 20 students selected for a very informative and worthwhile class. I suddenly became an "expert," the one asked to do staff development on sexuality topics, something I have continued to do for more than two decades. In doing workshops for parents and staff at residential, educational, vocational, and counseling centers, I found myself exposed to complex and disturbing family and interpersonal situations. In fact, this book is comprised of some "true stories" I heard from participants at workshops or from consultations with people who had heard of my expertise.

Although my nurturing seemed to originate from instinct, my interest in fertility control stemmed from family. My parents were advocates for family planning. As a teacher, my mother was aware of difficult family situations among her students and was convinced that every child should be planned and wanted. My family also worried about overpopulation. They were naturalists, to some extent, and wanted humans to balance with—and not destructively dominate—the nonhuman environment. On trips, family attention was inevitably directed to situations in which "the number of people undermined human dignity." Related to my parents' interest in population control was a sincere respect for the autonomy of individuals. Population control was an educational, and not a political, undertaking.

Fertility also had a personal implication. I had trouble getting and staying pregnant. Our first son's gestation was not an easy one, and after his birth, we decided that I was not ideally suited to pregnancy and would adopt. This decision was consistent with my husband's and my concern about over-population and, more important, about children in need of homes. We adopted a daughter the year after the birth of our first son and a son two years later. Soon after, when in his early thirties, my husband got a vasectomy. I would have insisted on being the one to get a tubal ligation, but at that time, if it was not done immediately after childbirth, it required a hospital stay.

I have been open about personal experiences in an attempt to situate my formal research in the context of my own concerns and interests. In writing this book, however, I found sources that endorse various perspectives on the controversial issues I address. My library search was truly multidisci-plinary: I went to the schools of medicine, physical and health education, public and environmental affairs, law, and education. Issues related to reproduction and mental retardation span these fields, but I integrate and synthesize the perspectives as much as possible. Even though I sought out respected scholarly works, personal perspectives were typically apparent, regardless of how objective the author tried to be. That, in fact, is why I preface this book with a summary of my biases and background. At this point, I must confess that I am not always sure of my position on a number of issues. The more research I did, the more complex the topic became. Thus, I hope to be comprehensive and inclusive, but the reader should not expect tight arguments or easy answers.

Acknowledgments

If I were to adequately acknowledge all of the people who have contributed to this book, the list would be very long. First, it would include the students, family members, and the many professionals that I interviewed. Next, I would have to recognize the contributions of people who attended my workshops and shared stories about their situations with me. Some of these stories are included in the book. Then, it would include the colleagues, support staff, and graduate and undergraduate students at Indiana University with whom I have often discussed topics related to this book. I would have to say a special thanks to the librarians who eased me into new technologies to find the references I researched for the book. There are a few professional colleagues at other universities that I will mention by name. Vivian Correa, Paul Sindelar, and Barbara Ludlow of *Teacher Education and Special Education* have encouraged my work. Thomas Good, editor of the *Elementary School Journal* has been generous with his support. James Halle, editor of the *Journal of the Association for Persons with Severe Handicaps*, not only supported an early publication of my research on sterilization of individuals with mental retardation, but also gave me valuable advice about dealing with the mounds of data I had collected on the subject. I am also appreciative of the patience and editorial support extended by James Sabin, John Harney, Marcia Goldstein, Sherry Goldbecker, and Catherine Lyons of the Greenwood Publishing Group. Last, I am fortunate to have family members and friends who, through their willingness to discuss issues with me, helped me become acquainted with various perspectives on topics. I must thank my mother, Rose Nott Anderson; my sister, Wilda Anderson Obey; my friends, Pam Lohmann and Mamie Merrifield; my children, Andrew, Susan, and Jeremy, and my husband, Patrick Brantlinger for sharing their widsom and their time.

Introduction

This book includes issues, perspectives, and cases related to the sterilization of people with mental retardation. Two inevitable subtopics are sexuality and reproduction. Engaging in intimate relations, getting married, establishing households, and having children are expected of adults in all societies. Youths with intellectual disabilities aspire to marriage and parenthood (Brantlinger, 1985a, 1988a, 1988b), as do adults (Craft & Craft, 1978; Heshusius, 1981; Hingsburger, 1988; Koegel & Edgerton, 1982; Zetlin & Turner, 1985). Yet there is little consensus among the general public, families with a member who is mentally retarded, or professionals who work with people with retardation about whether the domestic activities expected of nondisabled people are appropriate for those with retardation. Setting general goals for sexual expression, marriage, and parenthood for people with intellectual disabilities remains more controversial than endorsing their right to literacy or full employment. Given the general silencing of controversial issues, sexual topics—and especially sterilization—are less often addressed than those in vocational and educational domains (Brantlinger, 1992a; Elkins & Andersen, 1992; Ferguson & Ferguson, 1992; Fine, 1988).

Historically, laws have prevented marriage and childbearing among people judged to be retarded (Burgdorf, 1983; Corbett, 1989; Finger, 1990). Part of the rationale for the extensive development of public institutions with large open wards and constant surveillance during the nineteenth and twentieth centuries was control of "undesirable populations" (Bogdan, 1993; Foucault, 1973; Green & Armstrong, 1993). During the early part of the twentieth century, more than half of the states enacted laws that required people to be sterilized prior to release from institutions (Haavik & Menninger, 1981). Some states still have laws that establish retardation in parents as adequate cause for removing offspring (Thurman, 1985a). Only a few progressive courts refuse to treat disability as prima facie evidence of parental unfitness and as a detriment to the child (Gilhool & Gran, 1985).

DISABILITY DEFINITIONS

Before proceeding to the issues involved in sterilization, it is essential that "mental retardation" be defined, although this is no easy or neutral task. Although the terms are used synonymously and interchangeably, impairments, disabilities, and handicaps can be distinguished. *Impairment* is an abnormality or a loss of psychological, physiological, or anatomical structure or function. *Disability* is a restriction of ability (due to the impairment) to perform an activity within the range considered normal for a human being. *Handicap* is a disadvantage resulting from disability that limits or prevents the fulfillment of normal roles within a culture. The difficulty in describing and measuring disability arises partly from the fragmentary evolution of our current system of benefits and services (Dalley, 1991).

Mental retardation (mental handicap, and previously mental deficiency) is applied to individuals whose intellect develops at below-average rates. The official definition is as follows:

Mental retardation refers to substantial limitations in present functioning. It is characterized by significantly subaverage intellectual functioning, existing concurrently with related limitations in two or more of the following applicable adaptive skill areas: communication, self-care, home living, social skills, community use, self-direction, health and safety, functional academics, leisure, and work. Mental retardation manifests before age 18. (Smith, 1994, 179)

The mental retardation classification applies to a continuum of individuals subdivided into four functioning levels: mild, moderate, severe, and profound; these subcategories are roughly synonymous with the previous educable, trainable, and custodial classifications. People included at each level have distinct, although often overlapping, characteristics and capabilities. Individuals with profound mental retardation have essentially no motor or verbal skills and may be medically fragile and in need of constant care and supervision, whereas those classified mildly handicapped are capable of independent living and competitive employment and may be identified only during their school years because of academic difficulties in that setting (Mercer, 1973). Severe levels of retardation (moderate, severe, profound) fall under the general classification of developmental disability,

which includes cerebral palsy, autism, and seizure disorders. The connect-
ing theme of these conditions is that their impact is substantial, it occurs
early, and it has lifelong implications; people have common needs for
special services from early childhood to death. It must be noted that
heterogeneity within groups is often as great as differences between groups
and that diagnoses, hence prognoses, vary among individuals and over time.

Haavik and Menninger (1981) maintain that mental retardation is an
ambiguous, impractical, and potentially discriminatory classification because it includes such a broad spectrum of people who share so few
characteristics. One of the few common factors among people with mental
retardation—the essence of the disability—is the social (and economic)
consequences of being different from the majority (Stubbins, 1991). Many
(e.g., Gartner & Lipsky, 1987; Skrtic, 1991) have shown that disability is a
social construct that varies historically and situationally. Yuker (1988)
recommends that ways be found to talk about conditions without using
demeaning and disempowering labels.

Social competence is an important component of the construct of mental
retardation because it is individuals' incompetence that draws attention to
them (Edgerton, 1967). Competence is evaluated by comparing everyday
(adaptive) behavior with normed age-level expectations (Grossman, 1983).
Adaptive behavior is part of the 1983 American Association on Mental
Retardation (AAMR) definition of retardation; poor results on adaptive
behavior scales, as well as low scores on intelligence tests (i.e., below 70),
are required for classification as retarded. In an attempt to disentangle
noncognitive components (affect, context) from cognitive components of
the definition, some (Greenspan & Granfield, 1992; Greenspan, Granfield,
& Becker, 1991) recommend that the term "adaptive behavior" be dropped
because it implies character disorders or mental illness and be replaced by
"social intelligence," which they define as ability to understand and deal
with social and interpersonal objects and events. Siperstein (1992) recommends a lifespan approach, which acknowledges that competency results
from complex interactional processes with others and from self-percep-
tions.

Retardation is also defined by ideas about its prevention. Drash (1992)
makes a case for a distinction between biological and functional (cultural
familial, mild) retardation. The latter comprises approximately 80 to 85
percent of mental retardation (Bijou, 1983, p. 224). Prevention of functional
retardation involves providing quality environments (quality education,
nutrition) from birth onward, whereas prevention of biological retardation
involves eliminating genetic abnormalities as well as diseases and trauma
that cause damage to a biological organism. Scott-Jones (1984) points out

problems in distinguishing between environmental and genetic influences on intellectual performance. Much of our knowledge of comparative contributions comes from early childhood education projects and twin studies. Garber and Heber (1982) examined the impact of early intervention on low-income children and found that in spite of significant early IQ gains, follow-up tests of experimental and control subjects showed no significant differences. Schweinhart and Weikart's follow-up (1981) revealed that subjects provided with early educational programs had an advantage in achievement (teacher ratings, grade placement, standardized achievement test scores), but not IQ measures. Based on studies of adopted children, Scarr and Weinberg (1978) placed heritability of IQ at from .4 to .7 and warned that by assuming that all variance in behavior is attributable to environmental influences, social scientists have "fallen into an intervention fallacy" (p. 690). Similarly, Luster and Dubow (1992) found that mother's IQ was a better predictor of a child's IQ than was home environment. Clearly, the nature/nurture controversy lingers.

The most important caveat regarding classifications and causes is that people with disabilities are people first. Regardless of functioning level or degree of impairment, they share many of the same feelings, characteristics, and goals as people without disabilities. Because they are people first, it is important to speak about them as individuals and not just members of disability groups. For convenience and brevity, however, I resort to using "MR" as an abbreviation for "mentally retarded."

PERCEPTIONS OF PEOPLE WITH
MENTAL RETARDATION

Early studies of social perceptions primarily focused on attitudes or complexes of feelings, desires, fears, convictions, and prejudices that structure people's perceptions and play a powerful role in determining behavior (Allport, 1967). Attitude research distinguishes between interpersonal behaviors determined by individual characteristics and intergroup behavior based on category memberships, labels, and stereotypes (Doise, 1990). Wright (1988) discusses a "fundamental negative bias" that steers thoughts about MR people along negative lines (p. 3). Similarly, the "fortune phenomenon" refers to members of devalued groups being regarded as unfortunate even if they do not view themselves so (p. 8). Negative attitudes retain barriers between MR people and others and keep them from things crucial to a dignified life: jobs, housing, relationships, and independence (Lusthaus, 1985).

Livneh (1988) elucidates the determinants and origins of negative attitudes by pointing out the psychodynamic contributing factors. She claims that social ostracism is a guilt-based mechanism for the "able-bodied" to justify their good fortune in reaping the rewards of able status by pointing out MR persons' inferiority and unworthiness (p. 36). The public may expect disabled people to suffer as a sign that the assets they lack are valuable and important (Katz, Hass, & Bailey, 1988).

Assigning individuals disability status designates them "Others"; that is, objects of the viewers' experience, but not individuals with whom one might identify (Sherwin, 1992a; Wendell, 1992; Wolfensberger, 1992). People project rejected aspects of themselves or fears of what they do not want to be onto "Others" (Griffin, 1981). As "Others," "the disabled" evoke pity, fear, and patronizing attitudes—praise may be heaped on them for carrying out normal acts (Barnes, 1991, pp. 199–201).

Although stereotypes supposedly result from ignorance and lack of contact, direct-care workers have been found to have less favorable perceptions of MR people than the lay public (Geskie & Salasek, 1988; Spicker, 1984; Yuker, 1988). Attitudes in the workplace are affected by symbolic overtones of role expectations as well as asymmetry of power relations (Wiseman, 1979). The stigma of residents is generalized to care providers; those who work with MR people (mainly women) are overworked and underpaid, and there is a delicate relationship between worker and client (Finch, 1991; Spicker, 1984). Based on Foucault's (1973) theory that the technical knowledge of social science professionals has taken the place of brute force in controlling people, Stubbins (1991) observes that as surrogates of their agencies, staff are allowed by a "mesh of power relations" to define problems, set agendas, and regulate social reality to serve their own interests rather than those of their MR clients (pp. 22–25).

The minority-group paradigm compares how the conditions of segregation, discrimination, and subordination of MR people are similar to those of certain ethnic, racial, social class, and gender groups. As with other inferiorized groups, collective action, public awareness, and advocacy campaigns result in recognition of rights as well as improved community access and accommodation (Biklen, 1986; Bogdan, 1988). Yet, in spite of antidiscrimination campaigns, much of the general public retains ambivalent and conflicting feelings about MR individuals (Yuker, 1988). They are suspicious about MR people living among them—especially in group homes in their neighborhoods—and hold to the idea that they are not really normal (Dartington, Miller, & Gwynne, 1981; Lusthaus, 1985; Nelson, 1988). Underlying positive statements about MR people are unverbalized rejecting thoughts (Katz, Hass, & Bailey, 1988). Unlike other minorities, problems of MR people cannot be completely externalized (Dalley, 1991). Even if prejudice were eradicated, someone with Down syndrome, for example, might not be entirely pleased to have the condition.

Certain writers (e.g., Barnes, 1991; Boylan, 1991; Goffman, 1963; Livneh, 1991; Lusthaus, 1985; Wiseman, 1979; Wright, 1988; Yuker, 1988) externalize disability, attributing its existence to sociopolitical factors rather than individuals' problems. Others (e.g., Gliedman & Roth, 1980; Hahn, 1987, 1991) concur that external factors connected with prejudice may be more debilitating than disability itself. Dalley (1991) separates radicals, who stress the excluding role of disabling societies and resist seeing disability as a problem in itself, from reformers, who accept that impairments may be problems in their own right, although they acknowledge society compounds them.

As serious as others' attitudes, the negative associations of labels are internalized by those classified, so that stigma becomes part of their conscious and unconscious intrapsychic life (Edgerton, 1967; Goffman, 1963; Wright, 1959). Davis, Anderson, Linkowski, Berger, and Feinstein (1991) observe exaggerated self-consciousness and obsession with others' reactions to themselves among MR people. Wright's (1988) theory of the "spread effect" of labels is pertinent to insiders' and outsiders' perceptions. Labels apply to specific inabilities, but spread to imply global incompetence. Status depends on productivity and achievement; marginalization, degradation, and personal guilt for being a burden to others result from lack of success (Finch, 1991).

Language perpetuates bias. Derrida's (1976) deconstruction of technical terms and Foucault's (1973) semantics approach make us aware of the subjective character of knowledge formation about disability (Stubbins, 1991). Psychological terms structure and dominate disability meanings and reduce individuals to disability definitions (Hahn, 1991). Wendell (1989) urges an understanding of the degree to which medicine has constructed social attitudes that lead people with certain biological conditions to feel alienated from their bodies and leave them frustrated by a socially supported sense of failure.

Countering the predominantly negative literature about disability, Gleason (1989) maintains that some institutional staff are sincerely interested in the purposeful actions of MR residents, and Alaszewski and Ong (1990) find they become genuinely fond of MR individuals and get pleasure from caring for them. Taylor and Bogdan (1991) refer to this as the "sociology of acceptance," and Wright (1988) calls it a "constructive view of living with disability" (p. 19). Currently, the belief that MR people should have freedom of choice, autonomy from interference, and independence in goal setting pervades the scholarly and lay literature (e.g., Dalley, 1991; Turnbull & Turnbull, 1979, 1985; Wolfensberger, 1992). Trends in care providing incorporate such principles as self-determination, the maintenance of environments that do not impose excessive restrictions, arrangements that bring persons as close as possible to the social and cultural mainstream, and protection of human and legal rights (Neufeld, 1979). Although the normalization principle predominates in the scholarly and lay literature, Boggs (1978) suggests that some like the idea because it "glosses over realities of difference" (p. 52). Rejecting it as the appropriate goal for her profoundly MR son, Boggs tries to see the world from his point of view and think of the kind of environment that would minimize boredom and loneliness and enhance his sense of dominance.

Attitudes Toward the Sexuality of MR Individuals

The controversial nature of issues related to sexuality and birth control, embedded in various views of MR people, produces attitudes about the sexuality of MR people that are discordant and strongly felt. Many see disability and sexuality as incompatible concepts—the first automatically precluding the second (O'Toole & Bregante, 1992). An argument used by those opposed to sterilization of MR people is that they should not be engaging in sexual intercourse—that mental incapacity keeps them in a juvenile, hence asexual, status. Because sexual expression is denied, need for contraception is ignored. Not only does this stance ignore the desires of MR people, but also it is unrealistic. Suppression of sexual expression may negatively affect social behaviors (Abelson & Johnson, 1969).

Although MR individuals' right to sexual expression and social intimacy has been established by laws, litigation, and special codes, their sexual lives are inevitably governed by the feelings and behaviors of those who care for them. The negative and controlling attitudes that shape the supervisory styles and decision making of those who work with MR people are as important as any written policy or enacted legislation in influencing practice (Brantlinger, 1983, 1985a, 1987a, 1992a, 1992b; Dalley & Berthoud, 1992; Ducharme & Gill, 1991). Agencies rarely have stated policies about sexual behaviors (Dalley, 1991; Fleming, 1979; Humm-Delgado, 1979). Only 23 percent of staff members from private residential facilities for MR persons report having guidelines, although 70 percent want them (Saunders, 1979). Often direct-contact staff think there is a policy when there is none (Brantlinger, 1983; Deisher, 1973). Without administrative guidelines, an influential factor in determining sexual policy in supervised settings for MR people continues to be direct-contact workers' attitudes about sex and their clients. If there is a cultural or educational lag among care providers, or if MR people are restricted in sexual expression because of either real or perceived contextual constraints, rights continue to be denied.

There is, in fact, considerable evidence of ignorance and bias about sexuality among professionals and care providers (e.g., Brantlinger, 1983, 1988a, 1988b, 1992a; Geskie & Salasek, 1988; Katz, Hass, & Bailey, 1988; Stubbins, 1988; Wright, 1988). Administrators are unduly cautious in developing policy governing sexual behaviors and avoid responsibility for providing sexuality education programs (Brantlinger, 1991, 1992a; Dalley, 1991; Fine, 1988; Gordon, 1976); hence, sexual behaviors are suppressed (Birenbaum & Re, 1979; Mitchell, Doctor, & Butler, 1978; Nigro, 1977; Scheerenberger & Felsenthal, 1977). Attitudes toward sexuality vary according to personal characteristics as well as type of residential setting in which staff work (Brantlinger, 1983). Group home staff are more liberal (i.e., they believe that sexual expression is positive and MR individuals have the right to be sexually active) than institution staff, and nursing-home employees are the most conservative. Generally, older workers are more conservative than younger ones, workers with more education are more liberal than those with less, and people who judge themselves to be very religious are more conservative than their less religious counterparts.

Attitudes change in a liberal direction as a function of in-service workshops (Brantlinger, 1987a). In addition to changes measured on an attitude scale, through personal communication I learned that many practices had changed as a result of training: Masturbation by clients in their beds at night was no longer stopped or punished, staff arranged for private times for clients on certain wards and provided them with contraception, a more tolerant attitude toward homosexuals had been adopted (instances of homosexual behavior were not always penalized by sending clients to the punitive "behavior modification ward"), and clients suspected of being unwilling participants in sexual activities were encouraged to reject unwanted advances.

STATUS OF STERILIZATION FOR MR INDIVIDUALS

The pendulum has swung away from compulsory sterilization of MR people. Nevertheless, there still is discrimination. Bias now resides in restrictions of access to sterilization. Numerous phenomena prevent access, including physicians' concerns about legal or publicity repercussions, a conservative judicial system, and a far-reaching federal regulation issued by the Department of Health, Education, and Welfare (now the Department of Health and Human Services) in 1979, which prohibits the use of federal money for sterilizations of persons under age 21, institutionalized persons, and persons declared mentally incompetent (Levine & Veatch, 1984). According to Petchesky (1979), the regulation was passed in recognition of the danger that caretakers, including parents, might choose sterilization to avoid the more difficult responsibilities of sex education. Petchesky believes the regulation prevents sterilization irrespective of the best interests of the individual and could lead to abuse.

It must be countered that people choose to be sterilized because it is a relatively safe, cheap, long-term birth control method. In other words, it has advantages. At the same time that the general public is increasingly selecting sterilization (Sloan, 1988), MR people are denied access to it. In *In re Nietro* (1985), the California Supreme Court maintained that prohibiting sterilization of all MR persons denied their right to privacy (Elkins & Andersen, 1992). Principles of normalization provide armature to arguments for access to sterilization. In opposition to restrictions, others prefer an approach that takes into account particular situations of MR individuals.

AUTHOR'S PERSPECTIVE

Modern trends in caring for MR individuals incorporate principles of normalization and sensitivity to safeguarding civil and human rights of MR people. Concurrently, laws regulating sexual behaviors have been less frequently enforced in recognition of individuals' rights to engage in behaviors in which there is mutual consent and in which there is no victim; there is greater tolerance for personal choice in values and orientations (Grant, 1992; Nathanson, 1991; Reiss, 1970; Sloan, 1988). In spite of almost universal affirmation of the goal of normalization for MR persons, a persistent problem remains of how to achieve it in the field. Literature about life circumstances of MR people reveals that supervision continues to be restrictive and suppressive about sex even when other facets of the people's lives are fairly normalized. Care providers determine unwritten policy by encouraging and discouraging sexual behaviors according to their own tastes, personal morals, and convenience. It is essential that those in contact and control be made aware of the basic human, sexual, and birth control needs and rights of MR individuals. A major goal of this book is to get pertinent information about sexuality and sterilization to professionals, parents, and others who, in some way, influence MR individuals.

SCOPE AND PLAN OF THE BOOK

With the hope of filling the gaps left by the avoidance of the controversial issue of sterilization of MR people, this book includes issues, perspectives, and cases related to sexuality, relationships, parenting, birth control, and sterilization. This chapter has addressed definitions of mental retardation and common attitudes toward MR people. Although the cases involving sterilization of MR individuals in Part III may comprise the most important part of the book, it is necessary to ground these cases in a thorough understanding of the theoretical and practical issues surrounding sexuality and sterilization. In an attempt to round out knowledge of the topics, a variety of research and theoretical reports from a number of disciplines is considered.

Part I includes four chapters that introduce issues related to sterilization. Chapter 1 consists of an overview of the growth and decline of the eugenics movement. In addition to examining eugenics movements explicitly related to genetic control of heredity, this chapter explores the types of modern thought and actions that fall within the realm of eugenics thinking. Chapter 2 covers constitutional law, special legal codes, federal and state legislation, and case law as they relate to MR people, and especially to sterilization of MR individuals. Legal developments in the United States document a rich history of thinking about disability, sexuality, childbearing, and child rearing. This chapter includes ideas about determining consent for sterilization when someone is too cognitively limited to understand the issues and make decisions.

In Chapter 3, ethical issues related to health care, birth control, and sterilization are addressed. Debates in medical ethics and feminist analyses of control over decision making, informed consent, and access to medical services are summarized. The feminist discourse on health care is pertinent because it addresses power relations that affect MR people. Chapter 4 delineates the most common forms of birth control and types of sterilization. An evaluation of the benefits and drawbacks of these methods for MR individuals is included.

Each of the four chapters in Part II describes a different perspective related to sexuality, reproduction, and sterilization of MR people. Chapter 5 covers family adjustment and family members' reactions to the member with disabilities. Although much of the discussion in this chapter is not directly related to sexuality and procreation, it provides background information about the impact of an MR member on family life. Chapter 6 reviews postschool and postinstitution adjustment studies, particularly, but not solely, focusing on the findings related to sexuality, fertility control, marriage, and parenting. It also reviews studies of parenting competencies of MR individuals as well as parenting interventions for those who experience problems in parental roles. Chapter 7 includes the results of my own studies of mild MR adolescents and teachers of secondary MR students. Similarly,

Chapter 8 presents a study that examined the extent of professionals' involvement with MR people and their awareness of cases in which MR persons were sterilized.

Part III consists of two chapters, each including five cases in which decisions were made about sterilization. Descriptions are based on actual circumstances of MR people. The cases are presented as they occurred; hence, they reflect current practice related to sterilization in a particular geographical area. The discussions of issues and perspectives in Parts I and II provide the background for readers to form their own opinions about the appropriateness of decisions about sterilization in each case.

Chapter 9 first describes two quite different women, supposedly classified mildly MR. It also includes three cases of individuals who not only were mildly MR, but also had emotional problems. When possible, sufficient background is supplied about their early socialization to allow the reader to make judgments about the causes of their problems as well as prognoses about their futures. Chapter 10 includes three individuals who tested in the moderate range of mental retardation, but were fairly well adjusted in their respective situations. In these cases, the families' roles in decision making about sterilization come to the fore. The last two cases involve the distinct circumstances and rationales for sterilization of MR adolescents with autism.

Part I

ISSUES

1

Historical and Theoretical Overview of the Eugenics Movement

The science of eugenics developed and eugenics movements proliferated during the latter half of the nineteenth century and continued through the middle of the twentieth century. Although the word "genetic" was not coined until 1905, the term "eugenics" was adapted from the Greek word *eugenes* (meaning "wellborn") by British scientist Francis Galton in 1883 to encompass the social uses to which knowledge of heredity could be put in order to achieve the goal of "better breeding" (Stepan, 1991, pp. 1, 11). Later, eugenics became a movement to improve the human race or to "preserve the purity" of certain groups (Mazumdar, 1992).

Stepan notes that the growing economic competition among nations and the rise in demands from previously marginalized working class and women's groups during the last three decades of the nineteenth century caused the early optimism of the mid-Victorian period to give way to widespread pessimism about modern life. During the Boer War (1899–1902), the "discovery" that many enlisted men were "unfit" for military service because of low scores on screening tests heightened eugenicists' fears (Abbott & Sapsford, 1990). Science, a highly social activity, is not sealed off from the values of the society in which it is practiced (Harding, 1993). The science of eugenics figured prominently in recommending solutions for the social ills of modern life. Darwin's theories of evolution with their concepts of "survival of the fittest" and "natural selection in breeding" (1871, 1898) resulted in, or at least coincided with, beliefs about biological determinism in heredity (social Darwinism) and fears of individual and societal deterioration.

Different theories about the nature of genetic influence have been endorsed over time. Dugdale (1877) popularized "familial" social inefficiency by noting the interconnectedness and probable heritability of "feeblemind-edness," "insanity," and other undesirable traits (cited in Cranefield, 1966, p. 12). Mid-nineteenth-century scientists hypothesized that negative conditions resulted from a progressive loss of "vital energy" from one generation to the next (Cranefield, 1966). Half a century later, Tredgold (1903) conjectured that deterioration of germinal plasm, diminishing the general physical and mental health of offspring, was caused by such harmful parental conditions as consumption, syphilis, and alcoholism. Eugenics created and gave scientific and social meaning to new objects of study—unfit or "dysgenic" groups (Stepan, 1991, p. 11).

Fernald (1896), founder and director of an institution for MR individuals in Massachusetts, described a particular dysgenic group:

The feebleminded are a parasitic, predatory class, never capable of self-support, or of managing their own affairs. Feebleminded women are almost invariably immoral and if at large usually become carriers of venereal disease or give birth to children who are as defective as themselves. Every feebleminded person, especially the high-grade imbecile, is a potential criminal, needing only the proper environment and opportunity for the development and expression of his criminal tendencies. (p. 67)

Referring to a chart showing the defectives in Isadore's family tree, Goddard (1914) somewhat more positively noted:

Isadore was always cheerful, never quarrelsome, was active and obedient, affectionate, truthful, good tempered, not destructive, and was rather mischievous. This boy ran away [from the institution] some time since, and his whereabouts are now unknown. It is safe to say that if he gets into trouble no judge or jury is likely to believe that he is not thoroughly responsible for anything he may do. No one but experts in the field of feeble-mindedness would suspect anything wrong with him. He is the kind of case that makes the skeptics believe that the Binet tests are absolutely wrong, but ten years experience with him in an institution proves beyond a shadow of a doubt that he is as truly mentally defective as any boy in school. He will undoubtedly marry or become a father and the consequences are easily guessed by reference to the chart. (p. 112)

About Mary, Goddard said:

Mary is a splendid illustration of that type of girl that is most dangerous in society. Pretty and attractive and with just enough training to enable her to make a fair appearance she deceives the very elect as to her capacity. Responsibilities would be placed on her which she could never carry. In institutional life she is happy and useful. Unprotected she would be degraded, degenerate, and the mother of defectives. (p. 93)

Dugdale (1877), Estabrook (1916), and Goddard (1912) used scientific analysis of family genealogies to document the inheritability of such degeneracies as alcoholism, illegitimacy, sexual immorality, prostitution, criminality, feeblemindedness, and epilepsy. There was widespread fear that these conditions were on the rise, they would spread perniciously, and their unchecked growth would place an insurmountable burden on others; that degenerates would swamp society and pull others down with them.

Historical reports highlight the writings of individual eugenicists. From a modern perspective the bias and paternalism blatant in the writings of Goddard seem ludicrous. It is easily assumed that bizarre notions were unique to quoted individuals; however, a personalized approach villainizes certain writers by implying that these beliefs were peculiar to them or that they unduly influenced social institutions and practices. A closer look at the period reveals the ubiquitous popularity of eugenic ideas (Kevles, 1987; Mazumdar, 1992; Stepan, 1991) and suggests that those quoted, if not actually spokespersons, were highly representative of the thinking of their time. Literally dozens of journals with eugenics-related titles published during the late nineteenth and early twentieth centuries line library shelves. Some of these changed names after World War II; for example, the *Eugenics Quarterly* became the *Journal of Social Biology* (Spallone, 1989, p. 143).

In order to understand social trends such as the eugenics movement, it is important to consider the nature of "widespread beliefs" and similar concepts that dominate academic disciplines under a variety of names: "myth" from anthropology, "norm" from sociology, "collective mental representation" and "social construct" from social psychology, and "stereotype" from psychology (Bethlehem, 1990; Fraser & Gaskell, 1990). Widespread beliefs sanction, justify, and undergird particular cultural practices. "Intergroup attribution" theory clarifies how members of social groups explain the behavior and social conditions of members of their own ("normal") and other ("abnormal") groups (Jaspars & Hewstone, 1990). Beliefs about the nature and causes of disability influence social systems and public policy (Pascoe, 1990). In the name of eugenics, powerful groups sought to encourage reproduction among "fit" individuals and groups (people like themselves) and prevent the "unfit" from doing the same. Instead of protecting the rights of minorities, governments in the United States acted to protect dominant groups from them. Barnes (1991) maintains that the philosophy of social Darwinism served the purpose of dispelling and allaying qualms of the rich about their not helping the poor by assuring them that suffering was inevitable and the fault of those who suffered.

Although "institution" in this book usually refers to large residential and treatment facilities designed to train, care for, and contain MR people

(Stone, 1985), other definitions are relevant. Jasso (1991) defines institutions as patterned individual and/or social behaviors—the prevailing ways of doing something—that vary across space and time (p. 155). Somewhat narrowing this focus, a social welfare institution is one purported to promote the welfare of the population. It is essential to note the relativity of the idea of "promoting the social welfare of the population," because, as illustrated by the eugenics movement, ideas about what promotes social welfare look radically different now than they did 100 years ago. In *The Hour of Eugenics*, Stepan (1991) documents how the eugenics movement took different forms in Latin America than in England and the United States. Certainly, even when eugenic sterilization was at its prime, it looked different to someone forced to be sterilized than it did to those who advocated and controlled sterilization.

New and old ideas get assembled and reassembled, modified, and elaborated on by specific groups of people for specific purposes and become part of the complex fabric of social and political life (Stepan, 1991). The eugenics movement was not just in the minds of a few writers of the period, but was a social phenomenon thoroughly entrenched in the beliefs of society. A broad base of people—not only those responsible for running the government and social institutions, but also those served by them—held views of retardation, heredity, and the future that made it possible to override the rights of freedom of movement and procreation of MR individuals and to incarcerate and sterilize them not only without their consent or even their knowledge, but also usually with no attention given to their own preferences or best interests. In retrospect, it seems reasonable to assume that even families whose members were sterilized must have condoned—or at least tolerated—eugenics practices. At this time, at least on a conscious level, ideas that smack of eugenics are promptly dismissed.

EUGENIC INFLUENCES ON MR INDIVIDUALS

When eugenics notions were canonized into law, they produced coercive environments for MR people. In 1913, the British Mental Deficiency Act made provisions for lifelong institutional segregation of the feebleminded (Abbott & Sapsford, 1990, p. 141). Predominant solutions for counteracting such undesirable inheritable traits as mental retardation were gender segregation—accomplished through widespread institutionalization—and involuntary sterilization. Justifications for eugenic control were partly based on the paternalistic notion that some people have to be controlled for their own well-being (Beauchamp & Pinkard, 1983). As Goddard (1914) said: "Mollie has not much intellect and if out in the world would undoubtedly be the victim of bad men just as her mother and grandmother were" (p. 143), and "Tamar had a strong tendency toward immorality and only by careful custodial care was she saved" (p. 156). Sterilization and incarceration were also based on the idea that MR individuals were detrimental to others and so had to be managed for the good of society. Goddard concluded case descriptions with the warning that, if unchecked by institutional care or sterilization, this person would become "criminal" and the "parent of defectives." Pascoe (1990) points out that the urge to impose middle-class authority by containing the underclasses was prevalent in the form of creating reservations for Native Americans, settlement houses for wayward women, and poor farms for the unemployed.

During the first half of the twentieth century, it was typical for children with moderate and severe forms of retardation to be institutionalized at birth and for those in the mild ranges to be committed during adolescence when they showed signs of interest in sexual expression. State hospitals ensured separation of the sexes by housing inmates on single-gender wards and then reinforced this tactic by installing elaborate lighting arrangements on the grounds and fortifying with fences to keep men and women apart (Gordon, 1976). Morris (1969) quoted a British psychiatrist in charge of a mental subnormality hospital who had strong misgivings about rehabilitation hostels (group homes):

These hospitals should in every case be separated for sexual problems loom high in the lives of these patients; homosexuality, child assault, rape, exposure with the men, prostitution and some perversion with the women. Ideally the men's hostel should be in one town and the women's in a neighboring one. They should be at least two or three miles apart. Social contacts between the two hostels should be discouraged to prevent illicit affairs and marriages among the subnormal. (p. 20)

In addition to enforcing physical separation, hospital staff utilized psychological methods of convincing residents of the wrongfulness of sexual relationships (Carruth, 1973; Heshusius, 1981; Mattinson, 1971; Morris, 1969). As Kratter and Thorne (1957), superintendents of a training school, admitted: "Basically boy and girl relationships for many years within the institution had been frowned upon. A moral code prohibited and enforced through punishment the holding of hands, having secret conversations together, and kissing was almost regarded as an unforgivable sin" (p. 47).

At least half of the states had legislation enabling involuntary sterilization not only of MR people, but of criminals, epileptics, and promiscuous people as well (Gilhool & Gran, 1985). Moreover, involuntary sterilizations occurred at the same rate in states with no legislation (Haavik & Menninger, 1981).

The annual rate of involuntary sterilizations of MR people peaked in the 1930s (Smith, 1989), but the practice continued to be prevalent through the 1950s (Bass, 1978; Whitcraft & Jones, 1974). Between 1907 and 1945, 70,000 individuals were sterilized (Kevles, 1987, p. 111). Sterilization could be initiated by parents, but state-level legal decrees often required it during MR persons' childbearing years as a precondition for release. It was reasoned that with their reproductive capacity controlled, MR individuals might succeed in communities and that would allow the termination of expensive institutional care. Even when sterilization supposedly involved free and informed consent, there was little chance of noncoerciveness in the context of MR persons tempted with offers of freedom and intimidated by threats of extended confinement (Beauchamp & Pinkard, 1983).

EUGENICS RATIONALE IN CURRENT THINKING

A major theme in this book is that social conscience and social movements are neither universal nor static, but are contested and often superseded by opposing movements that at some point seemed inconsequential and benign. Individuals or groups have fairly distinct reasons for advocating eugenics. In 1935, Alva Myrdal, a Swedish pioneer in population policies, called for strengthening sterilization laws not as a method of preserving Swedish racial quality, but as a means of protecting against individual suffering caused by bad heredity (cited in Trombley, 1988, p. 159). The Swiss and Danes also had eugenics programs prior to the Nazis, but their rationales seemed motivated by a desire to make societal living conditions tolerable for everybody rather than by a racist belief in Nordic superiority (Stepan, 1991, p. 30). Currently, people may not readily admit that they actually do believe in some form of eugenics because of a worry that such ideas are politically incorrect. Although eugenics advocates are not dominant or very visible, there are remnants of old movements or starts of related movements today. And there may be wisdom to certain aspects of eugenics positions. Six grounds can be envisioned for restricting procreation: transmission of disease, unwillingness to provide proper prenatal care, nonmarriage, inability to rear children, likelihood of psychological or physical harm to children, and overpopulation.

Genetic Diseases and Improper Prenatal Conditions

Brody (1987) delineates arguments for genetic engineering, including the utilitarian position that benefits would accrue to humans from lessening genetic disease. By keeping people with inherited diseases alive and allowing them to reproduce, the gene pool is gradually polluted, or at least undesirable conditions are not eliminated. An extension of this is that active measures are needed to counteract genetic deterioration of the species. Brody maintains that a decision to prevent certain people from reproducing would be using advanced technology and medical knowledge rationally, rather than in a willy nilly fashion.

Society's right to control the transmission of disease has been expressed in quarantining individuals with contagious diseases, preventing immigrants with certain diseases from entering the country, and arresting and prosecuting individuals who knowingly infect others with dangerous contagious diseases. Carriers of inheritable diseases have not been legally deterred from childbearing, but there is social pressure not to reproduce.

In preventing the transmission of mental retardation to offspring, it first must be questioned whether mental retardation is a disease. Although the medical model that conceptualizes retardation as a pathological condition within individuals predominates, many (e.g., Gartner & Lipsky, 1987; Skrtic, 1991; Sleeter, 1986) argue that it is instead a social construct that evolved to deal with differences in intellectual competence. To undergird their assertions, these writers point to the evolution of disability classification systems and varying responses to human diversity over time. Nevertheless, it seems that mental retardation should, if possible, be prevented. Federally sponsored early childhood programs have the explicit goal of preventing school failure and handicap classification by better preparing children for school (Garber & Heber, 1982; Ramey & Campbell, 1984). Genetic counseling and prenatal screening also are based on the assumption that people want to prevent defects in offspring and/or prevent the birth of defective offspring.

Whether or not mental retardation is viewed/construed as a disease, approaches to prevention remain problematic. In the first place, most MR children are born to parents of normal intelligence, and the offsprings' retardation cannot be predicted prenatally (Andron & Tymchuk, 1987; Paul & Simeonsson, 1993). Second, only a small percentage of identified cases of mental retardation have known genetic causes (Thoene, Higgins, Krieger, Schnickel, & Weiss, 1981). Third, MR parents often have children of normal intelligence (Reed & Reed, 1965; Thurman, 1985b). Hence, eugenics practices are likely to be less effective in preventing retardation than proponents would have us believe.

Although the Supreme Court's 1992 *Planned Parenthood v. Casey* decision upheld women's right to abortion by reconfirming the 1973 *Roe v. Wade* decision, a few recent cases indicate that the law can be interpreted such that states have an obligation to protect fetuses by prosecuting women in situations in which they decide to proceed with pregnancies and then act in ways that damage the fetus (Colker, 1992; Sandmaier, 1992). Legal intervention against pregnant women can be argued on two grounds. First, because the state will probably shoulder some or all of the costs of children injured by their mothers' behaviors during gestation—perhaps even having to take custody of the children and provide for them their entire lives—the state has the right to regulate mothers' behaviors in order to prevent costly damage (Berkowitz & Berkowitz, 1985). The nonmonetary argument is that the state must protect even potential citizens from harm from others (Sutherland, 1990). Harmful conduct during pregnancy (smoking, drinking, taking drugs) might be perceived as child abuse. Failing to get prenatal care or refusing to eat a balanced and nutritious diet might then be seen as child neglect. These arguments are based on the assumptions that children have the right to be born healthy and that states have the right to avoid financial or social burdens—and that these rights override a woman's liberty to do as she pleases during pregnancy. In the absence of legal mandate, the social pressure of advertisements against smoking and drinking during pregnancy exerts control over individuals. Some feminists argue against any notion of states' right to control pregnant women's actions.

Inability to Rear Children and Likelihood of Doing Harm

At the time that involuntary sterilization was commonplace, states had laws preventing MR people from marrying. Readers may recall questions about mental retardation, epilepsy, and criminal conviction on applications for marriage licenses. Such laws were based on the premise that preventing marriage would impede childbearing; hence, children born out of wedlock were illegitimate. As of 1981, 38 states had regulations pertaining to marriage of MR individuals (Haavik & Menninger, 1981). Undergirding these regulations was the belief that retardation was prima facie evidence of parental unfitness (Harris & Wideman, 1988; Reilly, 1991). As Hill (1950) wrote:

It has been the policy of the state of Oregon to sterilize mentally deficient persons before releasing them from its institution and this program has been of benefit from economic, social, and eugenic standpoints. It assists the individual in his transition to a non-institutional life, and relieves the state of financial burden.

A mentally deficient person is not a suitable parent for either a normal or a subnormal child, and children would be an added burden to an already handicapped individual, who does well to support himself. It would be unfair to the state, to the individual, and particularly to his potential children, to permit his release without the protection of sterilization. (p. 403)

In an attempt to confine sexual activity and reproduction to marriage, numerous laws criminalize cohabitation, fornication, and sodomy. Given the high percentage of children born to single women (Beller & Graham, 1993), such laws are illogical. Although the classification "illegitimate" for children born out of wedlock may be dated, the ideal of children being born within the confines of heterosexual marriage is certainly prevalent. The assumption that preventing marriage might impede procreation also lingers, especially in the case of MR people.

Few states allow marriages between members of the same gender. Even when single-gender marriages occur, such benefits of heterosexual couplehood as being a recipient of the spousal health-care benefits and retirement pensions are disputed and denied by state, federal, and private agencies and institutions. Lesbians can become impregnated by artificial insemination or by sexual intercourse with a male. Some agencies and states allow adoptions, particularly of hard-to-place children, by homosexual couples or by single people. Although permitted, they are not universally condoned (Ethics Committee, 1986).

In utilizing genetic screening, parents choose to prevent avoidable suffering by replacing a child who would have been born handicapped with one who will not through either subsequent conception or adoption. Children cannot replace defective parents so easily (Harris, 1988). Unless parents voluntarily give up custody, abuse or neglect must be detected before children can be removed from parental care. Although adequate predictive tools to distinguish beforehand between suitable and unsuitable parents are lacking (Vitello, 1978), child abuse and neglect laws provide the framework for defining (un)acceptable parenting. By stating what parents cannot do, laws indirectly set minimum standards of parental behaviors. If it is surmised that certain individuals, retarded or otherwise, are likely to abuse or neglect potential children, it stands to reason that they should be discouraged—perhaps even legally or forcibly prevented, such as through involuntary sterilization—from having children. Studies indicate that MR women have significantly more problems parenting than nonretarded females (Koller, Richardson, & Katz, 1988; Schilling, Schinke, Blythe, & Barth, 1982). At the same time, adolescents in special education have higher rates of pregnancy than nonclassified counterparts (Kleinfeld & Young, 1989; Muccigrosso, Scavarda, Simpson-Brown, & Thalacker, 1991).

In the absence of refined techniques for judging parental adequacy, care must be exercised in order not to discriminate against MR parents. Established parents are screened by social service professionals who may be biased against MR people because of their labels, the presence of mannerisms or stigmata, or their inability to deal in a credible or dignified manner with the stressful prospects of losing custody of children (Andron & Tymchuk, 1985, 1987; Payne, 1978; Sovner & Hurley, 1989; Wayment & Zetlin, 1989). It is common for those in caring professions to have negative and patronizing attitudes toward the recipients of their services (Abbott & Sapsford, 1990; Abbott & Wallace, 1990; Brantlinger, 1983); there is a stigma attached just to receiving services (Spicker, 1984). Bias also occurs in the legal system because of the devalued status of MR individuals as well as their inability to cope with the system's complexities and effectively represent themselves as either victims or defendants (Calnen & Blackman, 1992; Ellis & Luckasson, 1985).

Perhaps it is better for children in extremely problematic circumstances to be moved from the care of their biological or adoptive parents, but questions of who makes decisions and on what grounds and what to do with removed children remain (Janko, 1994; Wolfe, 1989). According to Habermas (1986), care-providing systems create a "therapeutocracy" in which professional expertise increasingly substitutes for family preferences. Illich (1977) uses the phrase "disabling professions" for the official undermining of individual and family autonomy. Referring to the biopolitics of normalizing the health of individuals and populations, Foucault (1973) explores the ways in which Western society has become increasingly disciplined, regulated, and under surveillance. Welfare agents, typically women, intervene as "soft police" to reinforce patriarchal state authority and maintain order (Abbott & Sapsford, 1990; Abbott & Wallace, 1990). Pascoe (1990) claims the benevolent activities of middle-class white American women a century ago, done in the name of purity and piety, were directed toward impoverished women, particularly those of color. Controllers are members of the dominant culture—in this country, European-American middle-class, middle-aged males; those controlled are youthful members of minority racial and ethnic groups (Bell, 1992; Bowser, 1991; Davis, 1981; Stepan, 1991), females (Nathanson, 1991), and those with disability status (Boylan, 1991; Dalley & Berthoud, 1992).

Overpopulation

The United States Supreme Court has reviewed the right to reproduce primarily in two contexts: the sterilization of criminal or MR persons and public access to contraception (Ethics Committee, 1986). In the landmark 1965 *Griswold v. Connecticut* case, the Supreme Court declared a Connecticut statute that prohibited the use of contraceptives unconstitutional because it restricted the right of married people to privacy in their own bedrooms; that is, to practice birth control free from government interference (Sloan,

1988). The right to privacy recognized in *Griswold* was later expanded to a variety of values in personal, associational, family, and sexual matters, ultimately encompassing the right to abortion in *Roe v. Wade*. In *Eisenstadt v. Baird* (1972), the Court held that unmarried persons have the same right of privacy.

Any law limiting nonhandicapped married couples' right to have children when and as they choose would probably be struck down as a violation of the fundamental right to procreate (Ethics Committee, 1986). People's right to bear children is well established, yet there is social pressure against large families, especially for the poor. Although the pressure to combat teenage pregnancy is contested (Hudson & Ineichen, 1991; Nathanson, 1991) concern about it appears regularly in the popular press. News reports have ambivalently covered the provision of free Norplant implants for high school students who are at high risk for pregnancy. China's strict population control measures, including the necessity to have government permission to have a child and the forced abortion of fetuses conceived without permission, are viewed with abhorrence in this country as violations of individual liberties. Yet Americans are rarely aware of the context of these policies—of the ravishing effects of overpopulation.

There is not always consensus about what constitutes overpopulation. There would be fairly high levels of agreement that parts of China, India, Africa, and Mexico have populations that exceed what can be sustained by their land base. Desperate acts of emigration (boat people, risky border crossings) give evidence of "surplus population." Many maintain that even within the United States there are more people than the land can sustain in health and dignity and with protection of endangered species. Problems with the disposal of garbage and sewage—not to mention hazardous wastes—are critical, although Hartmann (1987) contends these problems have remedies other than population control.

A conservative rallying point is that public assistance has allowed—even encouraged—women to have babies at an early age without personal financial support. Although the rhetoric of welfare dependency, abuse, and fraud is frequently used in campaign speeches, there has been no significant push for states to set and enforce limits on reproduction or to withhold support from needy families. There is no legislation pertaining to population control in the United States, although perhaps a case could be made for such legislation.

ARGUMENTS AGAINST EUGENICS

A major argument used to refute the ethics of birth control and steriliza-tion is the slippery slope or wedge (foot in the door, small beginnings lead to . . . , setting precedent for) idea, which makes the case that although a particular action may seem reasonable and appropriate, it inevitably leads to undesirable actions or outcomes. Applying the slippery-slope logic to the sterilization of MR people, it is argued that although it is appropriate for those at some functioning levels, it is not appropriate for others. Therefore, because it is difficult or arbitrary to distinguish between levels (and delineate the grey area), sterilization should be disallowed for any MR individuals. There are two versions of the slippery-slope position: The logical conceptual declares an absence of defensible lines between certain acts (e.g., abortion and infanticide) unless there are clear distinctions sustained by moral reasons; the psychological associations version connects neutral positions with renown unacceptable positions (e.g., sterilization with eugenics with genocide with Nazi atrocities).

Although a rationality position can be used to support a eugenics position, it also can be used to oppose it. An argument against genetic engineering is that resources allocated to it might better be spent on other kinds of projects (Beauchamp & Pinkard, 1983). Another is that the short- and long-term outcomes of eugenic actions cannot be predicted (Brody, 1987). Indeed, there is mixed evidence on genetic deterioration. Using a genealogical method for heredity studies as Goddard, Dugsdale, and Estabrook had done many years earlier, Reed and his colleagues (Reed, 1955; Reed, Reed, & Palm, 1954) found that the incidence of mental retardation was not growing as had been feared; that the proportions of people of various IQ levels remained stable over time. Reed concluded that MR people's childbearing would have little effect on future gene pools. Later, Reed and Reed (1965) qualified this conclusion by cautioning that this was true only as long as reproduction was not encouraged for previously nonproductive members. Similar to Reed's initial conclusion of no general decline in intelligence, Preston and Campbell (1993) estimated that a relaxation of natural selection by enabling people with "bad genes" to survive produces very little change in average gene frequency. Coleman (1993) found fault with these conclusions about population drifts and cautioned against a dismissal of common beliefs about negative population changes.

Another rational argument against selective breeding is that it may have undesirable consequences. Eugenic actions are typically based on valuing some human traits more than others and on reducing the numbers of people with certain traits; that is, increasing human homogeneity and decreasing human diversity. Yet diversity may benefit society; diverse types of people are needed for various societal roles.

Arguments against eugenics include the view that restricting reproduction is unnatural or based on bad values. Although officially defined as the science of improving the human species, Spallone (1989) calls eugenics "the dumping ground for racial, sexual, and class prejudice—as a way to get rid of those identified as inferior" (p. 134). In pointing out the essential fuzziness of racial concepts, Gould (1981) explores ways that race was created in eugenic theory during the nineteenth and twentieth centuries. Gould also gives evidence that scientists exaggerated and even distorted data to fit their theories. By directing services primarily toward curbing the birth rate of poor women, family planning organizations have been accused of having a hidden racist and classist agenda (Davis, 1981; Diskin, 1992; Jasso, 1991). Identifying social class as central to worldwide eugenics thinking, Mazumdar (1992) asserts that the "reforming middle class persists in seeing others as inferior and in believing that heredity is a factor in social class status (p. 5). Stepan (1991) concurs with this position, adding women to the list of "dysgenic" groups. Relatedly, this book examines how mental capacity figures in eugenics thought and movements.

THE WANING, BUT SUBTLE, PERSISTENCE OF EUGENICS MOVEMENTS

Immediately following World War II, the status of eugenics sharply declined in reaction to Hitler's genocidal practices. Ideas linking race to cognition became unmentionable—condemned and silenced by strong public sentiments. Even before the war, genetic explanations had been increasingly countered with theories about the influence of environmental circumstances on mental and moral development, and environmental explantions began to take precedence. New types of biological and psychological research provided a different—and presumably more accurate—framework for perceiving the transmission of human traits. Studies (e.g., Skeels, Updegraff, Wellman, & Williams, 1938; Skodak & Skeels, 1949; Spitz, 1946) documenting the effects of maternal stimulation on the intellectual and emotional growth of infants born in institutions supported an environment position. By 1969, the social milieu was of such a different mind about the comparative places of the environment and genetics in human development that Arthur Jensen became a pariah in both the scholarly and the lay communities for publishing an article that attributed differences in measured intelligence to heredity.

The ascendancy of views stressing the importance of environmental influences on intelligence, the momentum of civil rights movements, and the negative views of eugenics and containment that resulted from Nazi atrocities triggered reactions to and eventual rejection of indiscriminate incarceration and involuntary sterilization of MR people. Although a few years earlier the Supreme Court in *Buck v. Bell* (1927) upheld the constitutionality of compulsory sterilization, in *Skinner v. Oklahoma* (1942) the Court articulated that procreation was a basic civil right, thus challenging state statutes mandating sterilization. During the 1970s, compulsory sterilization laws were declared unconstitutional (Burgdorf & Spicer, 1983).

The growing repertoire of new genetic technologies related to reproduction, although not developed under the rubric of eugenics, often focuses on detecting flaws in genes. Ultimately, then, many are eugenic in that they incorporate the thinking that better genes make better people. Furthermore, the new genetics identifies some genes, and some people, as unfit. According to Spallone (1989), the growth of reproductive technologies is based on an "arrogant belief in scientific and social control" and "a desire to assert more social/biological control over women, pressuring them to have the perfect baby" (p. 112). Spallone believes that fertility interventions presume that "only genetically related children are authentic children," hence ignoring acts of love, bonding, and caring (p. 113).

2

Legal Systems that Affect Sterilization

Developments at all levels and in all kinds of legal systems in the United States document a rich history of thinking about disability and sexuality. There are four legal sources that influence the daily lives of people with disabilities and their families, as well as others in the community: the United States Constitution, state and federal legislation, litigation or case law, and special statements of rights.

CONSTITUTIONAL LAW

The Constitution of the United States lays down fundamental principles for the organization and administration of society. The concepts of equal protection and due process contained in the Fourteenth Amendment embody basic moral principles of fundamental fairness by stating that laws must be applied equally to diverse groups and that when deliberate classifications or exclusions occur in state or federal legislation, a "compelling government interest must exist to justify them" (Mayer, 1979, p. 75). Hence, Haavik and Menninger (1981) challenge:

Can our society legitimately and legally prevent retarded people from marrying and having children when no such prohibitions have been placed on others who are judged to be unfit parents, such as alcoholics and child abusers? While procreation may be inadvisable for some severely involved individuals, the same proscription may be quite unfairly and inappropriately applied to other individuals who may be capable of parenthood but happen to be labeled mentally retarded. (p. 67)

Other constitutional provisions such as the Eighth Amendment's prohibition against cruel and unusual punishment and the Thirteenth Amendment's proscription against involuntary servitude have been invoked in lawsuits on behalf of MR people. The Fifth Amendment guarantees that no person shall be deprived of life, liberty, or property without due process of law. Due process, or the regular administration of the law, according to which no citizen may be denied legal rights, is an important safeguard against arbitrary or abusive government action and is the only legitimate way by which individuals can be dealt with against their wills (Neville, 1981, p. 67).

SPECIAL PROCLAMATIONS OF RIGHTS

The International League of Societies for Persons with Mental Handicap, founded in 1960 by professional and parent groups, recommended a set of rights for MR people to the United Nations General Assembly that was adopted in 1971. To prevent limitations of rights due to retardation, the proclamation specifies that rights for MR people are the same as for other citizens. Yet, to account for circumstances particular to MR individuals, their rights extend beyond those of ordinary citizens. The League's list includes the rights to proper medical care and physical restoration; education, training, habilitation, and guidance to develop full potential; economic productivity and security; a decent standard of living; family and community participation; a qualified guardian to protect them from exploitation, abuse, and degrading treatment; and proper legal safeguards to protect against denial of rights.

Hoffmaster (1982) questions the logic of separate rights by reminding that having the same rights as anyone else precludes requests for special rights. He notes that the right to perform productive work or other meaningful occupation is not of a universal nature because it is not guaranteed other citizens. Distinguishing between "the right to" and "the opportunity to," he maintains that the latter implies the right to compete with everyone else, which is more consistent with normalization principles. Hoffmaster acknowledges that achieving normalization requires imbalanced expenditures on MR people and recommends that degree of retardation be considered in allocation formulas.

Debate about unique treatment applies to the MR offender. In *In Re Penry* (1988), it was argued that MR criminals do not possess the "level of culpability" essential for capital cases—that categorical disqualification is required because of their limited cognitive abilities. MR defendants may lack the ability to perform the tasks required at trials and detract from fact finding about their case. Differential treatment also has been argued on the grounds that professionals within the criminal justice system do not understand the nature of mental retardation and so MR persons are subject to abuse by the system (Calnen & Blackman, 1992). Therefore, because of vulnerability, MR defendants are entitled to certain protections (Ellis & Luckasson, 1985).

Some MR citizens slip into mainstream life without help, but most find that in order to get into educational, health care, and income systems (jobs or government income maintenance), they must submit to special processing, which may be complex and humiliating (Varela, 1979). Rights are conferred by the common consent of the governed—a consent that largely depends upon the "prevailing social conscience" (Mayer, 1979, p. 68), which has consistently been "uninformed, negative, or ambivalent" (Richman & Trohanis, 1979, p. 85). Therefore, MR people face limitations imposed not only by their condition, but also by social and legal systems that use labels of dependency and incompetence (Weinberg, 1988). Neville (1981) urges a critical check on "the totalitarian impetus lurking in social policies that require people to 'be good,' in this case, to submit to involuntary restrictions (sterilization) in order to have a decent sex life" (p. 69). Although reputed to be objective and detached, the legal system is structured on an adversarial model, which essentially polarizes rights by establishing the rights of one party while placing duties on another (Weinberg, 1988).

Advocacy Needs of MR Individuals

Partly because of their condition and partly because of prejudice against them, MR people need advocates to speak in their behalf. Advocacy initiates confrontation with authorities who are wrongfully withholding benefits or excluding MR citizens from community life and provides supports for MR individuals and their families. Turnbull and Turnbull (1979) delineate such characteristics of effective advocates as willingness to examine assumptions about disabilities and to sharply focus on and move toward goals. They caution against "true believers" who "have lost sight of goals" (p. 65).

As a result of the 1975 and 1978 Developmental Disability Acts, state-level legal advocacy groups were developed with the functions of (1) providing legal aid attorneys with specialized knowledge in the areas of law affecting individuals with disabilities, (2) working with consumer groups to formulate training programs for lay advocates, (3) maintaining close liaisons with legislators, (4) providing continuity in relations with state agencies and bar organizations, and (5) evaluating legislative and administrative proposals (Mayer, 1979, p. 74). Although these defined roles allude to broad functions, the actual roles of Protection and Advocacy commissioners seem limited to advice giving—and then only when someone from outside initiates interaction (Brantlinger, Klein, & Guskin, 1994). Moreover, because appointments to the Commission are political, they may depend more on professionals' connections than competencies.

LEGISLATION

Over the years, legislation specific to MR people has had both restrictive and beneficial effects. In the early part of the twentieth century, specialized legislation primarily imposed barriers and denied freedoms. One restriction was on reproduction. The first state law making sterilization of nonconsenting MR people legal was passed in Indiana in 1907 (Brakel & Rock, 1971). Within a few years, more than half of the states had enacted laws enabling involuntary sterilization (Allen, 1969). Even in the absence of legislation, such as before the first statute went into effect, sterilizations were routinely performed (Brakel & Rock, 1971), as they were in states without enabling legislation (Haavik & Menninger, 1981). These statutory measures coincided with the prevalent public conviction that insanity, promiscuity, criminality, and low intelligence were closely linked and that prolific breeding among defectives would eventually swamp society with undesirables (Tyor & Bell, 1984).

During the past two decades, legislation to establish rights and provide services for MR people resulted from the powerful efforts of advocacy groups. Discrimination against persons with disabilities in the work force and community was prohibited by Section 504 of the Rehabilitation Act of 1973 (Pub. L. 93–112): "No otherwise qualified handicapped individual in the United States . . . shall, solely by reason of his handicap, be excluded from participation, be denied the benefits of, or be subjected to discrimination under any program or activity receiving Federal financial assistance".

The 1975 Education for All Handicapped Children Act, Pub. L. 94–142 (updated by Pub. L. 101–476, the Individuals with Disabilities Education Act (IDEA), which went into effect in 1990) ensured the right to free, appropriate public education. The passage of the Education of the Handicapped Act Amendments of 1986 (Pub. L. 99–457) extended services to preschool children with special needs and their families. In 1978, Comprehensive Services for Independent Living was added to the Rehabilitiation Act, authorizing grants to states to provide transportation, attendant care, interventions for preschool children, and provisions to enable severely handicapped persons to live independently in their own communities. The Americans with Disabilities Act (ADA) of 1990 (Pub. L. 101–336) went further in making it illegal to discriminate against individuals with disabilities in public accommodations, public services, employment, and telecommunications and mandated the removal of architectural and communication barriers that restrict access to employment and to community activities.

LITIGATION

Advocacy groups can take credit for a number of court cases that set precedent for the delivery of services to MR people. The case that laid the groundwork for Pub. L. 94–142, *Pennsylvania Association for Retarded Citizens v. Commonwealth of Pennsylvania* (1972), established that a child with a disability cannot be excluded from school without due process. This enabled children with disabilities to have a viable, community-based alternative to institutionalization and allowed parents enough support so that they could consider keeping MR children at home. At the same time, by supplementing the education of identified children with federal funds, Pub. L. 94–142 stimulated a burgeoning of classified school-age populations. Because children of color and those with limited English proficiency were disproportionately identified and excluded from regular education classrooms, a number of court cases attempted to prevent the overlabeling and overplacement of certain children in special education. *Larry P. v. Riles* (1979) set precedent for diagnosis that adequately takes into account different cultural and linguistic backgrounds.

Litigation in the seventies also focused on institutional conditions. In the landmark *Wyatt v. Stickney* (1972) decision, the Supreme Court formulated guidelines for the use of aversive or deprivation treatment as well as involuntary sterilization and mandated institutions to provide privacy for heterosexual relationships. *Haldeman v. Pennhurst* (1981) addressed the right to treatment and decent conditions and the alternatives to institutions for MR individuals.

Litigation Specific to Sterilization

In the notorious *Buck v. Bell* (1927) case, Supreme Court Justice Oliver Wendell Holmes upheld the Virginia law that authorized sterilization of institutionalized people (Smith, 1989). Carrie Buck was the 17-year-old illegitimate daughter of an institutionalized MR woman who herself had been sterilized involuntarily immediately after she had given birth to Carrie. At the time of Carrie's court hearing, Carrie's infant daughter was assumed to be retarded. Yet, shortly before she died of smallpox, Carrie's daughter was judged to be a brighter-than-average second grader. Holmes' justification of his decision to permit sterilization provides a classic eugenicist's viewpoint:

In order to prevent our being swamped with incompetents, it is better for all the world if instead of waiting to execute degenerate offspring for crime or to let them starve for their imbecility, society can prevent those who are manifestly unfit from continuing their kind. The principle that sustains compulsory vaccination is broad enough to cover cutting the fallopian tubes: three generations of imbeciles are enough. (p. 200)

It is not surprising, but it is significant, that in *Buck*, Holmes spoke of fallopian tubes and the prevention of procreation by females, emphasizing that sterilization has traditionally been aimed at the potential childbearer rather than the sperm donor. The reproductive consequences of women's sexual activity have received more attention from the courts than any other aspect of sexuality and social life (Oakley, 1984, 1985; Smith, 1989). *Buck* made sterilization of MR persons without their consent a legitimate public health measure and made preventing the birth of undesirables a national goal. Following that notorious case, 20 states passed sterilization laws, and the annual rate of sterilizations peaked (Burgdorf & Spicer, 1983).

Another Supreme Court case, *Skinner v. Oklahoma* (1942), involved sterilization of nonconsenting thrice-convicted habitual criminals who had committed felonies involving moral turpitude. In *Skinner*, it was successfully argued that there was no evidence that children of larcenists were more dangerous to society than children of embezzlers, who were not subject to sterilization (Gilhool & Gran, 1985). *Buck* upheld the constitutionality of compulsory sterilization; *Skinner* overturned *Buck* on the grounds that *Buck* violated the basic civil right to procreate. During the 1970s, in state after state, compulsory sterilization laws were declared unconstitutional (Burgdorf & Spicer, 1983). The Indiana statute was repealed in 1975. Yet, under a Department of Health and Human Services regulation and a federal court order (*Relf v. Weinberger*, 1974), a moratorium was placed on the use of federal funds for sterilizations of minors and incompetent individuals.

Not only was Indiana the first state to enact an involuntary sterilization statute, but also the infamous *Stump v. Sparkman* (1978) case took place in the state. Known for setting precedent for judicial immunity, *Stump v. Sparkman* coincidentally brought sterilization into the spotlight. The case involved a 15-year-old "somewhat retarded" girl named Linda. Linda's mother requested sterilization on the grounds that Linda had been "staying overnight with men." In spite of the fact that Indiana had recently repealed the half-century-old involuntary sterilization legislation, not only was Linda not seen in court, but also she was not informed of the court order for sterilization, and the surgery was performed on false pretenses—Linda was told she was having an appendectomy. A few years later, when Linda and her husband wanted a baby, they discovered that Linda had been sterilized. At that point, Linda Sparkman and her husband sued Linda's mother, the attorney who drafted the petition for the sterilization order, the doctors who performed the tubal ligation, the hospital administration, and Judge Stump.

Judge Stump argued that he was protected by judicial immunity, which holds that judges cannot be liable for damages resulting from acts within the scope of their jurisdiction (i.e., their power as defined by the legislature). When the case went to the United States Supreme Court, Stump was criticized for his reprehensible handling of the case, but he was granted judicial immunity on the grounds that he did not act in the absence of jurisdiction even if he acted in excess of it. It was noted that the Indiana law gave broad powers to judges and no statute specifically prohibited the consideration of sterilization petitions. Because Judge Stump was protected by judicial immunity, no one else sued by the Sparkmans could be held liable.

The *Stump* decision has been criticized for expanding judicial immunity to the point that it potentially sanctions almost any malicious, erroneous, or destructive judicial act, yet the case did not affect statutes enabling sterilizations, nor did it overturn statutes in states that prohibit sterilization in the absence of enabling legislation. Although it had no official impact, *Stump* did serve as a reminder to judges hearing cases involving MR individuals to consider the evidence carefully.

In *In re Simpson* (1962), after an 18-year-old unmarried girl with an IQ of 36 had given birth, the judge ordered her sterilized on the grounds that she would probably have more children that she would be unable to care for and all would be a drain on public funds. The judge felt he had authority to take action to prevent the pregnancy of a "feeble-minded" person when the institution could not. In contrast to *Stump*, in *Simpson* the judge was criticized for "unauthorized judicial action" and "perversion of the law" (Haavik & Menninger, 1981, p. 134).

In England, *In re B.* (1987) involved a 17-year-old with a "mental age of five or six." Expert testimony indicated that she was unable to grasp the relationships among sexual intercourse, conception, and childbirth and that she would be incapable of consenting to marry. Unlike Sparkman, who, if retarded at all, was mildly so, B. was moderately to severely retarded, had behavioral problems, and was taking medication that would put her or a fetus at risk if she were to become pregnant. B. was known to be sexually active. Unanimous support was given for sterilization at all court levels because it was judged to be in B.'s best interest. It was felt that the severity of her disabilities would prevent her from making an informed decision about sterilization even as an adult (Sullivan, 1992).

Whereas *Stump* and *Simpson* in the United States and *In re B.* in England granted sterilization, a landmark Canadian case, *Eve v. Mrs. E.* (1986), denied it. Eve, classified moderately retarded, was 24 years old in 1979 when the case first arose. To avoid becoming responsible for a child, Eve's mother sought sterilization for Eve. The first-level court challenged Eve's mother's right to substitute consent and prohibited the sterilization procedure, maintaining that parental consent does not make it voluntary consent from the offspring's position (Soskin, 1977). In *Eve*, the relief of child-rearing responsibilities for Eve's mother did not become a factor even though the court recognized that Eve was not capable of rearing a child herself. The court felt it had the authority to provide parental protection to Eve as a vulnerable person regardless of her mother's preferences. The rationale for denial was that, if Eve could not consent because of a lack of intellectual capacity, it could never be safely determined whether such a procedure was for her benefit. The judge took the view that sterilization would deprive Eve of her basic human right to reproduce if at some future date she would be able to appreciate the significance of reproduction and would have the capacity to marry. The court argued that the potential to violate Eve's mental and physical integrity through nonconsensual, nontherapeutic sterilization was greater than the risks of childbirth, which had not been shown to be traumatic for her. The appeals court upheld the mother's request, but the Supreme Court of Canada held that sterilization could not occur for nontherapeutic purposes under the jurisdiction of the court as parens patriae, that is, under the court in its role of protecting the rights and interests of a minor or an incompetent person. Like *Skinner,* *Eve* endorsed procreation as a human right. The well-publicized, protracted deliberations in *Eve* stirred up a range of professional and popular commentaries on sterilization and resulted in an Ontario regulation that prohibits nontherapeutic sterilization of minors under 16 years of age in public hospitals (Sullivan, 1992).

The New Jersey Supreme Court also relied on a process of substitute consent by the court in *In re Grady* (1981). The Gradys sought a sterilization order for their daughter, Lee Ann, a woman with Down syndrome, arguing that because Lee Ann lived in a community setting that was less restrictive than an institution, certain safeguards were necessary for her protection. The Gradys felt that Lee Ann's independence in the community would be enhanced by sterilization—that some of the barriers to autonomy would be removed if she were free from worry about contraception and childbirth. The request was denied on the grounds that the interests of the petitioners (the parents) must be separated from those of the subject (the MR adult) because they cannot be presumed to be identical. The decision stressed that only the best interests of the incompetent person, and not the interests or convenience of the parents or the state, should be considered. Furthermore, it was argued that it was the duty of the court, under the doctrine of parens patriae, and not the parents to determine the need for sterilization (Weinberg, 1988).

An opposite conclusion was reached by the British House of Lords in the late 1980s in the case of Jeanette, a 17-year-old mentally disabled and epileptic girl who had shown signs of being vulnerable to sexual approaches. Jeanette's mother, and the local borough council in whose care she was, applied to the High Court for wardship so that Jeanette could be sterilized to avoid pregnancy. It was argued that a fundamental right to reproduce was not valid because Jeanette could not understand the links among sexual intercourse, pregnancy, and birth (Cusine, 1990). Those opposed to the decision felt that Jeanette, who could handle her periods, would be capable of handling birth control. They claimed the assumption that she would not mature intellectually was faulty and complained that sterilization was done for convenience and cost-cutting purposes because centers were understaffed and sterilization allowed release from institutional care. The case set precedent for sterilization of MR women in England (Lee & Morgan, 1989a).

Other litigation granted sterilization of adult MR women on the grounds that, for reasons connected with their retardation, temporary forms of birth control were not feasible. *In re Anderson* (1974) established that the "least drastic" birth control should always be tried first, yet expert witnesses gave evidence that MR women were usually unable to reliably keep to the schedule of taking birth control pills or could not combine the pill with other medication. Barrier forms of contraception were judged unsuitable because MR women could not reliably use a diaphragm or recognize the signs of an IUD becoming dislodged (Cusine, 1990; Sloan, 1988). More recently, it has been argued that because of the availability of Norplant and Depo-Provera, nonconsenting sterilization should not be allowed.

North Carolina Association for Retarded Children v. State of North Carolina (1976) offered five reasons for sterilization of MR individuals: (1) if it can be determined that the mental retardation is inheritable and that there is a significant probability that offspring will be retarded; (2) if it can be predicted that the person will be incapable of handling the responsibilities of parenthood; (3) if the person cannot understand the consequences of sexual activity; (4) if the person is incapable of using contraceptives; and (5) if involuntary sterilization is in the best interests of the state or the person, or both. It might be noted that reasons 1 and 5 have eugenics overtones. The case was underinclusive in not applying to people who, although not retarded, would have genetically defective children and/or would not be good parents and was overinclusive in not recognizing that some MR people have normal children and are good parents (Haavik & Menninger, 1981).

Guidelines for involuntary sterilization also were included in the *In re Hayes* (1980) decision, in which it was determined that the courts can order sterilization if there is no statute prohibiting such orders. *Hayes* specified that individuals must be (1) incapable of making any decision concerning sterilization in the present or future, (2) capable of procreation, (3) likely to engage in sexual activity, (4) disabled in a way that renders them incapable of caring for a child, and (5) unable to use other birth control alternatives. In contrast to *North Carolina*, *Hayes* rejected the eugenics rationale for sterilization.

Eroding of Parental Authority

In the past, it was assumed that parents had certain natural rights that enabled them to act for their children (or MR adults) until they were capable of governing themselves (Sullivan, 1992). Recent court decisions have overridden parents' wishes in recognizing minors' constitutional rights. Courts can act in the capacity of parents, and extensions of their role in protecting vulnerable persons have included protection from parents (Cusine, 1990). Regardless of parental preference, with preadolescents and adolescents, involuntary sterilizations are rarely permitted because of recognition that their intellectual functioning might improve with maturity (Craft & Craft, 1978). Regarding abortion, the United States Supreme Court, in its decisions in *Planned Parenthood of the State of Missouri v. Danforth* (1976), *Bellotti v. Baird* (1979), and *H. L. v. Matheson* (1981), has stated that there are situations in which parents do not have to be consulted or informed; that minors have constitutionally protected privacy interests that allow them to make procreative decisions free of parental control (Sullivan, 1992). In *In Re B.* (1987), *In Re Grady* (1981), and *Eve v. Mrs. E.* (1986), there was a significant shift of authority from parents to courts. In *Eve*, the state protected the individual's right to choose (although she was incapable of choosing); in *In re B.*, the courts protected B. from the physical harm likely to result from pregnancy. Even the court cases that granted parents' requests for sterilization did not give authority to parents to make those decisions. Indeed, the power of the courts in controlling access to sterilization for MR individuals has been firmly established, whether or not states have legislation enabling sterilization. Courts recognize parental authority, but the weight of authority remains with the courts (Cusine, 1990; Haavik & Menninger, 1981; Sullivan, 1992).

In England, *Gillick v. West Norfolk and Wisbech Health Authority* (1985) represented another strike against parental authority. Local health officials issued a circular outlining the circumstances under which they might provide children under 16 with contraceptive advice and treatment without parental consent. Mrs. Gillick sought a declaration from local authority that material in the circular was unlawful because it amounted to doctors' encouraging sexual intercourse for a girl under 16, which constituted a criminal offense. Mrs. Gillick contended that giving contraceptive advice or treating anyone under 16 without parental consent was a violation of parental rights.

The lower court judge held that parents' rights were more accurately described as duties and that, accordingly, there was no interference with parental rights when advice or treatment was given to girls under 16. The judge also concluded that, by giving contraceptive advice or treatment, doctors would not be committing the criminal offense of encouraging unlawful sexual intercourse. The court of appeals granted the declaration sought by Mrs. Gillick on the grounds that a child under the age of 16 cannot validly agree to contraceptive treatment without her parents' consent; therefore, the circular was unlawful. On the next appeal, the House of Lords supported the lower court's decision, maintaining that, provided they had the capacity to understand what they were doing, children could consent to such advice and treatment independently of their parents and that parental rights were not infringed by a competent child's exercising his or her capacity to make an informed choice. The addendum of "capacity to understand," as a precondition for children to act on their own, calls into question the provision of services to MR individuals. Sullivan (1992) claims arguments that apply to adolescents overlap with persons who lack capacity.

Lee and Morgan (1989b) believe "age of maturity" for consent in *Gillick* is determined by a clinical judgment by doctors and not by an arbitrary age cut-off, whereas Mason (1990) maintains that *Gillick* means that parents' rights terminate at puberty. According to Smith (1990), in *Gillick*, contraception was a "damage limitation exercise" that served the purposes of protecting the health of a person for whom childbearing would be dangerous, preventing the birth of a child who could not be looked after by the mother, avoiding pregnancy, and facilitating sexual self-fulfillment (p. 13). The outcome of *Gillick* gave authority to adolescents judged to be competent minors, privileged doctors' roles, authorized the courts to act as protectors, and diminished parental authority.

AUTONOMY, COMPETENCY, AND CONSENT

Autonomy (self-governance, liberty) constitutes a central theme in legal interventions with MR people. The principle of respect for autonomy recognizes capacities and perspectives, including the right to hold views, make choices, and take actions based on personal values and beliefs. To be autonomous, people must be competent to act intentionally and with under-standing. The components of competence include the ability to give evidence of preference or choice, understand the situation and disclosed information, and give rational reasons for choices. Incompetence due to illness, immaturity, ignorance, irrationality, or intellectual deficit results in restrictions to autonomy.

In questioning external intervention in individuals' choices, the field of ethics has mainly considered the autonomy of competent persons (Bucha-nan & Brock, 1989). People whose independence and decision-making abilities are hindered by mental retardation or mental illness constitute a complex challenge to interpretations of autonomy. Locke, the philosopher whose statements on autonomy are regarded as canonical, states that children who have not reached the age of reason and adults whose powers of reason are severely impaired do not have rights of self-governance because they are incapable of governing themselves; thus, others must act in their behalf (cited in Deigh, 1989). Nonautonomous decisions—or pa-ternalistic actions—occur when there are constraints on autonomous choices. In medical contexts, paternalism refers to physicians' making decisions on behalf of patients without the latter's full understanding or consent. In a critical analysis of paternalism, Sherwin (1992a) states that the person in control believes he knows what is right for others and rationalizes that patients, especially when their reasoning capacity is dimin-ished, make irresponsible choices. Sherwin contends that women cannot rely on the subjective judgment of doctors because they hold stereotypes of women—especially minority women—as irrational or stupid.

On the other side, Mappes and Zembaty (1986) contend that proponents of paternalistic interventions feel that MR people's condition renders them incapable of realizing their own long-term interests. Hence, a conflict arises for significant others about whether to allow the maximum independence in self-determination or to consider the likelihood of a decision's negative implications for the decision maker and others. Involuntary sterilization, for example, was rationalized partly by the judgment that MR people were ineffective or dangerous parents. Mappes and Zembaty (1986) believe that when people are temporarily or permanently incapable of making decisions about their own well-being, there is no usurpation of autonomy because the conditions for acting autonomously are absent. Similarly, Buchanan and Brock (1989), believe that in these cases, it is "incorrect to hold that the individual's autonomy has been infringed upon, interfered with, or limited" (p. 283). In response to the lack of clear standards for judging competence in MR individuals, Buchanan and Brock have formulated considerations that include specifying competency standards and reliable operational measures for ascertaining competency, determining who ought to judge competence, and developing institutional arrangements to assure that judgments of competence are made responsibly (p. 9).

Discussions often use binary reasoning, creating a dichotomy between those capable and those incapable of consent. Yet there is a range of decisional capacities among MR individuals, as well as a variety of decisions to be made. Competence is situation-specific and hence involves the adequacy of a person's decision-making abilities for particular decisions. Whether a person is competent to make a given decision depends on features of the decision as well as of the person. Often an MR individual can make (or is allowed to make) decisions about everyday matters—especially those that involve simple preferences and no great risks—but may not be able to make the more encompassing decisions that involve complex issues and serious consequences. It is important, then, to gauge the degree of competence needed for any particular decision.

Competence may be intermittent—a person may be temporarily depressed or lacking finances—so the variably impaired must be distinguished from the chronically impaired (Buchanan & Brock, 1989). Determining competence involves establishing a threshold standard necessary for making particular decisions. McCullough, Coverdale, Bayer, and Chervenak (1992) outline a continuum of three representative groups: (1) people who are chronically and irreversibly below thresholds of autonomy; (2) people who are irreversibly near thresholds of autonomy; and (3) people who can achieve thresholds of autonomy.

Competence depends on the opportunities someone has had to make decisions and be independent. As with any other skill, to some degree, proficiency depends on training and practice. Decision-making abilities develop incidentally through the processes of making decisions. McCullough, Coverdale, Bayer, and Chervenak (1992) note that many people are responsive to ameliorative interventions to improve decision-making capacity. Unless a degenerative condition exists, competence typically becomes greater over time; adults usually are more mature and capable of making complex decisions than are adolescents or children. An effort must be made to ensure that the actual practice of decision making reflects the fact that competence is decision-relative, fluctuating, and remediable.

Decision making depends on capacity for understanding as well as capacity for reasoning and deliberation; that is, affect and intelligence. Hence, it is important to distinguish between actual cognition of issues and evaluative understanding of the importance of pertinent issues to oneself. The former involves the mental capacity to understand, while the latter is based on an integrated, accurate, and rational sense of circumstances and self, which is related to individuals' mental health.

Informed Consent

Although the constructs of "competence for decision making" and "informed consent" (autonomous authorization of procedures) are integrally linked and sometimes seem indistinguishable, the term "informed" implies that others have a role in providing MR individuals with information relevant to certain decisions. Lilford (1988) details the elements of informed consent: (1) disclosure; (2) capacity to understand information; (3) voluntariness and freedom from coercion, manipulation, and persuasion; (4) competence for decision making; and (5) ability to authorize consent. Lilford believes that a professional's role is not just to present choices, but also to teach clients about the variables and consequences related to choices.

The contractual model of doctor-patient relationships requires that patients be involved in making decisions by being informed about the risks and benefits and by being allowed to make voluntary choices (Brody, 1987). Faden and Beauchamp (1986) delineate a model of informed consent that involves thorough disclosure of all aspects of decisions, evaluations of the comprehension of the disclosure by the recipient, and provision of conditions conducive to voluntary consent. Brody (1987) cautions that "the doctrine of omniscient decree" (that patients must be given complete information on anything possibly relevant, must use facts in a logical reasoning way, and must be emotionally stable and that physicians must be completely neutral) may extend the contractual model to "ridiculous extents" (p. 60).

Ensuring informed consent requires that information be given in ways that MR individuals understand. Informing is likely to involve more than simply telling—it may involve setting up experiences that give a feeling for situations. In facilitating decisions about parenting, for example, it would be important to provide exposure to children of various age levels over long periods of time. Some MR individuals make reasonable decisions once information has been adequately provided, whereas others' ability to process and retain information is perpetually limited by cognitive and attentional deficits and the comprehension needed for giving truly informed consent may not be attainable.

One of the problems in ensuring informed consent among MR individuals is that they may be abnormally weak, dependent, and surrender-prone. By definition, people with mental retardation have limited knowledge and reasoning power. Because MR women may lack finances, they may be in contexts that are not conducive to independence. Subordinate and dependent status and a protected life style result in limited assertiveness, undifferentiated trusting, and habitual overcompliance (Kleinfeld & Young, 1989). Bell (1992) observed the "subtle coercion" for desperate women in poor economic circumstances to choose sterilization because they feel they have no other choice (p. 301). Just as for other women, MR women's reproductive freedom depends on the economics of decent wages, accessible public health systems, sufficient welfare benefits, good housing, and adequate child care (Ditzion & Golden, 1992). There is a need to develop arrangements that allow MR individuals the freedom to make decisions without interference, duress, or manipulation (Buchanan & Brock, 1989).

Whereas a problem for MR people in earlier years was forced sterilization, a current problem may be lack of access to it. In the past few decades, there has been a growth in acceptance of sterilization as a birth control method, so that it is now the leading contraceptive method among married women in the United States (Gold & Daley, 1991). If competent people recognize its benefits, there are likely to be benefits for MR people. The equal protection clause of the Constitution means that if others are allowed to choose sterilization, unless the state has a compelling reason, it may not be appropriate to deny its use to individuals who are not competent to evaluate its benefits. Yet *Relf v. Weinberger* (1974) determined that, because of sterilization abuse, the Department of Health and Human Services would develop regulations for the use of federal funds for sterilization. These require voluntary informed consent using standardized forms, an explanation of other birth control methods and the irreversibility of sterilization, and a wait of 30 days between consent and sterilization; they prohibit overt or implicit threat of loss of welfare or Medicaid benefits, consent while a person is in labor or under the influence or alcohol and drugs, and the use of hysterectomies for sterilization and put a moratorium on federally funded sterilization of people who are under 21, who have been declared incompetent, or who are institutionalized. People with mild mental retardation should be perfectly capable of understanding what sterilization is, how it is done, and what the risks and benefits of the surgery are; that is, they are capable of consent. Lacking ways to judge incompetence, people at social service agencies sometimes may be forced to use the criteria of anyone classified by public schools as needing special education services, thereby including individuals with mild disabilities (Brantlinger, 1992a). In reaction to *Relf v. Weinberger*, in *In re Nietro* (1985), the California Supreme Court decreed that prohibiting sterilization of all persons with disabilities denies their right to privacy.

Elkins and Andersen (1992) believe that when an MR person with decisional capacity requests sterilization, the majority of doctors would consent to perform the surgery—that it would be discriminatory if they did not. In contrast to this conviction, my interviews with doctors reveal that they often have trouble determining whether or not certain individuals have decisional capacity and they tend to refuse the surgery in unclear cases, assuming that patients do not. (See Chapter 8.) Consent decisions are complex for the consenter, those who facilitate consent, and those who judge consent. Buchanan and Brock (1989) suggest that self-determination issues be included in the preparation of health-care professionals. They also discuss the need to develop techniques to ensure that MR individuals are properly informed about decisions they are entitled to make.

INVOLUNTARY STERILIZATION

At present, many states have no statute authorizing sterilization. Some interpret the absence to mean that courts have no authority, whereas others see the court's parens patriae power as authorization to approve sterilization. *Buck v. Bell* (1927) has not been formally overruled by the United States Supreme Court, yet the rights to procreation in *Skinner v. Oklahoma* (1942) and to privacy in *Griswold v. Connecticut* (1965) have meant that sexual activity and reproduction are seen as fundamentally protected constitutional rights. As a result, the routine involuntary sterilization that took place earlier in the twentieth century has been replaced by individual appeals to courts and compliance with strict procedural safeguards.

Elkins and Andersen (1992) recommend that sterilization be done only after a thorough burden versus benefits analysis and that it never be done punitively. Sterilization may be perceived as humane when it restores normality. It may be a least restrictive alternative in allowing individuals freedom in community and interpersonal relations (Mappes & Zembaty, 1986). Mason (1990), too, believes the comparative evil of nonconsensual treatment is justified by personal liberty benefits, but repudiates the general dispensing of contraceptive hormones for the supervisory convenience of health-care workers. Others (e.g., McCullough, Coverdale, Bayer, & Chervenak, 1992) contend that precisely because of the recent availability of effective, long-term, reversible contraceptive devices such as Norplant, forced sterilization is not justifiable.

Some parental requests for sterilization of minor or adult MR offspring are carried out with the cooperation of a doctor and hospital without court review (Brantlinger, 1992a; Elkins & Andersen, 1992). In other situations, parents' requests may not be granted by doctors, and/or hospital administrators may not allow the surgery without court appproval, and some doctors and hospitals refuse sterilization surgery even with court permission (Brantlinger, 1992a; Brantlinger, Klein, & Guskin, 1994). A search of the literature reveals a dearth of large-scale surveys of present hospital or physician policies and practices related to the sterilization of MR individuals.

In terms of judicializing decisions about sterilization, as of 1988, 14 involuntary sterilization laws survived, 7 of which specifically mentioned MR people (Smith, 1988, p. 77). Even in states without laws, the practice continues to be found legal by courts. Haavik and Menninger contend that courts' refusal to eliminate involuntary sterilization indicates that there are still valid reasons for the practice or that there may be disguised prejudice against MR persons in this society (p. 123).

Lee (1988), a Canadian, favors tightening the law in sterilization cases by taking decisions away from parents, doctors, and social workers, all of whom, he believes, feel they have the right to decide for someone under their care. Lee perceives the court as "disinterested authority" (p. 251). Nevertheless, Lee criticizes such decisions as *In re B.* (1987) on the grounds that "the courts were unimpressed by the argument that there is a fundamental right to procreate with which no law can interfere except where medically necessary for the sake of the girl's present health" (p. 249). Opposed to sterilization himself, Lee seems to prefer court decisions because in Canada they mainly disallow sterilization. More neutral, Buchanan and Brock (1989) list strengths of judicialization of sterilization decisions for incompetents: (1) They are public; (2) they must be supported explicitly by principles; (3) efforts are made at impartiality; and (4) proceedings are adversarial, which means more than one position will be taken into account (p. 141).

On the other side, when decisions are made by courts, the costs of court proceedings are entailed, and obtaining a court decision is a cumbersome and slow process. Judicializing decisions fails to address the special moral relationship that exists between incompetent people and their families and ignores the legal and moral presumptive authority of the family (Buchanan & Brock, 1989). Increasing the constraints on family decisions adds a layer of complexity to the already demanding task of parenting. Sullivan (1992) believes that court decisions about sterilization are mere transfers of author-

ity from parents, through courts, to the helping professions. Opposed to
routine use of the judicial system for such medical decisions as sterilization,
Beauchamp and Childress (1989) claim that reliance on courts makes
procedures costly and creates adversarial relationships between individuals
and governments. Powerless people may be intimidated by the idea of going
to court. Constitutionally protected rights allow procreative choices to be
free of state control; therefore, legal routes should be turned to only as a
last resort.

When courts do consider involuntary sterilization for an incompetent
person, the following due process steps are recommended: (1) The person
is represented by a disinterested guardian ad litem; (2) comprehensive
medical, psychological, and social evaluations of the individual are brought
as evidence; (3) the views of the individual are taken into account; (4) the
individual's incapacity to make decisions about sterilization is demonstrated; (5) evidence is given that the individual is unlikely to develop
sufficiently to make an informed judgment in the future; (6) the person is
shown to be physically capable of procreation and likely to engage in sexual
activity now or in the near future; (7) evidence is given that the person is
not capable of caring for a child even with reasonable assistance; (8) there
is documentation that less drastic (less invasive and more reversible) birth
control is unacceptable and that science is not on the threshold of finding
other treatment for the person's disability or other birth control procedures;
and (9) evidence is given that appropriate supervision, education, and
training have been available (adapted from Elkins & Andersen, 1992, pp.
20–21).

Substituted Consent

The right to self-determination in health care is widely acknowledged,
but questions about how decisions should be made for those not mentally
competent to decide for themselves remain open. Because of the nature and
extent of intellectual disability, some MR individuals are clearly unable to
give informed consent about any number of things. When a person has been
adjudicated as "legally incompetent" by a court of law, there must be a
legally mandated substitute for consent (Committee of Bioethics, 1988). A
parent, guardian other than a parent, or court may be in a position to give
substituted consent for MR persons, although they become wards of the
state if there is no one to assume responsibility for them.

Guidance principles provide substantive direction as to how decisions
are to be made for incompetent people. Imputed judgments involve acting
according to what it is assumed the incompetent individual, if competent,

would choose. In imputed judgments, it is necessary to locate and follow valid advance directives, or, in the case of MR individuals, to observe carefully in order to discern what their choices might be. Best interests involve acting to promote the maximum well-being of the incompetent individual. Substituted judgment is always to some degree speculative— being based on hypotheses developed from evidence about the person's interests, preferences, and values (Buchanan & Brock, 1989). In *In re Hayes* (1980) and *In re B.* (1987), it was argued successfully that sterilization was in the MR person's best interests. Best interests and imputed judgment requirements are difficult to meet, and requests for sterilization are denied in judicial hearings if neither is made clear (Weinberg, 1988).

Before any action is taken, suitable surrogates, or proxy decision makers, for the incompetent person must be identified, and it must be ensured that surrogates understand their role in relation to decisions. Some guardians, such as guardians ad litem who are appointed by the court to determine and act in accordance with the interests of the MR person, are assumed to be neutral or impartial because they have no personal connection with the MR person and no particular stake in the outcome of decisions. Some believe that uninvolved guardians are able to make the most objective decisions; however, neutrality is never readily attainable, and even outsiders bring their values, preferences, and prejudices to decision making.

Guardians who are relatives or who have lived closely with the MR person have been referred to as "bonded guardians" (Elkins & Andersen, 1992, p. 23). Because bonded guardians know the MR person's tastes and preferences, they may be truly able to choose for him or her. As with Karen Quinlan (*In re Quinlan* 1979), who became severely brain-injured, life-sustaining treatment was eventually withheld because her parents convinced the court that that was what Karen would have decided (Mason, 1990). It cannot be assumed that bonded guardians will automatically act in the best interests or according to the preferences of the MR individual. Family members have their own needs, concerns, and perhaps vested interests in certain outcomes, which they often communicate persuasively to doctors and judges. Being compassionate, such professionals may comply with parents' wishes. Professionals are more likely to be swayed by family members, with whom they more readily identify, than by MR individuals (Brantlinger, 1992a). Elkins and Andersen (1992) maintain that sterilization abuse most frequently happens when parents are excessively protective of their MR child. For that reason, Elkins and Andersen believe an MR person should be represented in court by a guardian ad litem.

Institutional Ethics Committees (IECs), also known as Medical Ethics Committees, Clinical Ethics Committees, or Hospital Ethics Committees and similar to Human Rights Committees, provide a mechanism for groups to follow ethical procedures in treatment (Sichel, 1992). IECs can be communicative networks involving everyone concerned with a moral dilemma and hence may be ideal vehicles for contextualized problem resolution. Because IECs make the rationales for decisions explicit, they provide education and consultation for staff, patients, and family as well as a forum for complaints (Buchanan & Brock, 1989). A 1981 survey indicates that such committees existed in only one percent of all hospitals (Beauchamp & Childress, 1989), but by 1985 59 percent of the nation's hospitals had working ethics committees (G. P. Smith, 1990).

3

Ethics of Health Care and Reproduction

The mainstream tradition of ethics has been preoccupied with principles articulated in highly technical language (Fry, 1992). Kohlberg's hierarchical model of moral dilemma resolution (e.g., 1969, 1981) dominated the field of ethical reasoning, but, by reexamining reactions of subjects, Gilligan (1982) found that boys and men apply abstract principles not necessarily relevant to situations, whereas girls and women attend to details of circumstances, and, in their reasoning, all parties retain life histories, identities, and emotions. Because women experience relations as asymmetrical interdependencies, they are likely to consider individuals' positions in situations (Sherwin, 1992a). Feminists (e.g., Noddings, 1993; Sichel, 1992) resist seeing ethics as abstract rules that can be specified apart from context. Also criticizing prevailing medical ethics as too formal and rational to contribute to the resolution of concrete cases, Christie and Hoffmaster (1986) prefer a contextualist morality in which preoccupation with deontological reasoning is abandoned. Practice is based on understanding, coping with, and muddling through problems as they arise. To show that a priori decision making does not fit, Hoffmaster observes that when confronted with the risk that any child they conceive will be disabled, parents in genetic counseling tailor decisions about childbearing to their particular circumstances. Joffe (1986) shows how conflicting ideologies of family planning—as a medical service, a political issue of women's rights, and a profamily moral issue—get translated into workable policies. Clinical work causes counselors to reject simple views of abortion in response to the complex realities of those who seek abortions.

FEMINIST ETHICS OF HEALTH CARE

The profusion of recent feminist writings on health care is relevant because of their emphasis on the effects of decisions on the least privileged members of the community. An interest in disability has arisen among feminists partly because 16 percent of women are disabled, but also because treatment of females and people with disabilities is linked to "cultural oppression of the body" (Wendell, 1992, p. 64). Seeking to empower individuals to pursue nonexploitative relationships, feminist ethics fosters the human agency often restricted by patriarchal medical institutions (Sherwin, 1992a). In spite of the supremacy of human rights thinking, women and MR people still face limitations because their gender or labels start a proceduralization of educational, legal, medical, and social services (Weinberg, 1988). There is a convergence of stereotypes of dependency, passivity, and incompetence for women and disabled people (Altman, 1985; Russo & Jansen, 1988). Examining the phenomenology that arises from being assigned a disabled position in a society that demands perfection from its members, Wendell (1992) claims that medical professionals' authority allows them to distort and silence personal body knowledge. It is paradoxical that attempts to alleviate suffering by making people "normal" yield damaging effects through covert messages that something is missing and wrong (Harris & Wideman, 1988; Holmes & Purdy, 1992).

Feminists are concerned about occupational roles in, access to, and relationships in health care (Warren, 1992). Unequal job status is highly visible: Men hold positions that are lucrative, prestigious, and powerful; women dominate the lower-status roles of nurse and nurse's aide. Disproportionate funds are spent on medical research benefiting males. Actual priorities for funding are set by federal agencies, not Congress, but the descriptors "white, upper class, and male" characterize the medical hierarchy, scientific establishment, and governmental posts (Rosser, 1992, p. 129). Researchers and practitioners authoritatively define women's mental and physical normalcy according to male-defined interests (Sherwin, 1992a). Feminists see women's depression as a natural reaction to oppressive circumstances. By situating the problem in women and medicating depression, physicians perpetuate women's status and deflect attention from injustices. Male researchers emphasize female sexuality as out of control (unwed pregnancies, spreading disease) (Rousso, 1988). Feminists propose methods in which researchers identify and form bonds with subjects (Harding, 1987; Sherwin, 1992a).

Regarding relationship issues, Warren (1992) contends that physicians are educated to believe that decisions are technical and they have final authority regarding treatment. Perceived as crises handled by persons in charge, health-care decisions rarely address psychological subtleties or intricacies of long-term needs. They routinely ignore "housekeeping" problems, which are ongoing, rather than resolved once and for all, and are embedded in complex life experiences. As a "domestic" issue, conditions that foster informed consent are created. Surgery and "saving lives," done by males, bolster the illusion of importance much more than does the patient, ongoing process of rehabilitation or the management of long-term illness, equally important to well-being, but less dramatic, and typically done by females (Wendell, 1992).

Based on the belief that discrimination on the basis of race, class, gender, sexual orientation, age, size, or disability is insidious, pervasive, and morally wrong, feminist ethics is committed to eliminating all manifestations of oppression, or the interlocking restrictions, barriers, and coercive environments that reduce the options available to members of devalued groups and interfere with their protection from exploitation (Frye, 1983; Harding, 1987; Sherwin, 1992b). Its features are hierarchical structuring of social patterns and personal perspectives, either/or thinking that posits normative dualisms as exclusive and oppositional rather than complementary and similar (able/disabled, mind/body, male/female), and logic justifying domination of "inferior" groups (Warren, 1989). Activists seek to eliminate laws, practices, institutional structures, and social attitudes that reduce people to gender or disability. Like gender, disability is not a biological given, but is socially constructed from biological reality (Fine & Asch, 1988; Gliedman & Roth, 1980).

Underlying ethical medical decisions are respect for self-determination, concern for well-being, and equity in access to services. Yet medical care is affected by supply, demand, and such characteristics of patients as insurance coverage, financial resources, age, gender, general health, and value placed on them. Health-care reform focuses on such allocation formulas as giving treatment (1) equally; (2) according to need; (3) based on personal effort, contributions, and merit; or (4) according to free-market exchanges. An "equal share" alternative might not meet the extensive needs of some MR people. Treatment "according to need" results in those with special needs receiving more than others. In Rawls' (1971) model of distributive justice, disparities are permitted if they benefit the least advantaged. Yet differential valuing of people relating to race, social class, gender, age, sexual orientation, and intelligence means that allocation of research efforts, scarce resources, and medical interventions are often inequitable (Veatch, 1987).

QUALITY OF LIFE

Ideally, individuals should make decisions, governments should be impartial, and doctors should act as fiduciaries, protecting and promoting patients' choices (Brennan, 1991). The ideal, however, is far from the reality. Those most in need of medical resources are often most unable to exert authority over them. Many MR people depend on others, so their claims to rights implicitly acknowledge that such claims cannot be vindicated without support, as in families' or neighbors' acceptance of them as members of the community (Burt, 1984). Although MR people depend on the benevolence of others, quality-of-life considerations cause some care providers to believe that the negative aspects of a disabled life outweigh the benefits; that life is so diminished for some MR people that death is preferable.

Selective Nontreatment

Some medical resource distribution practices deliberately exclude people with substantial disabilities through "selective nontreatment." The major rationale undergirding nontreatment is that, if kept alive, individuals would suffer a diminished life. The complexities of ethical decision making related to quality-of-life judgments were illustrated in the well-publicized Baby Doe case. This case challenged medical judgment, hospital practices, and institutional rules and created conflicts among local, state, and federal governments (Beauchamp & Childress, 1989). In the spring of 1982, Baby Doe was born with Down syndrome and a tracheoesophageal fistula (an opening between the breathing and swallowing tubes that prevents passage of food to the stomach). His parents were informed that corrective surgery for the fistula would have an even chance of success, but if he were left untreated, he would starve or die of pneumonia induced by stomach secretions reaching the lungs. Baby Doe's parents, who had two healthy children, chose to withhold treatment and let nature take its course. Court action to remove the infant from parental custody (and permit surgery) was sought by the county prosecutor, but was denied. The Indiana Supreme Court declined to review the lower court's ruling. Observing that the mother was with Infant Doe until he died at six days of age, the parents' lawyer stated: "It wasn't a case of abandonment. It was a case of love" (cited in Beauchamp & Childress, 1989, p. 423).

To prevent future withholding of medical treatment from MR infants, Richard Schweiker, then Secretary of the U.S. Department of Health and Human Services, issued letters to 6,800 hospital recipients of federal funds, reminding them that under Section 504 it was unlawful to withhold nutritional sustenance or medical treatment required to correct life-threatening conditions if withholding was based on the infant being handicapped. This regulation mandates routine care regardless of the severity of an infant's condition (Mason, 1990; Walker, 1979; Wells, 1989). Whereas formerly parents and doctors had discretionary powers about providing treatment, by making quality-of-life judgments in neonatal treatment dilemmas unacceptable, the regulation gives power to courts and governments and undermines the positions of parents and local health-care workers.

Rigid rules disallowing nontreatment may oversimplify complex circumstances. Proponents of reinstating quality-of-life judgments call the Baby Doe exclusion inhumane because prolonging life may subject individuals to burdens disproportionate to any benefit of living (Buchanan & Brock, 1989; Weir, 1984). Competent people may choose not to prolong their lives at the expense of other things they value—medical treatment can deplete family funds and can be painful and undignified (Veatch, 1987). Treatment is optional with patients who are irreversibly comatose or whose treatment would only prolong dying, would be futile, or would be inhumane or too expensive. Dalley and Berthoud (1992) question routine processing of decisions through rule-bound systems and advocate that professional judgment be based on a contextualized, discursive, and reflective morality.

Because of the dire consequences of either nontreatment or treatment, attempts have been made to establish criteria for quality-of-life judgments. Fletcher (1971), a theologian and professor of medical ethics, proposed criteria to indicate personhood: (1) has minimal intelligence (an IQ below 40 was questionably a person, below 20 was not a person); (2) has an awareness of self, time, past, and future; (3) has some control of existence; (4) is capable of relating to others; (5) has curiosity, rationality, and feeling, a recognizable identity; and (6) has neo-cortical function. Bromham, Dalton, and Jackson (1988) maintain that children should have physical and mental health, freedom from pain and suffering, brain function sufficient for sentience and cognition, potential to develop human relationships, and ability to be independent.

The Bioethics Committee (1986) of the Canadian Paediatric Society set criteria for exceptions to sustaining and prolonging life: (1) irreversible progression of disease and imminent death, (2) treatment that is potentially ineffective or harmful, (3) severely shortened life even with treatment, (4) greater comfort with nontreatment, or (5) life filled with intolerable and intractable pain. The Committee did distinguish between active (euthanasia, mercy killing) and passive (nontreatment) approaches. Believing that doctors are not entitled to withhold treatment on the grounds of "letting nature take its course" because that is what they are employed to prevent, Jackson (1988) goes on to claim that it does not follow that doctors must do all in their power to save or sustain patients' lives. Ordinary means are obligatory, whereas extraordinary means are morally optional. Campbell (1990) recommends that doctors assume the primary responsibility when not treating patients to relieve families of guilt they may feel if left to make decisions on their own.

Genetic and Prenatal Screening

Similar to selective nontreatment in that they ultimately involve quality-of-life issues, genetic screening and prenatal screening monitor the presence of defects in potential offspring or, as Harris (1988) writes, consider "characteristics and qualifications of potential children for their adequacy as children" (p. 156). Genetic screening examines evidence of inheritable conditions in the family histories of potential parents, and genetic counseling conveys the risk of occurrence of genetic disorders, provides facts about the course of disorders and management of them, and describes the benefits and risks of amniocentesis and the availability of therapeutic abortion. Amniocentesis, a method of obtaining amniotic fluid, which can be tested for genetic defects, is done under local anesthesia 15 weeks after conception. In approximately 1 out of 100 cases, it causes complications such as bleeding, infection, inhibited fetal cell growth, and abortion.

Disabling conditions and infant deaths result from over 1,500 genetic diseases; 1 family in 10 has a child with a serious, identifiable disease such as cystic fibrosis, sickle cell anemia, hemophilia, Down syndrome, or Tay-Sachs disease (Fraser, 1974). Genetic diseases do not always appear at birth or in childhood; diabetes mellitus is often not detected until people are in their fifties. Diseases may occur regularly in every generation, skip generations, or occur for the first time in family memory in a newborn child. Fraser recommends that the following high-risk groups receive genetic counseling: (1) members of an ethnic group prone to a certain disease (African Americans to sickle cell anemia; Ashkenazic Jews to Tay-Sachs disease; Greeks to thalassemia); (2) women over 35 because of the risk of Down syndrome; (3) people with a relative with a genetic disease; (4) couples who already have a child born with a genetic disease; and (5) women who have had multiple miscarriages.

Tort law influences such medical procedures as the routine use of ultrasound testing because failure to screen for disorders can result in legal charges of negligence against doctors for not preventing a "wrongful life" of pain, suffering, and financial hardships (Lee, 1989). The case is made that if parents had known about defects prior to conception or early in pregnancy, they would have made sure the child would not have been born. Parents receiving information about impairment do not always choose abortion. Although healthy children are preferred to disabled ones, the latter are sometimes judged to be better than none at all (Harris, 1988). Potential parents are not legally obliged to undergo genetic screening—not even those in high-risk categories—nor do laws require that defective fetuses be aborted. In fact, the Hyde amendment (1976) to Medicaid entitlements bans Medicaid funds for abortion unless the mother's life is endangered. Brody (1987) hypothesizes that if Congress passed a compulsory health insurance act, it might discourage irresponsible parenthood by denying reimbursement to parents who received a prenatal diagnosis of defect and still chose to have the child. Revealing the inherent flaws of contractual models of social relations if power is not equally distributed among citizens, Brody warns that, given the reality of the above scenario, the rich could afford to have children with severe disabilities, whereas the poor could not. Social pressure exerts bipolar influences: by some, to abort; by others, not to, regardless of the nature of the fetus. Some (e.g., Asch, 1990; Blatt, 1988; Finger, 1990; Koop, 1989) believe disability in a fetus is not an appropriate reason to abort. Fine and Asch (1988) believe people falsely assume that children with disabilities are too costly to families and society, that they contribute nothing to family life, and/or that life with a disability is not worth living. Wolhandler and Weber (1992) might rebut that the option to abort if serious defects are found should not conflict with the commitment to improve life for people with disabilities.

Burdens of MR Childbearing on Families

Until about 30 years ago, the greatest-happiness principle was the standard for judging laws and policies (Deigh, 1989). Perceived as hindering the rights of the majority, MR people's admission to public schools could be blocked, as could access to community life and their reproductive capacities. Compulsory sterilization was routine, and, depending on the type of surgery performed, other aspects of sexuality affected by hormonal and menstrual cycles often were diminished. Human rights arguments started to take precedence, and concern was expressed about the justice of segregation and prohibition of procreation. In 1974, the United Nations' World Population Plan adopted the position that all people have the right to decide freely and responsibly the number and spacing of their children (Deigh, 1989).

Some insist quality-of-life considerations apply only to the family member with disabilities. Bromham (1992) calls the "distortion that quality-of-life ideas mean worth in utilitarian terms of costs to others" and the "false interpretation of nontreatment of seriously abnormal infants as a general policy of discrimination" against MR individuals "hyperbolic propaganda" (p. 11). Although not recognized in recent court decisions, concerns can be expanded beyond MR infants to the burden on their parents. External (to MR individuals) interpretations are controversial, but pertinent, at a time when regulations require prolonging the lives of individuals who, in the past, would not have been treated. Even if children's lives might be meaningful, support for abortion and nontreatment of fetuses and newborns with substantial disabilities can be based on the argument that their presence would unduly burden other family members, usually mothers. Individuals' rights are limited by rights of others—a caveat that becomes particularly relevant when people's lives are closely linked, such as when some are dependent on others. Even if governmental costs of MR infants are not considered, costs to families are a legitimate concern (McCullough, Coverdale, Bayer, & Chervenak, 1992). Acknowledging the need to be responsible for decisions (Lilford, 1988), it is reasonable to assume that if parents are denied choices about the fate of offspring with substantial disabilities, governments should finance the rearing of such offspring.

Regarding parenting by MR individuals, infringements of rights extend in two directions: with the previous generation (with parents who may have to assume care for their MR children's offspring) and with the next generation (with offspring who have the right to proper care). Through genetic screening and prenatal intervention, parents replace children who would have been born disabled, but children cannot replace defective parents so easily. Children suffer from less than adequate parenting; thus, a dimension of "wrongful birth" is being born to inadequate parents (Harris, 1988). To prevent suffering from the perspective of the child, parents could be screened. Under the caption "harm to others," Jackson (1988) maintains that anyone's rights are circumscribed by others' rights; hence, there may be occasions in which MR individuals' rights to procreation are legitimately overridden (p. 126). Arguments against an MR (or any other) person becoming a parent can be based on proxy consent (deciding for someone incapable of making decisions) and judgment as to the best interests of potential offspring (Harris, 1988). This dimension of wrongful birth raises questions about the right to found a family and about suitable criteria and methods for screening parents (Wolhandler & Weber, 1992).

In addition to earlier practices of subjecting MR women to compulsory sterilization or abortion or requiring them to relinquish custody of children, attempts have been made to restrict reproductive rights of known child abusers and chronically unemployed mothers on welfare. At this point, collective and legal sentiments support reproductive freedoms and condemn limiting procreation. On the other hand, considerable public pressure to intercede to protect children in problematic family situations exists. Agencies and governments continually make post hoc judgments about the quality of people's parenting after abuse or neglect has occurred, yet suitable arrangements for children removed from families remain elusive (Janko, 1994). In spite of outcries about abortion and nontreatment, no commensurate offers of nurturing environments or movements for restrictive policies on reproduction are evident. If criteria to judge parental adequacy and effective methods to screen potential parents were developed, perhaps some abuse and neglect could be prevented.

There is a higher incidence of abuse, neglect, and inadequate parenting among MR people (Sobsey, Grey, Wells, Pyper, & Reimer-Heck, 1991), but some MR individuals are good parents. Members of other groups (smokers, substance abusers) endanger offspring, but are not prevented from parenting (Pincus & Swenson, 1992). Parenting resulting from teenage pregnancy inflicts social costs, but adolescents are not prevented from childbearing. Beller and Graham (1993) detail the economic plight of father-absent families, and Bronfenbrenner and Neville (1994) state that in 1990, in the United States, one child in four lived with only one parent and 17 percent of children lived with families whose incomes fell below the poverty line. Any attempt to avoid the costs of childbearing by MR individuals must be broadened to include other individuals and groups that present childbearing burdens (Kingdom, 1989).

INDIVIDUAL RIGHTS AND PUBLIC POLICY

Arguing that sterilization decisions legitimately involve criteria other than MR persons' right to procreate, Brody (1987) cites the public health model in which each patient is considered, but social values compete for priority, and individuals may be requested or coerced to promote chosen program goals. A public health model might screen for communicable diseases, health hazards, genetic carriers, and treatable diseases before allowing reproduction. Viewed from a patient's perspective, this might seem an invasion of privacy and a coercive limitation of freedom; seen as a greater public good, it is ethical to control diseases and make patients responsible for the best reproductive conditions. Given the extreme shift in opinion about human rights in this century, it is not surprising, as Kasachkoff (1989) notes, that there is neither public consensus nor philosophical agreement on the role of government in the lives of citizens. Bromham (1992) feels that any rationale for limiting procreation based on preventing burden to others is illegitimate. Petchesky (1990) calls involuntary sterilization abusive because it "subverts people's need to control their bodies in fully informed and conscious ways" (p. 71). Recommending that state power be used only to serve the interests of MR individuals, Szasz (1991) condemns coercion as based on false assumptions of social inferiority. Petchesky and Szasz couch their arguments in an autonomy framework and caution about acknowledging the boundary between justifiable protection and unjustifiable paternalism. Actions based on MR individuals' threat to others should document that antisocial acts warrant coercion (Buchanan & Brock, 1989; Wolfensberger, 1992). Although most see paternalism as at odds with individual rights, paternalism can protect persons from self-inflicted harm; hence, protecting the welfare, needs, and interests of coerced persons may be justified (Deigh, 1989).

Human rights encompass human well-being and needs for food, shelter, personal security, health, tranquility, and comfort. Compared to deprivations of these needs, limiting procreation or family size may not bring misery or seriously hinder individuals' prospects for happiness. In civil societies, zoning ordinances and building codes restrict (and protect) people's health and allow them to enjoy property. When individuals require public support to care for their offspring, perhaps governments, as citizen collectives, should have a role in decisions about reproduction. Tolerance of irresponsible and untimely reproduction, especially when combined with expectations that mothers and children should be supported by public funds, may be unrealistic and detrimental to society as a whole. Given the competing needs of individuals in society, it is essential to examine whether the right to procreate should be stated as strongly as it is in the United Nations' World Population Plan, which allows complete freedom of choice about reproduction. There is a need to balance rights and social obligations (Brody, 1987; Lee & Morgan, 1989a, 1989b).

Wolfe (1989) contends that citizens in liberal democracies prize individualism and freedom, but do not recognize the personal sacrifices and social obligations that made freedom possible in the first place and that are necessary to extend present benefits to future generations. Governmental institutions carry out services once provided by families such as pensions, welfare and medical benefits, child protection, and socialization of children in schools. Yet the emergence of the welfare state created an atmosphere of moral uncertainty that takes the form of distrust of authority and an unwillingness to contribute to the communal pot. Wolfe believes that, although they are uncomfortable with explicit discussions of obligations, middle-class people are in a position to make the kind of social world they desire. Wolfe makes a case for a "sociological approach" to civil society in order to reintegrate people into the moral process of decision making by encompassing such ideals as "organic solidarity," "collective conscience," and "the gift of relationship" (p. 17).

In contrast to Wolfe's view of "the state" as a social collective, others see it as an authority aligned with industry, with aims that run counter to the interests of common citizens. Governments intrude into family and community life by employing professionals in such low-status management areas as teaching, social service, and criminal justice work (Yalnizyan, 1988). With ambiguous status and power, this professional class reaps advantages in managing the social order and mopping up market casualities (Walker, 1979). Professional expertise increasingly substitutes for family autonomy (Habermas, 1986). Edelman (1977) asserts that, although the "language of help" evokes a world in which the "weak and the wayward" are controlled "for their own good," this discourse disguises the "authority and repression in which the powerless are abused by the powerful" (p. 60).

4

Sexuality and Reproduction

This chapter reviews the benefits and drawbacks of common birth control methods, including sterilization, for MR individuals. Concerns of care providers in protecting clients from sexually transmitted diseases (STDs) and the disability status of HIV-positive individuals are addressed. Barriers preventing unconstrained decisions for MR women are identified. Finally, the chapter includes findings about positive aspects of sexual expression for MR individuals as well as their vulnerability to sexual abuse.

CONTRACEPTION

It is important to review common forms of sterilization as well as contraceptive alternatives to sterilization.[1] In the interest of voluntarism and free choice, MR people should have the opportunity to select from the widest variety of contraceptive options (Shelton & Speidel, 1983). For those too cognitively limited to choose independently, others should make decisions based on what best suits MR individuals' needs.

Choosing contraception depends on effectiveness, safety, convenience, need for protection from STDs, reversibility, and cost. When considering effectiveness, there is a difference between the lowest expected failure rate, which is based on consistent and correct use of the method, and the higher typical user failure rate, which is based on records of actual use over time. User failure rates include instances of forgetting to take pills, failing to use condoms correctly, and removing diaphragms too soon after intercourse; they also reflect frequency of intercourse. Because effectiveness depends on correct usage, methods will be evaluated in terms of their use by MR persons.

Natural Birth Control

Abstinence has two definitions: to abstain from sexual interaction and to make love without sexual intercourse. With the second type of abstinence, pregnancy can result without actual penetration of the vagina by the penis if sperm are ejaculated close to the vaginal entrance. Moreover, STDs spread with close physical contact, and particularly with an exchange of body fluids. If used consistently, abstinence is an effective contraceptive that has been practiced for centuries. It has no adverse effects as long as prolonged arousal is followed by orgasm to relieve pelvic congestion. Just as with others, some MR individuals may be expected to abstain—may even intend to abstain—but may not actually abstain.

Withdrawal or coitus interruptus consists of withdrawing the penis from the vagina prior to ejaculation. It requires control by the man, and mistakes happen because of false anticipation of the exact moment of ejaculation. Moreover, preejaculatory fluid may contain sperm. Accurate failure rates are not available; the lowest expected rate is 4 percent, but a typical rate is likely to be around 18 percent. Withdrawal does not protect against STDs. For reasons related to mental slowness, withdrawal may be even less effective for MR men. *Douching* after intercourse may even increase the chance of pregnancy by forcing sperm through the cervix. *Avoidance of female orgasm* does not prevent conception. *Breastfeeding* prevents ovulation in some women, but not all.

Fertility observation or ovulation prediction makes use of our knowledge of the hormonal changes linked to fertility by observing cervical mucus, basal body temperature, and cephalad shift (cervix changes). The method relies on astute observations and accurate records. *Rhythm* used to be practiced by abstaining from intercourse for a few days in the middle of the monthly cycle. Because of variation in ovulation times, to be effective it must be combined with the temperature or mucus observation techniques.

Some health professionals rate all natural methods of birth control as poor, but Bell (1992) maintains they can be effective when understood thoroughly and used correctly. Because of the need for technical knowledge (reading a thermometer, charting, judging body conditions) and consistency in usage, natural methods are probably inappropriate for many MR people.

Barrier and Intrauterine Devices

A *diaphragm* is a piece of soft rubber in the shape of a shallow cup. Used with spermicidal cream or jelly, it is inserted into the vagina over the cervix. It has a failure rate of 6 percent if used correctly, but the typical failure rate is 18 percent. Presenting no risk of death, the diaphragm can cause discomfort if it is the wrong size or in the wrong position, urethritis or cystitis if it pushes against the bladder or urethra, and yeast infections if it is not washed thoroughly; spermicidal cream can cause irritation. A diaphragm costs about 20 dollars and lasts about two years.

The *cervical cap* is a thimble-shaped rubber cap that fits snugly over the cervix, blocking sperm from entering the cervical opening. It usually contains a small amount of spermicide. It has about the same effectiveness as the diaphragm. It creates the same health problems as other barrier methods inserted into the vagina. If left in place for long periods, it increases the possibility of toxic shock syndrome. Because the diaphragm and the cap are distributed by health practitioners, the cost of the examination should be included in the price.

The *vaginal pouch* (or *female condom*) is an over-the-counter device made for one-time use. It consists of a soft, loose-fitting polyurethane sheath with flexible rings located at either end of the pouch, one at the closed cervical end (which serves as an internal anchor) and one at the open end at the external edge of the vagina). It is about as effective as the cervical cap and the diaphragm in preventing pregnancy, but offers more protection against STDs and HIV infection. Some find the pouch cumbersome because it is noticeable during intercourse.

The *contraceptive sponge* is a disposable, one-size (two and one-quarter inches in diameter) sponge that is inserted into the vagina to cover the cervix. It is intended for one-time use and is available over the counter. It contains a spermicide, to which 2 percent of women have allergic reactions. Some women find it difficult to remove and complain it has an unpleasant odor. Some have more yeast infections while using the sponge. Its effectiveness rate is similar to that of the diaphragm. It offers little protection against STDs.

Jellies and *creams* are designed for use with a diaphragm or a cervical cap and are available without prescription. They are inserted into the vagina with an applicator tube shortly before intercourse. The lowest expected failure rate for spermicides used alone is 3 percent; the failure rate among typical users is 21 percent. Jellies and creams provide some protection against gonorrhea and chlamydia. They can cause allergic reactions.

The *male condom (rubber, prophylactic,* or *safe)* is a sheath, usually made of thin, strong latex rubber, designed to fit over an erect penis to keep semen from getting into the woman's vagina. Some condoms include lubricants or spermicides. Condoms are available over the counter, are fairly cheap, and have a failure rate of about 2 percent when used as directed, but a typical rate of 12 percent. They are good protection against some STDs when used in every instance of vagina-to-penis contact.

The reliability of barrier methods depends on consistent and correct usage; therefore, they may be inappropriate for many MR people. This judgment may stereotype MR people as irresponsible and inconsistent, but many who live or work most closely with MR individuals believe they would have trouble remembering to use these devices prior to sexual intercourse. On the other hand, extensive training in these methods may be advantageous because of the importance of protection against STDs. Condoms may be used in addition to the pill or sterilization to prevent STDs.

Intrauterine devices (IUDs) are small plastic, copper, or synthetic progesterone devices of various shapes and sizes that fit inside the uterus with a string attached that extends through the cervical opening into the upper vagina. They are inserted by a practitioner (at a cost of between $220 and $400) and replaced every four years. The IUD may cause inflammation or chronic low-grade infection in the uterus, which triggers the body's defense system to produce higher numbers of white cells that damage or destroy sperm or eggs. Another explanation is that they hinder the buildup of the uterine lining for implantation of a fertilized egg. It has a failure rate of 3 percent.

A major drawback of the IUD is its high expulsion rate (between 2 and 20 percent of users expel them within the first year). The IUD can harm fertility if it causes pelvic inflammatory disease, perforates the uterus, becomes embedded in the uterus lining, or results in ectopic pregnancy (which damages the fallopian tube). Other complications are infections, excessive bleeding and cramping during menstruation, and missing strings so women do not know if the IUD remains in place. IUDs offer no protection against STDs and increase the chance of pelvic inflammatory disease.

The IUD was considered a good long-term, reversible, birth control method for MR women because it did not require day-to-day decisions about its use. The difficulty of recognizing the IUD's expulsion and health problems were disadvantages. Nevertheless, the Dalkon Shield was withdrawn from the market as a result of the number of lawsuits related to problems in its use, and IUDs are rarely used in this country at this time (Grant, 1992).

Hormonal/Chemical Contraception

Birth control pills inhibit eggs from developing in the ovary by raising women's estrogen levels. The pill is almost 100 percent effective when taken daily, but has a typical failure rate of 3 percent. The pill is counterindicated for women with diabetes, hepatitis, breast cancer, gall bladder disease, sickle cell anemia, cardiac or renal disease, and any disease connected with blood clotting. Reported side effects are headaches, weight gain, depression, nausea, change in intensity of sexual desire and response, vaginitis and vaginal discharge, urinary tract infection, skin problems, gum inflammation, viral infections, cervical dysplasia, and chlamydia. The higher incidence of disease may be due to the pill altering women's nutritional requirements. Return of fertility after stopping the pill may take several months. The pill's advantages are that it regulates menstrual cycles, results in lighter flow and fewer cramps during periods, relieves premenstrual tension, reduces pelvic inflammatory disease (PID), and possibly clears up acne. It does not prevent STDs.

The pill was approved in 1960 based on little research, and, because of its generalized impact on women's bodies, it still has not been conclusively tested. A common belief in the United States is that risks increase with long-term use. Interviews with women and health-care workers in Australia and New Zealand revealed their belief that the pill could be taken indefinitely; hence, they are less likely to recommend sterilization. Because the pill can be dispensed routinely, it is frequently given to all MR women of childbearing age in institutions.

Norplant consists of six match-size, flexible, silastic rubber capsules, containing the synthetic progestin levonorgestrel (a hormone present in some birth control pills), that are implanted in the fleshy part of a woman's upper arm just under the skin by a qualified practitioner. It works by both inhibiting ovulation and thickening cervical mucus, which impedes sperm activity. The pregnancy rate for five years' continuous use is 3.9 percent. Because it has been used only a short time, the long-term effects are unknown. In the short term, there has been no evidence of cardiovascular, respiratory, or central nervous system problems. A possibility of interaction with antiseizure drugs exists. An implant costs about $350 and lasts up to five years, but can be removed at any time.

Depo-Provera ("the shot"), a long-acting (up to three months) synthetic hormone (progesterone), suppresses ovulation, increases cervical mucus, and alters the uterine lining, making it unsuitable for implantation. It has been used in over 90 countries. Because Depo-Provera and Norplant do not require daily attention, they may be effective for MR women who have access to treatment. Neither prevents STDs.

Sterilization

Voluntary sterilization increased rapidly during the last two decades and is now the contraceptive method used most frequently by married couples in the United States and by persons throughout the world (one-third of contraceptive use) (Sloan, 1988). The practicality and safety of female sterilization were improved by replacing inpatient procedures that used general anesthesia with outpatient surgery done with local anesthesia. The availability of vasectomy also accounts for sterilization's growth. Use expanded because donors such as the Agency for International Development (AID) increased funds for sterilization from a few thousand dollars in 1970 to over $25 million in 1981 (Shelton & Speidel, 1983, p. 1). In spite of the dramatic increase, there still is a large unmet demand for sterilization services. As with any birth control method, the factors used in selecting a method of sterilization include availability, safety, cost, ease of delivery of services, and individual and social acceptability. Sterilization is virtually 100% effective and is very cost-effective, considering the years of protection it provides.

A *vasectomy,* usually done in a doctor's office or clinic, takes 15 to 30 minutes and costs about $400 to $450. A local anesthetic such as Novocaine is applied, small incisions are made in the scrotum, each vas deferens (two tubes that carry sperm from the testes to the penis) is located, a piece is removed, and the ends are tied off. A vasectomy leaves the man's genital system basically unchanged, his sexual hormones remain operative, and there is no noticeable difference in his ejaculate because sperm make up a small part of semen. Also, experimental operations have placed plastic plugs or injectable chemicals into the vas deferens. Vasectomy and vas deferens blockage are considered irreversible; reversal surgery has a 50 to 90 percent success rate and costs $2,000 to $3,000. A vasectomy is a surgical procedure, but does not require entering the abdominal cavity and is not associated with a high degree of risk. Because the procedure is relatively straightforward, paramedical technicians have performed vasectomies in a number of countries.

A *tubal ligation,* female sterilization, requires abdominal entry because the fallopian tubes are within the abdominal cavity. It must be performed in a protected environment, and, even when using state-of-the-art technology, a surgeon's skills are required because vital internal structures close to the area may inadvertently be injured. Tubal ligations can be performed through a woman's vagina (colpotomy or culdoscopy) or cervix (hysteroscopy, an experimental procedure). They probably do not affect a woman's hormone secretions, ovaries, uterus, or vagina, although the menstrual cycle may become irregular. Eggs released from the ovary stop partway down the tube and are reabsorbed. A tubal ligation costs between $900 and $1,500; a reversal costs between $5,000 and $10,000 and has a success rate of 10 to 90 percent. Another option for getting pregnant is in-vitro fertilization.

Tubal ligation is essentially unavailable to much of the developing world owing to an inadequate number of physicians in rural areas where most of the population lives. Surgically trained physicians who practice in rural areas are overwhelmed with other pressing medical problems. Even with the use of new technologies in developed countries, female sterilization is an expensive procedure and absorbs a significant part of available health funds. A female sterilization procedure that is simple, inexpensive, nonmorbid, and nonsurgical would be a useful adjunct to the delivery of family planning services.

Laparoscopy, or "Band-Aid" surgery, is the most common female sterilization technique in the United States. The procedure, usually done with local anesthesia and a light sedative, takes about 30 minutes and involves making a small incision in the belly button and inflating the belly with carbon dioxide or nitrous oxide so internal organs are visible. A laparoscope (a thin tube containing a viewing instrument and light) is inserted through the incision, and an instrument to block the fallopian tubes by burning (electrocoagulation or cautery), cutting, clipping shut, or applying rings is introduced through the laparosope or a second tiny incision below the belly button. Afterward, some women feel pain in their shoulders from the gas.

A *minilaparotomy,* or minilap, involves making a small incision just above the woman's pubic bone, moving the tubes into view with a tenaculum (clamp) and ultrasound, pulling the fallopian tubes up through the incision, and blocking them (usually by tying and cutting). Women have more and longer-lasting pain than with a laparoscopy. The minilaparotomy and the laparoscopy have a failure rate of about 0.2 percent. Because surgery involves anesthetic, complications are possible, but depend on the skill and experience of the practitioner. Cardiac irregularity, cardiac arrest, infection, internal bleeding, and perforation of a major blood vessel are a few of the potential hazards. Some women experience a postlaparoscopic syndrome, including heavy irregular bleeding and increased menstrual pain, which may create the need for repeated dilation and curettages or hysterectomies. The surgery should be considered permanent, but recent advances in microsurgery have increased the possibility of reconstruction.

Nonsurgical sterilization involves injecting substances into the fallopian tubes, inserting pellets or plugs, or modifying surgical procedures by using new types of clips or rings rather than cutting tubes. Its advantages include less training needed by personnel, improved availability, and decreased cost and time. With the exception of the tubal plug, all are considered permanent methods with little chance of reversal.

A *hysterectomy* (total or complete) involves removing the uterus and cervix. The woman continues to ovulate, but does not have menstrual periods. An *oophorectomy* includes the bilateral salpingo-oophorectomy in which the fallopian tubes (salpingo) and (usually both) ovaries (oophor) are removed. In a *radical hysterectomy*, the upper part of the vagina and sometimes the lymph nodes in the pelvic area are removed. Removal of the uterus can be done through an abdominal incision or through the vagina. A number of risks and complications can result from a hysterectomy: (1) The death rate is between 1 and 2 women in 1,000; (2) as a sterilization method, it has 20 times the complication rate of a tubal ligation; (3) surgical complications include infection (which is sometimes severe), urinary tract complications (almost half of the women have kidney or bladder infections following surgery; sensory nerves may be cut, causing loss of the sensation of having to urinate and control bladder function), hemorrhage (1 woman in 10 requires transfusions), bowel problems (due to damage to the intestines during surgery), blood clots, death or paralysis from anesthesia, and postsurgical complications. Hysterectomies are done because of cancer, severe uncontrollable bleeding, blockage of the bladder, pelvic infection, and rupture of the uterus. Oophorectomies are done because of ectopic pregnancy, endometriosis, malignant or benign tumors, cysts on the ovary, and pelvic inflammatory disease. Crowe (1992) concludes that 30 to 50 percent of operations are clearly unnecessary and another 10 percent could have been avoided (p. 598).

Patients are readily reassured that there is no impact on sexual response from hysterectomy and that any problems women report have a psychological cause. However, 33 to 46 percent of women have difficulty becoming aroused and reaching orgasm after hysterectomies (Crowe, 1992; Zussman, Zussman, Sunley, & Bjornson, 1981). There are three plausible explanations for diminished arousal: (1) Uterine contractions contribute to arousal and orgasm by causing increased stimulation of the abdominal lining; (2) there is less tissue in the pelvic area to become engorged with blood, which adds to the sexual arousal sensation; and (3) when the ovaries are removed, ovarian androgens, which affect sexual response and cannot be replaced by estrogen replacement therapy, may be greatly reduced.

Sterilizations performed on MR women over the years were not always tubal ligations, but hysterectomies and oophorectomies, which prevent hormone production and development of secondary sexual characteristics. Visits to institutions reveal elderly people who retain the general appearance of children because their sex glands were removed prior to puberty. Through interviews with professionals, I learned that a local doctor did sterilizations of MR people by directing X-ray radiation toward the ovaries or testes. Although the method requires no surgery and left no scars, sterilization by radiation has never been selected for personal use by the general public because of the risk of damaging other organs. Its unique use for MR individuals illustrates how little value is placed on their lives. Just as this example documents a surreptitious, and it is hoped very limited, practice, it is likely that a history of involuntary sterilization would reveal that "local wisdom" resulted in various abusive practices in different parts of the country.

In making decisions about birth control, there is a need to strike a balance between the drawbacks and potential risks and the likelihood of positive consequences. Sterilization is chosen precisely because childbearing is not desired or advisable, and it is the preferred method of birth control. These same rationales should undergird decisions regarding sterilization of MR people. Three basic questions are pertinent: (1) Is the person sexually active or interested in being sexually active in the future? (2) Does the person want to prevent impregnation, or is it advisable that impregnation be prevented? (3) Are other less permanent, less invasive forms of birth control not preferable? If these cannot be answered affirmatively, sterilization is not recommended.

Credible arguments justify involuntary sterilization of MR people who are sexually active, yet too cognitively impaired to give informed consent, use temporary birth control effectively, or be adequate parents. In such cases, it is plausible to see sterilization as a least restrictive alternative (Mappes & Zembaty, 1986). Neville (1981) claims: "Paradoxically, to refrain from sterilization is to do them the violence of preventing participation in the community in one of the important respects of which they are capable" (p. 67). Yet, with the threat of malpractice suits, physicians shy away from the risks of sterilizing individuals perceived as incapable of giving consent (Brantlinger, 1992a).

SEXUALLY TRANSMITTED DISEASES

Given the risk of AIDS and STDs, Neville's recommendation for sexual freedom must be implemented cautiously. Crocker, Cohen, and Kastner (1992) admit little is known about HIV in MR populations, but warn that, in the absence of epidemiology information, residential facilities should take a proactive stand in testing clients for HIV. In a seroprevalence survey of 241 MR adults served at a clinic (Pincus, Schoenbaum, & Webber, 1990), none was HIV positive. A study of agencies for the mentally retarded and developmentally disabled in 44 states found 45 HIV-antibody-positive clients in 11 states (two-thirds lived in institutions and one-third in the community) (Marchetti, Nathanson, Kastner, & Owens, 1990). In spite of the high incidence of homosexual behaviors in residences that separate by gender, Fidone (1987) found little hepatitis B or AIDS among MR residents.

Fidone predicts an increased risk for MR people in the community because of their likelihood of interacting with HIV-positive individuals as well as their not understanding how to protect themselves. Even those with mild cognitive limitations lack the knowledge and social skills to prevent potentially dangerous situations (Bell, Feraios, & Bryan, 1991).

Fifty percent of the general population contact gonorrhea or syphilis by age 25 (Sugar, 1990); 94 percent of 19- to 25-year-old women are sexually active, but only 28 percent require sexual partners to use condoms (Grace, Emans, & Woods, 1989). In spite of ever-increasing risks of contracting serious STDs, students report the same absence of communication about sexuality in families in the 1980s as in the 1970s (Sarrel & Sarrel, 1990). Sexuality curricula mainly emphasize abstinence and ignore protection in sexual relations (Bell, Feraios, & Bryan, 1991; Llewellyn & McLaughlin, 1986). Educators must recognize the futility of making recommendations so frequently rejected by youth. Explicit and practical AIDS education on resisting social pressure to have sex and using a condom is available on videotape (Levy, Levy, & Samowitz, 1988).

Individuals who are HIV-positive are recognized as entitled to disability status by the IDEA and the ADA (Diamond & Cohen, 1992). AIDS dementia in adults resembles mental retardation, and prenatal acquiry of HIV is a major infectious cause of intellectual impairment (Rowitz, 1989). If individuals are HIV-positive, confidentiality and safe environments for infected individuals and others are to be guaranteed (Gerry, 1988; Kastner, DeLotto, Scagnelli, & Testa, 1990; Pledgie & Schumacher, 1993).

THE POLITICS OF FERTILITY CONTROL

While sexual activity does not have to lead to procreation, religious and cultural mores binding sexuality to parenthood have optimized its chances (Greenberg & Campbell, 1992; Lee & Morgan, 1989b). Nongenital sex, masturbation, relations between same-sex partners, and sex during menstruation have been considered unnatural, illegal, or immoral (Klein, 1992, p. 11). Orthodox Judaism bans sexual activity during menstruation, Catholicism defines contraception, abortion, and masturbation as sins; and various state laws against birth control, abortion, and sodomy demonstrate how equating sex with reproduction has been a central theme of Western culture (Greenberg & Campbell, 1992).

There was no law against abortion in the United States until 1821 (Sloan, 1988). Nineteenth-century antiabortion campaigns were successful, and, by 1900, abortion could not be legally obtained anywhere in the United States at any stage of pregnancy (Grant, 1992). In 1910, abortion after "quickening" (the time that fetal movement can be felt) could result in life imprisonment for both doctor and patient (Sloan, 1988, p. 6). The Comstock Law (1873–1938) banned interstate mailing of birth control devices. Campaigns against reproductive freedom tend to support patriarchal patterns of female dependency and spurn liberal policies allowing women permissive sexuality (Sherwin, 1992a; Wolfe, 1989). Many antiabortionists actively campaign to limit support for housing, child care, and education—the sorts of services necessary to make childbirth affordable for many women who choose abortion (Sherwin, 1992a). The World Health Organization acknowledges that poverty is the major health hazard to women and children and that concerted measures to promote social equity are needed (Spallone, 1989). Although more widely available than ever before, economic factors restrict the poor from access to contraception (Murphy, 1992).

Historically, children were an economic advantage, but during the Depression worry about excess population resulted in the overturning of the Comstock Law (Grant, 1992). Impetus for change also came from drugs (Thalidomide) and a German measles epidemic that caused birth defects (Sloan, 1988). Declaring unconstitutional a Texas statute that made abortion a criminal offense, *Roe v. Wade* (1973) essentially overturned all antiabortion statutes. *Roe v. Wade* was argued on women's "constitutional right to privacy," the same argument used in *Griswold v. Connecticut* (1965), the litigation that overturned laws forbidding contraceptives because it meant that the police would have to search bedrooms (Dworkin, 1993). Some (e.g., Colker, 1992; Dworkin, 1993; West, 1990) believe that in a male-dominated society, a woman's right to privacy is an illusion; that reproductive rights should be defended as an attempt to improve equality by allowing women to plan responsibly, develop strong ties to others, provide for family, and pursue work commitments.

At the same time that attention is directed to controlling fertility, women with physical impairments or medical conditions are lacking information, counseling, and care. Women with diabetes, epilepsy, and spinal cord injuries are frustrated by the lack of knowledge about sexuality, birth control, pregnancy, and childbirth pertaining to their special circumstances (Asrael, 1982). Because ignorance results in unsafe practices, women with these conditions need good advice and care from gynecologists, obstetricians, and rehabilitation counselors (LeMaistre, 1985).

CONFLICTING NEEDS OF MR INDIVIDUALS

Public opinion and policy seem divided between endorsing MR people's right to sexual expression and stressing their need for protection from sexual abuse. Advocates from both sides take strong stands and rarely address ambiguities or conflicts within their own positions. Rousso (1988) notes the ambivalence toward the emergence of sexuality among people with disabilities and the prevalent myths of their asexuality. Part of the problem in evaluating the legitimacy of sexual expression among severe MR people who are nonverbal stems from the difficulty of determining consent. However, such individuals routinely communicate consent or lack of consent through behaviors: Going into the kitchen and getting food can be interpreted as a sign of hunger or, at least, a desire to eat. Even severely MR and multiply handicapped individuals have been observed to initiate sexual interaction (Brantlinger, Klein, & Guskin, 1994). Perhaps actions can be interpreted as consenting to sexual relations. In more ambiguous cases, MR individuals comply with someone's lead, but interaction appears to be of a less consenting nature. A tenuous line may exist between intimacy and abuse in situations of dependency and limited communication (Weinberg, 1988).

Sexual abuse occurs when someone manipulates, forces, or tricks another into sexual contact or when one party is too young or cognitively limited to consent to relations (Cole, 1991). Due to their learning styles and life situations, MR people are especially vulnerable to sexual abuse (Bregman, 1984; Brookhouser, 1987; Chamberlain, Rauh, Passer, McGrath, & Burket, 1984; Garbarino, Brookhouser, & Authier, 1987; Green, 1988; Griffiths, Quinsey, & Hingsburger, 1989). Those in institutions are exploitable because they lack suitable models of intimate relations; learn to trust an ever-changing staff; have little wisdom to judge others' behaviors and little power to defend themselves or reject undesired advances; are subject to others' authority and must be compliant, regardless of what is done to them; may be too physically weak to ward off aggression; and may be unable to report abusive circumstances (Kempton & Gochros, 1986; Mulhern, 1975; Painsky, Katz, & Kravetz, 1986). Lengthy institutional stays result in confused self-concepts and lack of knowedge about sex (Hingsburger, 1988). Because of others' attitudes and the furtive nature of their sexual experiences, they view sexuality as negative and sexual expression as wrong (Heshusius, 1981). The incidence of sexual abuse is also high in community settings (Hewitt, 1987), especially for previously institutionalized people (Lakin, Prouty, White, Bruininks, & Hill, 1990; Levy, Levy, & Samowitz, 1988). Isolated from peers with whom they could have mutual relations, MR individuals agree to relations with inappropriate partners.

Finkelhor's (1984) model of preconditions for sexual abuse sheds light on why MR individuals are so often victims. First, the potential offender has to overcome the internal inhibitions against acting on their motives to abuse. The low status of MR individuals results in a potential abuser's devaluing them and feeling that they are unworthy of consideration. In overcoming the external impediments that deter abuse, the potential MR victim may be socially isolated, so actual instances of abuse go unnoticed by potential defenders. Rindfleisch and Bean (1988) found that willingness to report abuse among care providers is influenced by the nature of the abusive incident, the commitment to the clients, the organizational support for reporting, and the nature of the affiliation with the abuser. Another precondition for abuse is the undermining or overcoming of resistance. Whether in family homes or other residences, MR children and adults may be lonely, emotionally deprived, hungry for attention and affection, and unable to recognize the exploitive nature of acts. Because they have few positive outlets for sexual expression, they may willingly go along with something that is demeaning or painful. They may lack knowledge of such sexual taboos as incest or adult/child interactions (Eshilian, Haney, & Falvey, 1989; Griffiths, Quinsey, & Hingsburger, 1989; McClennen, 1988).

There is substantial evidence of MR individuals' problematic sexual behaviors with little focus on positive aspects of sexual expression. Although concern about the voluntariness of MR people's sexual relations is often genuine, restrictiveness may be evidence of a continuing taboo against sexual activity for MR people (Omenn, 1978; Weinberg, 1988). When care providers and families perceive social and sexual activity as threatening and constantly worry about the possibility of abuse, they send very negative messages about the appropriateness of sexual expression to MR children, adolescents, and adults (Abramson, Parker, & Weisberg, 1988; Brantlinger, 1983; Gardner, 1986; Kempton, 1977; Weinberg, 1988). Although mental disability makes the line between voluntary sexual activity and sexual abuse difficult to determine, that confusion should not result in suppression of all sexual expression. In order to develop helpful services, it is essential that those who work with MR individuals sort through their ideas about clients' sexual expression and make sincere attempts to distinguish between consenting and unwanted sex.

Although concerned with the rights of minors, Canadian writers Bearchell (1985) and Sullivan (1992) challenge standard views of youthful sexuality and critique the assumptions and implications of the prominent 1984 Badgley Report. Due to their unique incapacities, vulnerabilities, and needs, the Report recognizes youths' special legal status regarding sexual expression in relation to those who deal with them. At the risk of putting MR adults in the same category as children, the ambiguous domain of sexual expression of minors in many ways parallels the complexities of sexual and reproductive behaviors of MR people. In fact, Sullivan often alludes to MR individuals, for example, contending that abuse statistics are overestimated because of the assumption that they would not voluntarily consent to sexual relations. It must be made clear that MR adults are truly adults, not children, and although "special weaknesses" of immaturity gradually diminish with age until youth attain the age of majority, the weaknesses and vulnerabilities of MR individuals may never totally disappear. Nevertheless, developmental changes for anyone are gradual and erratic, so there are no clear-cut imperatives as to the age when "capacity" or "competence" arrives "except insofar as most people would agree that it happens during adolescence" for the majority of individuals (Sullivan, 1992, p. 16).

Adding to the complexity of children's (or MR individuals') status is the fact that needs and capacities are influenced by demographic and historic variables. The term "child abuse" has become increasingly more explicit even from 1968 to the present (Janko, 1994). The status of children, as can be observed in school attendance and child labor laws, varies from country to country. Similarly, children's relationships to father, mother, extended family, and state depend on cultural traditions.

Badgley (1984) established four considerations to justify legal intervention in situations involving minors: (1) protection against abusive or exploitive interference with bodily integrity, (2) entitlement to express sexuality on an equal and genuinely consensual basis, (3) deterrence of violations of the trust implicit in adult-child relationships by exploiting emotional and physical vulnerability or by involving developmentally immature persons in sexual acts which they do not fully understand and to which they cannot give informed consent, and (4) deterrence from involving persons in sexual acts that may be physically and emotionally harmful to them (p. 292).

Bearchell (1985) attacks the Badgley Report for not acknowledging children's sexuality, for confusing trivial instances of unwanted sexual acts with dangerous and assaultive acts, and for lumping consensual acts under abusive acts for those under 16. In the Badgley Report, sexual intercourse between peers under 16 is de facto abuse; it is pathologized and discussed almost exclusively in the medicalized context of the dangers of STDs and the risk of pregnancy. There is evidence that medical arguments about the dangers of birth to fifteen-year-olds is flawed (Lancaster & Hamburg, 1986). Bearchell notes the crisis mentality in media reports that teenage pregancy rates have increased when they actually have declined, although the number of adolescents bearing children without the support of cultural institutions such as marriage or the extended family has risen.

Noting that sexual impulse has been subjected to shifting codes of ascetic repression and erotic stimulation in virtually all cultures, Sullivan (1992) deconstructs discourses about youthful sexuality and children's rights by employing the notion of exchanges of power central to the work of Foucault

(1985). "Childlike" in sexual terms has meant "pure," "without sexual knowledge," "uncontaminated"—ideas that Sullivan contends are adult-centered and dated (p. 20). He believes it is more accurate to see the illicit as present alongside licit culture, even among youth, and states: "Children are not simply passive innocents in danger of being overtaken by their own precocious and harmful sexuality on the one hand or by predatory adults on the other" (p. 27). Sullivan separates protecting children from protecting their rights—a distinction that depends on children's rational wills and their capacity to be self-determining moral agents. Even if it is agreed that those "lacking capacity" should be guaranteed protection, there is no simple standard for judging their best interests (p. 18). He notes the lack of boundaries between children and adults in discourse—both receive the same messages through television and other media. Sullivan adheres to the notion that young persons should be allowed consensual sexual expression—that sex should not be medicalized or criminalized.

Few actual opponents of sexual expression and sexuality education for individuals with moderate and severe disabilities can be found in the scholarly literature. One exception, in reference to individuals with autism, is Elgar (1985), who wrote that explicit training in such sexual behaviors as masturbation was meaningless, confusing for them, and likely to instigate socially unacceptable behavior that would not be easily corrected. She also believes that an abstract, information-oriented sexuality education is not feasible for people with autism. Although the sentiments expressed by Elgar are rarely openly acknowledged in journal publications, they are fairly common among workers in direct-care facilities (Brantlinger, 1983). Perhaps the dearth of information about sexuality in publications relating to MR people accurately represents the general attitude that sexual expression is not appropriate for this population.

NOTE

1. The information in this section mainly comes from The Boston Women's Health Book Collective, *The New Our Bodies, Ourselves* (1992) and Bruess & Greenberg, *Sexuality Education: Theory and Practice* (1988).

Part II

PERSPECTIVES OF FAMILIES AND PROFESSIONALS

5

Families' Roles Related to the Member with Mental Retardation

In all families, each member influences others and, in turn, is influenced by family context. One member's disability affects the total family ecology—parents, siblings, and even extended family members. MR members challenge families by making demands on their time, psychological well-being, social relationships, economic resources, and freedom of movement. Mental retardation, physical or sensory impairment, or chronic illness in a family member can restrict the family's functioning and impinge on the other members' emotional well-being in ways the general public may not experience (Darling, 1979, 1980; Hoffmaster, 1982; Ursprung, 1990). The parents' decision to have a child was not the decision to have an MR child (Hauerwas, 1982). Although public perceptions of disability may be altered and the social stigma of disability reduced (Biklen, 1986; Bogdan, 1988; Gliedman & Roth, 1980; Yuker, 1988), parents inevitably prefer to have healthy, intellectually sound children (Paul, Porter, & Falk, 1993).

VARIATION IN FAMILY RESPONSE

In discussing family response to an MR member, distinctions can be made based on characteristics of the MR individual and the nature of the family. One influence is the degree of impairment and the prognosis for future functioning, such as the likelihood of independence (Konstantareas & Homatidis, 1992). Another involves financial circumstances, employment status, age, and health of affected family members (Gerstel & Gallagher, 1993; Paul, Porter, & Falk, 1993). Whether the disability is readily apparent (and intrusive or disruptive) or is mainly concealed in daily life also influences response (Barnes, 1991; Wright, 1959, 1988).

Children who are first classified by school personnel are almost always in the mild range of disability (i.e., learning disabled, mildly mentally disabled, emotionally disturbed). Such children have been called "6-hour-a-day," "situational," or "school-defined" disabled (Mercer, 1973). Children with mild disabilities tend to be from low-income families (Brantlinger, 1987b; Brantlinger, Majd-Jabbari, & Guskin, 1993; Weisz, 1990), and their "problems" are attributed to disadvantages in their home lives (Weisz, 1990; Zill & Schoenborn, 1990). School personnel and the general public hold negative beliefs about low-income parents—that they do not care about their children and/or education or have low aspirations for their educational and vocational attainment (Brantlinger, Majd-Jabbari, & Guskin, 1993; Lareau, 1987). Stereotypes tend to be reinforced because low-income parents do not have the resources or confidence to comply with school personnel's views of the proper parental roles (Lareau, 1987). Research findings actually reveal the similarities in educational ideals and aspirations for members of all classes (Brantlinger, 1985b; Brantlinger, Majd-Jabbari, & Guskin, 1993; Seginer, 1983), although expectations tend to be modified over time to reflect "corrective feedback" from schools (Rosenholtz & Simpson, 1984). Theories that attribute cognitive differences to family values or behaviors have been criticized as ethnocentric and failing to acknowledge the sociopolitical aspects of school and society (Keddie, 1973; Smith, 1993). Nevertheless, attempts to remedy children's functioning are usually family-focused interventions that involve parents more integrally with their children's schooling (Konstantareas & Homatidis, 1992).

Although the size of the population with severe disabilities has remained relatively stable, the school-defined disabled population has expanded (Gerber & Levine-Donnerstein, 1989) in spite of constant controversy about the legitimacy of labels and pull-out special education programs. Among severe MR children, all ethnic, racial, and socioeconomic groups are fairly evenly represented, whereas a disproportionate number of children with mild disabilities are poor, culturally different from school personnel, or of color or have limited English proficiency (Argulewicz, 1983).

Families whose offspring have disabilities that are fairly readily identifiable in all domains of their life (and offspring whose parents concur that they are disabled) are likely to have more pronounced reactions to the disability than those whose disability is mainly visible in school settings. The former tend to be in the moderate or severe range of disabilities, although they can include all functioning levels (i.e., mild, moderate, severe, profound). Often, intellectual deficit is accompanied by physical stigmata, and these children are mostly identified at birth by medical professionals or—because of developmental delays—within the first year of life by families.

Sociologist Bernard Farber's seminal study, "Effects of a Severely Mentally Retarded Child on Family Integration" (1959), laid the groundwork for a multitude of family studies. One of Farber's claims was that the social role of the MR person shifts to that of the youngest child—the one dependent upon others and subject to their authority. This pattern of familial roles can be noted in many of the case studies presented in Part III of this book. Farber examines how families balance the pressures of meeting the needs of the MR child with the pressures of interests outside the family or the needs of other family members. Again, such conflicts are apparent in the cases involving sterilization presented in this book. Farber's (1986) recent contribution to family studies is his historical breakdown of family dynamics through two centuries. This work is relevant to understanding the fluctuations in service delivery and the various positions on sterilization of MR people. Therefore, I will summarize Farber's work in some detail here, but will supplement his analyses with research relevant to the time frames and issues he delineates.

Farber maintains that during the mid-nineteenth century, the "century of growth," there was an emphasis on economic rationality in family life. Each member was to be useful to the family unit, and those who were not productive because of mental retardation or illness were "put away" in institutions. Indeed, up until only a few decades ago, the predominant response to having a child with moderate/severe disabilities was placement in large hospitals, which, because of a desire to isolate MR individuals and remove them from public view, were mainly in rural settings. The "crisis" was adapting to "discarding" a family member (p. ix).

The "era of the welfare state" (beginning in the 1920s) marked a decline in the entrepreneurial family and the onset of a companionship model in which the primacy of reciprocity among members was stressed. There was a corresponding shift from regarding retardation as cumulative hereditary degeneracy to the result of insufficiencies in environments. Attention was directed to problematic family interactional patterns and the departure of family life from the norm, such as the degree of family disintegration, role tension and conflict, personality disorders, and psychosomatic illness (Gallagher, 1993). Minuchin (1974) distinguished "highly enmeshed" families, characterized by overinvolvement and overprotection, from "disengaged families" (or family members), who display little involvement with children. Zetlin, Turner, and Winick (1988) distinguish supportive (close and warm, parents a stable resource for grown children), dependency-producing (close and warm, parental regulation of grown children allows little independence), and conflict-ridden (tense, lacking in warmth and support, but continuation of control) relations.

Much of this research identified parents as contributing to children's disabilities (Rutter, 1982; Sameroff & Chandler, 1975; Sameroff & Friese, 1990). Particularly mothers were accused of being the source of problems—of causing disabilities or of interfering with the adjustment of children (Ramsey & Hill, 1988). At the very least, parental noncompliance with professionals' agendas was said to defeat professionals' goals (Schaefer, 1991; Sewell, 1981). Glidewell (1961) described maternal neuroticism as control ranging from indulgence and overprotectiveness to ignoring and neglect and pinpointed mothers' acceptance of the maternal role, capacity to find satisfaction with dependent children, and consistencies in parenting as influencing children's adjustment. There is little actual empirical evidence that parents are responsible for emotional disturbances in children; nevertheless, they often are blamed for children's conditions (Reinert & Huang, 1987). The "schizophrenogenic mother" was said to have caused mental illness (Abrahams, 1958). Others have implied that "superparents" could cure disabilities such as autism. Only recently has opinion swayed away from such extreme environmentalist positions. Contemporary researchers often attribute mental and emotional differences to organic causes (Franklin, 1989; Silver, 1989).

The literature on the impact of MR children on families is also consistent with Farber's claims of preoccupation with the psychiatric causes. Three somewhat distinct theories about parental response to disability have been delineated: chronic sorrow, stage theory, and nonsequential stage theory (Seligman & Darling, 1989). Chronic sorrow accounts (Olshansky, 1962; Wikler, 1981) tell of unrelenting trauma, stress, fear, anger, loneliness, guilt, and self-doubt and of no escape, constant burden, and little joy in parenting an MR child (Voysey, 1975).

Stage theories describe intermittent down periods with the possibility of adjustment or even good times. Stage theorists draw a parallel between such reactions to the death of a loved one as denial, bargaining, anger, depression, and acceptance (Kubler-Ross, 1969) and parents' reactions to the birth of an MR child. Yura and Zuckerman (1979) define stages of denial, bitterness, rejection, and guilt; Costello (1988) writes about grief, guilt, search for cause, and bonding. Stage theories are chacterized by happy endings, such as resolution in bonding or acceptance. Stage theories illustrate the congruence of human response in varying situations and link the occurrence of disabling conditions with other events that have a stressful impact.

Some deny the validity of stage theories by stating that adjustment is not linear—that stress emerges or reemerges at critical periods of the family's or the MR member's life. Nonsequential stage theories have parental reactions fluctuating with chronological periods or key transition points in life cycles (Blacher, 1984; Turnbull, Summers, & Brotherson, 1986). At childbirth, parents attempt to get accurate diagnoses, inform others, and make immediate personal adjustments to the special needs of the child. When the child enters school, the atypical, and often limited, educational and social careers available for MR children become apparent. Adolescence brings home the chronicity of the condition and the limited future options of offspring. Parents must deal with their ambivalence toward the sexuality of the MR adolescent, interpersonal conflict over intimate social relations, and worries about pregnancy or STDs. As MR children reach adulthood, families must adjust to continuing responsibility and deal with the uncertainty of releasing the person to nonfamily care providers.

Although stage theories dominate the literature about family response to disability, Turnbull (1988) believes that it is counterproductive to dwell on particular stages or critical periods and suggests that professionals adopt a holistic approach to understanding families. Darling (1980) wrote of strong families being a refuge from hardships of everyday life and of the positive side of the entrepreneurship patterns that families develop to find services for their MR children. She also told of parents' ability to tolerate a lack of perfection in their children and their desire to find professionals who treat the child humanely and do not blame the family.

Hill's (1949) ABCX Family Crisis Model separates family reactions into four components: A (stressor event) interacts with B (family's crisis-meeting resources), which interacts with C (definition or significance the family attaches to the event), to produce X (the crisis). Hill's model accommodates the broad range of family reactions to disability and is useful for determining the appropriate focus for professional intervention at any particular point in time. One stressor event is learning of the disability. The amount of stress initially engendered is dependent on such factors as the severity of the condition, its prognosis and cause, and the physical appearance of the MR child. Ambiguous conditions such as autism and uncertain prognoses are the most emotionally stressful to families (Fewell, 1986; Martin, 1988). In such cases, parents extend their search for plausible diagnosis and appropriate treatment. Genetic disorders entail broad implications: Not only do family members have to cope with the member's disabling condition and perhaps intrafamilial blame, but also they may be carriers, so they will be faced with serious decisions about their own futures.

Families' crisis-meeting resources depend on members' coping skills as well as family configuration and interactional patterns (Farber, 1978; Gerstel & Gallagher, 1993; Jendrek, 1993). Parenting, like other forms of care giving, is always demanding, but having an MR child adds to the complexity of the task. There are often extreme pressures placed on families, and some become overwhelmed and fatigued by the time and energy required for effective parenting (Farran, Metzger, & Sparling, 1986; Zarit & Pearlin, 1993). Parents of MR children report higher levels of stress than other parents (Sexton, 1989) and are at risk for developing emotional and personality disorders (Blacher, 1984; Crnic, Friedrich, & Greenberg, 1983). The birth and rearing of an MR child often cause marital stress and family breakup (Bristol, Gallagher, & Schopler, 1988; Seligman & Darling, 1989).

The social networks of families, such as the support they receive from extended family members and friends, affect adjustment (Dunst, Trivette, & Cross, 1986). A number of sources of family support and satisfaction with support are associated with personal well-being and family integrity, more positive attitudes toward the MR child, parent-child play opportunities, and improved child behavior and development (Bailey & Winton, 1989). Yet parents of MR children are socially isolated and report fewer meaningful contacts with others than those with no disabled family members (Turnbull, 1988); therefore, they experience the stress common to socially isolated people (Wikler, 1981).

According to Hill's model, parents' subjective response to a child with disabilities and their cognitive appraisal of the situation affect their coping (McCubbin & Patterson, 1983) and the probability of crisis leading to chronic depression (Richards & Light, 1986). The significance of disability for a family depends on such factors as the family's religion (Webb-Mitchell, 1993), ethnic background (Smith, 1993; Thomas, 1993), previous exposure to MR people, and timely access to information (Winton & Bailey, 1993). It also depends on the quality of services from schools and agencies (Arcia, Gallagher, & Serling, 1992).

Even when services are available, parents and siblings of an MR family member may still worry about responsibility for the condition, whether it is transmittable, and implications for the future. They may be uninformed or have difficulty understanding the diagnosis, or they may be defensive and resistant to accepting it. They are likely to share society's stereotypes and negative attitudes toward MR people. Siblings may have concerns about their own interactions with the MR brother or sister and about talking about the disabling condition with others (Wasserman, 1983). They may also have to deal with discomforting feelings of anger, hurt, embarrassment, guilt, and resentment (Meyer, Vadasy, & Fewell, 1985). Families may benefit from sensitive intervention at any of the levels delineated in Hill's model.

In the 1970s, deinstitutionalization stressed normalized conditions and community integration. This movement resituated MR individuals with their families or in group homes in home communities. The relocation was associated with responsibilities for families and family stress (Ursprung, 1990). In subsequent years, community options increased and improved, although certain families still may not have access to adequate services for themselves or their MR children because of the services available in particular geographic locations (Brantlinger & Guskin, 1987).

The literature about families has expanded from Farber's scholarly analyses to the self-reports of parents, many of whom are themselves professionals (e.g., Comegys, 1989; Darling, 1980; Dougan, Isbell, & Vyas, 1983; Farran, Metzger, & Sparling, 1986; Featherstone, 1980; Fredericks, 1992; Greenfield, 1978; Park, 1982; Turnbull & Turnbull, 1979, 1985). Parents have had a powerful impact on professional practice by actively making their needs and feelings known and by their pivotal role in affecting the litigation and legislation that have expanded services for MR people (Hauerwas, 1982; Jordan, 1987; Wood, 1988). Yet, in spite of improved school and community services, families still have major responsibility for the MR member. Many (e.g., Barnes, 1991; Dalley, 1991; Dalley & Berthoud, 1992; Darling, 1979; Krauss, 1986; Washington & Gallagher, 1986) point to the extra expense and effort incurred by families as a result of a family member's disability. Turnbull and Turnbull (1985), parents of an MR son, see the family as the core unit in society within which individual needs are met. Regardless of community offerings and public support, the MR child, adolescent, or adult may have additional needs that can be met only in the home.

The field continues to be rife with analyses of families that are pertinent to thinking about sexuality, reproduction, and contraception for MR individuals. Indeed, one consideration that is addressed several times in this book is the conflict among family preferences, MR offspring's autonomy, and governmental regulations or interventions. Because most information about families of MR children states both that families face stresses due to the presence of the MR member and that comprehensive public funds and services are grossly lacking, it seems unfair that states can interfere with decisions about the fate of fetuses or MR infants and yet not provide sufficient support for them. Similarly, state and federal regulations control access to birth control methods for MR individuals, yet expenses likely to result from lack of access fall on families. Goldstein, Freud, and Solnit (1979) argue for family autonomy and privacy in the face of state interventionism.

To return to Farber's (1986) last stage, reactions to bureaucratic authority resulted in a paradigmatic shift from the companionship family model, which emphasized the importance of mutual support and consensus among family members, to the pluralistic family model, which emphasizes individual members' rights. Prior to the 1960s, few believed that MR individuals should be awarded full legal rights as adults. Currently, at least from professional and legal perspectives, the rights of MR persons take precedence over family stability, family ties, and parental preferences. Parental authority has eroded and has been superseded by an emphasis on the rights of the MR individual.

The family-centered era was characterized by stories of parents of MR offspring; the present period has witnessed a burgeoning of personal accounts by professionals with (physical) disabilities (Brown, 1990; Diamond, 1993; Hahn, 1991; Rousso, 1986); fine anthologies with diverse perspectives on disability, often written or edited by people with disabilities (e.g., Boylan, 1991; Browne, Connors, & Stern, 1985; Fine & Asch, 1988); and sensitive renditions of the views of MR individuals gleaned through interviews or observations (e.g., Brantlinger, Klein, & Guskin, 1994; Ferguson, Ferguson, & Taylor, 1992; Gleason, 1989; Murray-Seegert, 1989).

Conjecturing about the "age of robotics" as early as 1968, Farber projected that technological changes would result in a huge expansion in the size and diversity of surplus populations (poor, elderly, mentally retarded), who, as subcommunities, would gather in colonies and demand services. He predicted that this period would include a constructed family model in which people devise their domestic relationships in ways that address the particular hardships they face. In this paradigm, individuals negotiate with governments (in their parental/paternal role) rather than with family. As predicted, the "constructed family" group-home model has expanded exponentially over the past two decades.

In contrast to the automatic hospitalization of MR infants in the past, presently MR children are rarely institutionalized, yet birth parents may not rear them. Some MR children happen to be born to people who planned to place them for adoption before they were aware of the disability. Others, such as mothers addicted to crack cocaine, have children removed from their care by child protective services. Some parents choose not to raise these children because of their retardation and may relinquish them to external caretakers after they have kept the children at home for a number of years. Whether or not they are released officially from parental custody, some MR children are raised in group homes, foster care homes, nursing homes, and instititutions. A revision of the definition of child abuse after the Baby Doe case means doctors and parents are no longer permitted to withhold life-sustaining treatment and let children with substantial disabilities die. Prohibited from this option, parents may find giving up custody an acceptable alternative.

There are few studies of families who intentionally adopt hard-to-place, MR children. Existing studies show that the majority of adoptive parents do not experience the same stressful feelings about MR children that biological parents do and many report personally satisfying experiences (Gath, 1983). However, a proportion of parents who adopt children with severe problems—especially medical problems—feel they are adversely restricted and experience stress similar to that noted by birth parents. Glidden (1986) recommends further investigation to determine whether adoptive parents experience less stress because it was their choice to take on a hard-to-place child or whether people who adopt are high on such characteristics as family integration and responsibility—factors found to influence the coping skills of birth parents. Studies of adoption agency records reveal a tendency for persons adopting MR children to be less well educated, single, and working class. It is speculated that this might be the result of agency policy to give "less desirable" children to "less qualified" parents, but it could also be due to self-selection (Glidden, 1986).

Family Reaction to the Sexuality of the MR Member

Parents' inability to recognize and affirm the intimate social and sexual potential of MR offspring can be understood in terms of family dynamics and broader societal values. Parents are often uneasy about the sexual futures of their MR children (Fine & Asch, 1988), and autoerotic behavior, overt signs of sexuality, and physical change in MR adolescents produce intense concern (Bernstein, 1990; Boylan, 1991; Taylor, 1989). Zetlin and Turner's (1985) observational study of 46 mild MR adults revealed that parent-imposed restrictions of information and relationships not only inhibit sexual development, but also create a defiance of parental control. These authors stress the need for counseling parents about their MR offspring's sexuality.

Others (e.g., Begab, 1970; Bernstein, 1990; Dupras & Tremblay, 1976; Turchin, 1974; Wolf & Zarfas, 1982; Zetlin & Turner, 1985) found that parents admit to confused, ambivalent, and anxious attitudes toward the sexuality of their MR children and claim both limited knowledge about sex and feelings of inadequacy in providing sexuality information. Hence, parents favor their MR adolescents receiving school-based sexuality education (Goodman, Budner, & Lesh, 1979). Although MR females receive more sexuality education from parents than males (Alcorn, 1974; David,

Smith, & Friedman, 1976; Hammar, Wright, & Jensen, 1967), MR girls feel uncomfortable discussing sex with their parents and are eager to learn from other sources (Bennett, Vockell, & Vockell, 1972). Parents who broach sexual topics may emphasize the dangers of expression and the importance of abstinence rather than a more positive and realistic overview of sexuality. Rousso (1988) contends that affirmation of sexuality and womanhood requires that mothers identify with their disabled daughters; parents who view their daughters as defective feel that sexuality is dangerous for them. The impact of socialization is apparent in Rousso's finding that women disabled prior to adolescence have less active sexual lives than those disabled afterward.

Family Role in Decision Making

There is considerable disagreement about who has legitimate claim to speak for MR people. Regarding medical treatment, many patients no longer accept passive roles. Civil rights movements have shaped beliefs about the autonomous agency of human beings (variously referred to as rights of personhood, liberty, self-determination, freedom of choice, and noninterference), so that individuals expect to make decisions regarding their own medical care (Sichel, 1992). Problems arise, however, when individuals are too cognitively limited to make informed choices. Families traditionally have made decisions for such individuals.

There are reasons that families should take active roles in decision making. First, families are typically close to MR individuals and care about their well-being. Second, families bear the consequences of treatment choices for dependent offspring. Third, it is generally agreed that parents have the right to raise their children according to their own standards and values and to transmit these to their children. Fourth, it may not be wise to interfere with attachments and interactions among family members if family unity is to be maintained (Buchanan & Brock, 1989). In spite of the literature that espouses the importance of parents' roles in decision making (Konstantareas & Homatidis, 1992), over time, parents have lost discretionary authority over their children. In actuality, others have been reluctant to trust parents' benevolence to act in their children's best interests (Hauerwas, 1982). Supreme Court decisions have allowed situations in which children have rights of their own that override parental wishes. *Bellotti v. Baird* (1979) established that minors have constitutionally protected privacy rights that allow them to make procreative decisions free of parental control. Although the decision was carefully worded to ensure that it not be misunderstood as a general exception to parental authority, blanket parental veto of minors' abortion decisions is considered unconstitutional (Sullivan, 1992).

One concern with family decision making is that individuals may take actions for personal convenience and may act in ways that are not necessarily in the best interest of an MR member. Although nonretarded members may speak in their own behalf, MR individuals may not understand situations or may not feel entitled to express their views. Serious decisions that are not in the best long-term interests of MR members may be made in response to short-term crises. Parents may naturally desire to put concerns behind them and settle things for offspring, a desire that intensifies when offspring have a condition like mental retardation that interferes with their becoming independent (Mappes & Zembaty, 1986). Yet MR offspring's life circumstances will not remain static, and less final decisions may suit the second generation's needs at any point in time.

Arguments for or against parents assuming authority for decisions are based on some theory of family and moral roles that parents play vis-à-vis offspring. Some literature takes it for granted that paternalism and individual rights are necessarily at odds (Kasachkoff, 1989). The literature also views institutional paternalism negatively. Buchanan and Brock (1989) contend: "The long and dismal record of neglect, abuse, and outright exploitation of the permanently institutionalized supports the conclusion that—at least for the more serious decisions—the role of surrogate decision-maker should not be assumed by health care professionals or administrators of the institution" (p. 139). The conception of paternalism as benevolent on the one hand and coercive or restrictive on the other underlies most attempts at justifying paternalistic action (Deigh, 1989).

Gliedman and Roth (1980) argue that parents' rights take precedence over those of professionals, who exist to further parents' visions of their MR children's futures. On the other hand, Greenfield (1978), the father of a child with severe retardation, feels that parents are too busy with the practical aspects of life (e.g., getting the child to eat or sleep through the night) to concern themselves with the abstract ethical issues often considered in laws and in courts. It may be difficult to identify the appropriate family member to make decisions. A child may be in foster care while the birth parent retains some rights. An adult may be married or living with a significant other. Homosexual partnerships not legalized by marriage may cause conflicts about decisions for incompetent persons. Some disagreements among family members are so intractable that the family cannot function as a coherent decision-making unit, whereas, in other cases, there is no family, or no family member, willing to serve as surrogate (Buchanan & Brock, 1989).

Richards (1986) believes it is the parents' right to decide to have MR offspring sterilized. Turchin (1974) found that 70 percent of mothers felt that sterilization was the best method of birth control for their children. In a study of 73 parents of adolescents, Pueschel and Scola (1988) found about half wanted their children sterilized or on long-term birth control because of their children's interest in the opposite sex and desire to marry. Parents of girls feared sexual exploitation, but few had provided their daughters with sexuality education. Wolf and Zarfas's (1982) survey revealed that 67 percent of the parents surveyed approved of sterilization for MR individuals and 64 percent did not feel the need for a legally authorized third person or committee to be involved with sterilization decisions, whereas 25 percent wanted external input. These parents wondered about MR individuals' likely adjustment to sterilization, the predictability of parenting behaviors, the disadvantages of being a child of an MR individual, the nature of stresses caused by children and marriage, the availability of support for marriage and child rearing, and the success rates for marriages. Wheeless (1975) found that parents thought a hysterectomy would decrease the chances of unwanted pregnancy and lessen menstrual pain and inconvenience.

The Department of Health and Human Services' sterilization regulation opposes sterilization for MR persons, thus summarily dismissing parental needs and concerns. Petchesky (1990) approves of the regulation because it prevents sterilization "done irrespective of the 'best interests' of the individual that could lead to abuse," citing the "danger that caretakers, including parents, might be tempted to consent to sterilization" as a way of avoiding the responsibilities of sex education, training in other forms of birth control, and alternatives to sterilization (p. 69). Petchesky believes negative reactions to the regulation are an acknowledgment of such existing social realities as the lack of sufficient training and community support services for mentally incompetent individuals—a dearth that increases the burden on parents and pressures them to seek sterilization.

6

Lives in Institutions, Lives in Communities

Studies of MR adults in institutional and community settings provide information about the social, sexual, and parenting aspects of their lives. It must be noted that studies conducted at different times drew from populations identified by distinct classification systems. The standards for identification as MR (Doll, 1941; Grossman, 1973, 1983; Smith, 1994; Tredgold, 1937) have become more restrictive; tighter standards mean that those labeled are lower functioning; hence, recent follow-up studies may have fewer positive cases than in the past. Methods used to select subjects, such as studying parents referred to child protection agencies, result in samples not representative of the general population of MR adults (Andron & Tymchuk, 1987). It is necessary to acknowledge the vast differences in support services available and the impact of context on adjustment.

REASONS FOR INSTITUTIONALIZATION

Things done to MR people have "for their own good" rationales (e.g., they are placed in special education so instruction will be geared to their level and they will not feel inadequate, they are sterilized so they will not be burdened by children). Institutions are alleged to provide rehabilitation and training to cure "deviants" (Wolfensberger, 1974). A reason for institutionalization offered by doctors through the years was protecting the family from what was considered the overwhelming task and disruptive influence of raising an MR child. Parents were told their offspring would receive appropriate services in institutions (Ursprung, 1990). Once benevolent rationales are thoroughly embedded in the public conscience, their benefits to others surface. Furtive reasons for institutionalization were distancing the "socially unfit" from the rest of society, hiding them from public view, and relieving others from dealing directly with them (Gollay, Freedman, Wyngaarden, & Kurtz, 1978). Institutions took on custodial roles and served to prevent reproduction by segregating MR men and women not only from society, but also from each other (McCarver & Craig, 1974; Shafter, 1957; Wolfson, 1956).

Turnbull and Turnbull (1975) criticize the nature of admission to and release from institutions: "At no time in these decisions does the retarded person have a right, or even an opportunity, to make a decision for himself, to affect a decision being made for him by others, or to even participate in the decision-making process—when the decision vitally affects his lifestyle, his "best" placement, where he will be, and who will take care of him in what situations and surroundings" (p. 14). Turnbull and Turnbull point out that due process is granted only with respect to public school special education classrooms and not in the case of the far more confining, liberty-depriving placements in institutions or community-based 24-hour facilities.

Although the reasons for institutionalization were not always disclosed, a perusal of the literature reveals that sexual behaviors have been a primary cause (Badham, 1955; Edgerton, 1967; McCarver & Craig, 1974; Wolfson, 1956). The burgeoning of admissions of adolescents and young adults supports the hypothesis that problems were related to sexuality. Fear of pregnancy and inability to deal with sexuality resulted in the commitment of many MR individuals who would have been able to live in the community (Deisher, 1973). On close inspection, it becomes clear that the "sexual problems" of MR individuals were often in the eyes of the beholder. A minor reason for involuntary commitment was that MR people were guilty of—or suspected of—committing illegal acts such as rape or child molestation. Being sent to a state MR hospital, rather than prison, was feasible because of the (suspected) perpetrator's MR diagnosis. It was typical for no trial to ensue—due process enacted to protect the rights of the accused was not recognized; hence, MR individuals were incarcerated without being given a chance to testify against accusations. Then, they were "sent away" for indefinite lengths of time. If they had been found guilty by jury trial, they would have received a set sentence.

In addition to the small number of admissions due to misdemeanors or felonies—actual crimes—commitment resulted from behaviors that were seen as problematic, but were not crimes or, if crimes, were rarely enforced for the general public. MR people were institutionalized for such common infractions as fornication, homosexuality, and unwed pregnancy. When these behaviors occurred with others, incarceration was not an option; hence, community solutions were found. Institutions were there for MR people and could be used. Because of mental slowness, MR people were likely to be caught for problems. MR women exhibit more sexual problems (Goddard, 1914; McCarver & Craig, 1974; Penrose, 1950; Wolfson, 1956)—a disproportion likely due to dual standards for sexual behavior for males and females as well as the gendered nature of an important criterion problem—pregnancy.

A third category of admissions was the result of stereotypes and misperceptions of MR people as asexual, so that flirting, being attracted to the opposite sex, initiating relationships, and showing an interest in sex or marriage—behaviors expected, even encouraged, in others—were seen as problematic and forbidden to MR people. As Rousso (1988) states, "Situations that hamper the emergence of sexuality are rarely acknowledged as problems, whereas there is a myth in our society that disabled people are asexual" (p. 140). Markers of the transition to adulthood—becoming sexual, having the privileges of the twenty-first birthday—are ignored for MR people (Weinberg, 1988). Fine and Asch (1988) cite *The Glass Menagerie* and Laura's disqualification from courtship and marriage as an example. On the positive side, Fine and Asch conjecture that culture may "fail to leave its heavy sextyping brand" on disabled girls—an oversight that results in the liberation and lack of sexual repression apparent in many disabled activists (pp. 132–134). Self-sufficiency might also be due to others' avoidance and marginalization of them.

An opposite image was that MR people had an overabundance of sex drive; they were animalistic, sexual ogres, sexually driven, perverse, and oversexed, or at least they lacked restraint in inhibiting sexual drive. Even if MR people showed no unusual sexual behaviors, others assumed they were lurking and would just need the opportunity to be unleashed. The "hush hush" aura surrounding sex meant fears went unexamined and undiscussed, and solutions to problems were not found. Thus, MR individuals were incarcerated because of others' prejudices, imaginations, and fears (Brantlinger, 1983; McAfee & Gural, 1988).

Finally, commitments to institutions were made because of others' worries. MR people were seen as innocents who were not (or should not be) interested in sex, but were vulnerable to abuse or corruption by others. Thus, they were incarcerated for their own protection. It is true that exemption or exclusion from voluntary sexuality has not prevented disabled females from being sexually victimized. Because they tend to be even more dependent on others to survive than nondisabled women, they may confront serious psychological and social problems in ending abusive or exploitative relationships (Bregman, 1984; Brown & Craft, 1989; Fine & Asch, 1988; Koller, Richardson, & Katz, 1988; Satterfield & Sugar, 1990). Fine and

Asch (1988) believe sterilization has been done to keep the effects of rape from the public eye. But institutionalization was unlikely to deter sexual exploitation.

Related to the high rate of commitments of MR people during their sexual prime, concerns about sex and impregnation were incentives for continued incarceration and strict supervision (Adams, Tallon, & Alcorn, 1982; Edgerton & Dingman, 1964). Involuntary sterilization regulations specified sterility as a prerequisite for release (Sabagh & Edgerton, 1962; Shafter, 1957). Those who had been committed for sexual reasons or who had been implicated in sexual situations while in institutions were the last to be considered for release (Badham, 1955; Cate & Gegenheimer, 1950; Deisher, 1973; Kratter & Thorne, 1957; McCarver & Craig, 1974; Morris, 1969; Wolfson, 1956). To prevent "mistakes," in which someone residing in an institution was able to have sexual intercourse, even individuals with little chance of release were sterilized. If MR women became pregnant, their children were placed for adoption or were raised in orphan homes.

DEINSTITUTIONALIZATION

Because of the labor shortage during World War II, many MR individuals left institutions to join the work force. Following the war, a deinstitutionalization movement began to take hold of imaginations and practice. Postwar trends in treatment of MR people were based increasingly on principles of normalization (Payne, 1976; Wolfensberger, 1974) and on the safeguarding of civil and human rights. The necessity of institutionalizing disabled infants was questioned. A number of previously institutionalized MR adults and children reentered community settings. Between 1977 and 1987, MR people in facilities with more than 300 residents decreased from 143,000 to 69,000, and people in settings with fewer than 7 individuals increased from 20,400 to 80,900 (Lakin, Prouty, White, Bruininks, & Hill, 1990).

Families of MR individuals were initially distressed about their relatives' relocation from large institutions to community-based facilities (Heller, Bond, & Braddock, 1988). Many had a distorted image of institutions as safe, clean, pleasant places (Ursprung, 1990). Moreover, the transfer rekindled feelings of guilt associated with the original decision to institutionalize. Heller, Bond, and Braddock (1988) found that over time there was a dramatic reversal from strong resistance to positive attitudes; eventually, 94 percent were satisfied with the idea of community facilities and normalization philosophies of care.

Normalization is a difficult ideal to operationalize, yet there is evidence that people in community residential settings (foster care, family residence, group home) have more integrated and more typical life experiences than those in institutions (Conroy & Bradley, 1985; Felce, DeKock, & Repp, 1986; O'Neil, Brown, Gordon, Schonhorn, & Green, 1981). Nevertheless, MR people in community-based arrangements still may be socially isolated and may not participate in community life (Crapps, Langione, & Swain, 1985; Hill, Rotegard & Bruininks, 1984). Bachrach (1985) maintains that deinstitutionalization involves little more than a physical change of placement for MR people because community support is sparse or nonexistent. Bercovici (1983) observes that community living often resembles the most negative aspects of institutional living: routinized group treatment, social isolation, and lack of meaningful occupation.

ADULT ADJUSTMENT

Postschool and community adjustment studies offer important information about the daily lives of MR adults in the community. The studies have a vocational focus, but some report the intimate social, sexual, and domestic aspects of MR people's lives. In defining adjustment, Gollay and her colleagues (1978) note that it is not unidimensional, but a complex of multiple aspects of living and coping. They warn that standards for judging MR individuals should not be harsher than standards used to evaluate others. Studies report a broad range of adjustment patterns among MR adults as well as a variety of success rates. Rosen, Clark, and Kivitz (1977) put success at about 50 percent; others were reluctant to be specific, but similar figures slipped out. Many note that adjustment depends on personality and social variables, rather than measured intelligence, and stress its reflections of the appropriateness of MR individuals' previous environments and educational programs as well as current support in communities.

More meaningful than quantitative breakdowns are the thick descriptions of daily life in some excellent studies of community adjustment. One of the finest and best known postinstitution studies is Edgerton's (1967) *The Cloak of Competence,* and his 1984 follow-up, *Lives in Process: Mildly Retarded Adults in a Large City,* which took place in California. Mattinson's (1971) book, *Marriage and Mental Handicap,* is about British adults who had been released from long-term institutional care—many had been born and raised in institutions. The focus of Henshel's (1972) *The Forgotten Ones* is Anglo and Chicano graduates of public school special education programs in Texas.

As might be surmised from the title *The Cloak of Competence*, Edgerton emphasizes that the stigma of having been judged as MR was totally unacceptable to his informants, and their lives were directed toward denying mental incompetence and establishing themselves as the same as everyone else. Edgerton writes that retardation implies "lacking in competence"; thus, acceptance of the label is incompatible with self-esteem and renders independent life difficult or impossible (pp. 207, 212). His participants compared themselves to severe MR people in an institution and believed that they and their peer group (mildly to moderately MR people), who had few physical stigmata, were normal. They did call themselves backward and slow. Edgerton notes that release from institutions "seemed like long overdue justice," but they also experienced "release shock" (p. 150).

Henshel (1972) judged most of her special education graduates to be fairly unaffected by their labels, although negative feelings about special education were frequently expressed. Mattinson (1971) asserted that most MR adults seemed to accept themselves as they were, but later observed that feelings of inadequacy were evident in fears that children had inherited disability, denial of the necessity of institutionalization, and their keeping well away from neighbors because they were afraid to admit that they had been in a "mental house" or "put away" (p. 184).

Edgerton's (1967) subjects had been allowed work leave from the state hospital precisely because they demonstrated the ability to perform well on jobs. The incentive for continued vocational success may have been a fear that if they did not do well, they would be returned to the institution. Although the women had been successfully employed before marriage, all but three were housewives at the time of his study. Perhaps similar to the majority of woman in the mid-sixties, few married women remained employed outside the home. Mattinson's (1971) married women were also housewives. Of the males, 12 were regularly employed, 11 were erratically employed, and 6 were permanently unemployed. Henshel's (1972) participants were worse off than others of the same social class. Other studies of MR graduates of special education programs found they were likely to be unemployed (Becker, 1976; Dinger, 1961; Tobias, 1970) or in low-paying unskilled and semiskilled jobs (Crain, 1980).

With few exceptions, Edgerton's (1967) former state hospital patients had located benefactors—spouses, lovers, siblings, parents, neighbors, landlords, employers—who voluntarily helped with daily existence. He stressed the importance of benefactors' assistance and emotional support as MR individuals coped with the complexity of everyday life. Thirty-two percent also received aid from social welfare. Informal and formal care interfaced to meet the needs of MR adults (Zarit & Pearlin, 1993).

Mattinson's (1971) couples had spent long periods in institutions, and many had been committed because they were orphaned or because family units broke down. They did not rely on friends and neighbors as much as expected. Having no relatives on which to rely, her MR adults depended on social service agencies and each other. Marriages were complementary: Spouses pooled their resources, relying on the skill of one partner to compensate for the inabilities in the other. They were each other's benefactors.

Henshel's (1972) participants had lived at home and attended public school, and some continued to live with, and be dependent on, families. The singles were lonely and wanted relationships. Overprotected by parents, some said that even if they met someone they were interested in, their parents would not allow them to date. Mexican-American women received substantially more support from extended family than their Anglo counterparts, and their lives were also much more controlled; however, their families expected them to marry and have children.

Although family members, agency personnel, and benefactors enable community success, when MR people are dependent on others, the others' authority has a major influence on them (Bercovici, 1983; Burchard, Hasazi, Gordon, & Yoe, 1991; Gollay, Freedman, Wyngaarden, & Kurtz, 1978; Kennedy, Horner, & Newton, 1990). Zetlin and Hosseini (1989) felt parents engaged in a benevolent conspiracy that maintained their children's unrealistic job or relationship plans even though parents were ultimately frustrated by the uncertainty of their children's futures. MR adults tend to be "entrenched in an extended period of adolescence and continually test parental authority to achieve some measure of independence" (Mitchell-Kernan & Tucker, 1984, p. 188). Troubles between parent and offspring continue into adulthood (Kaufman, 1984).

Agency personnel and community professionals usually pay more attention to nondisabled individuals than MR individuals in negotiations (Brantlinger, 1983; Brantlinger, Klein, & Guskin, 1994). This phenomenon may be due to the (often fallacious) view that MR persons do not understand or have preferences or to professionals' lack of experience—and subsequent discomfort—in working with MR individuals or their valuing smarter people more than MR individuals. Whatever the cause, agency personnel feel compelled to please the benefactor or relative rather than the MR person.

Benefactors may pressure MR individuals, but they have no actual legal control. Legal guardianships must be established by courts. Guardianship is sometimes interpreted to mean absolute authority over the property and person of the ward, whereas it is really invoked only to ensure the ward's best interests. Turnbull and Turnbull (1975) feel that the entire guardianship law needs to be refined to provide for limited guardianship in which partial control is exerted over specified aspects of the MR individual's life. Because some MR individuals are able to manage property, money, and/or social freedom, the Turnbulls advocate a system of degrees of guardianship tailored to individuals rather than total guardianship based on invalid assumptions of total incompetency. Courts usually require parents to become legal guardians of adult offspring before considering sterilization requests from them.

FRIENDSHIPS, SEXUAL INTIMACIES, AND MARRIAGE

MR people have small social networks, have few close friends other than benefactors, and rarely participate in community activities (Bercovici, 1983; Edgerton, 1967; Hill, Rotegard, & Bruininks, 1984; Kennedy, Horner, & Newton, 1990; Lambert, 1974; Mattinson, 1971; Saenger, 1957). Mattinson's couples lived "cocooned" lives in which "friendship was relatively unknown to them"; therefore, their marriages were of particular significance because spouses were their only friends (p. 183). Gollay and her colleagues (1978) found that loneliness was a big problem—MR adults felt restricted by circumstances and wanted more social activities.

Because sex is a "perilous topic," Henshel (1972), and many others who conducted adjustment studies, chose not to ask about it. Nevertheless, participants' lengthy talks about sex and intimacy revealed they were experiencing a variety of problems and confusions. Similarly, Edgerton (1967) concluded:

Sexual behavior is of special importance in the everyday lives of these former patients because it has so often caused them trouble in their prehospital lives. For all of these former patients, sexual matters were an ever-threatening source of trouble in the community, and for many of these persons, real or fancied sexual misconduct was the ostensible reason for their original institutionalization. Moreover, sex remains potentially a highly troublesome matter for these people after discharge. (p. 111)

Zetlin and Turner (1985) note "excitement in boy-girl relations" as well as "lack of good judgment about relationships," "risky behaviors," and "vulnerability to abuse" (p. 576).

Among the early advocates for sexual expression for MR individuals, Edgerton and Dingman (1964) observed that MR people's need for affection was fundamental. They suggested that MR individuals be permitted to interact with peers with as little supervision as possible. In 1978, Craft and Craft reported that MR individuals tend to shift attention and affection rapidly and shallowly from one person to another. They believed that the lack of deep feelings resulted from having been kept from bonding with significant others because they had been institutionalized. Craft and Craft suggested that intimate relations and affection cure loneliness, as well as apathy; therefore, it is essential for parents and staff to agree that sex and intimacy are important.

In contrast to the large pool of peers in institutions, MR adolescents and adults in the community may lack contact with others similar to themselves. Loneliness has often been cited as a major problem for MR adults living in the community. Gollay and her colleagues (1978) found that fewer than half of the MR adults in their study had romantic relationships after leaving the institution and dating was rarely named as a leisure activity. Of those who had relationships, more than three-fourths were evaluated by family members to be handling them satisfactorily or very well.

Mattinson (1971) believed that many of her long-term hospitalized couples had platonic relationships similar to those between a brother and sister—an enormous need for each other, but little adult sexual expression. When first admitted to the institution, males and females were officially segregated, so they did their courting "behind the hedge" (p. 172). They were increasingly allowed more contact; nevertheless, much of their dating was done at the weekly hospital dance, at which they were allowed one dance an evening with the same partner. Mattinson's discussion of institutional life is particularly noteworthy:

In the best sense of the word the patients were offered asylum from the conditions and experiences which had not helped their intellectual, emotional, and social development. But care, supervision, and control were unimaginative and imbued with the concept of permanence, reflecting the theory of that time, that regarded the mentally deficient as untrustworthy children who were to be excluded from the community for a protracted period of time and segregated from members of the opposite sex. The dependent and tractable patients were more able to adjust to the situation which, for them, remained overprotective and continued to deprive them of the opportunity for further development of independence. (p. 37)

Institutions and sheltered workshops offer access to peers—potential friends, lovers, and spouses. Although competitive employment carries higher prestige than workshop settings, the latter offer more social opportunities for reciprocal friendships and romantic partnerships (Kaufman, 1984).

Postschool and postinstitution studies show that in spite of MR adolescents' and adults' desires for friends of the opposite sex, marriage, and children, training was not geared toward their expressed needs and preferences (Hamre-Nietupski & Ford, 1981; Hewitt, 1987; Hingsburger, 1988; Hirayama, 1979; Kempton & Gochros, 1986; Schultz, 1981). An interviewer in the Gollay (1978) study summed up:

Again and again comments were made about the lack of training given to mentally retarded persons about getting along with people. The females all want to get married, have a hard time separating boys as friends and boyfriends—either way, they want marriage out of the relationship. This struck me as a rather desperate plea for some sort of real, deep, profound experience in their lives rather than living on the fringes of activity and experience. Family lives assume such mammoth importance in the life of a mentally retarded person and they want that same opportunity to create what they have been living with. Given the fact that women in . . . do marry young and seem to be programmed for it at every turn, it is understandable that marriage for mentally retarded adolescents is seen as a prime goal—yet the supportive services available for that type of relationship are pitifully lacking. (p. 92)

Instead of learning about adult sexual relations, reproduction, and contraception, MR individuals received information about grooming and nonsexual aspects of hygiene and health.

Edgerton (1967) reports that "desires for marriage and children were vital concerns and cherished goals" (p. 111). Henshel's (1972) MR participants had "internalized society's visible and highly valued goals related to family living" (p. 247). Rosen, Clark, and Kivitz's (1977) institutional discharges wanted relationships and marriage, but singles were at a loss about how to make appropriate social contacts with the opposite sex. Only 20 of the 65 (mean age of 28.8) were married—11 to others from the institution. Of the marriages of 80 deinstitutionalized people in the Floor, Baxter, Rosen, and Zisfein (1975) study, 65 percent married former residents approximately 19 months after release. A large proportion marry others from their institution (e.g., Edgerton, 1967; Mattinson, 1972; Gollay, Freedman, Wyngaarden, & Kurtz, 1978).

Henshel (1972) notes a randomness in her participants' choices of spouses as well as in their decisions to marry. In contrast, Mattinson's (1971) MR adults showed persistence and determination to be married when faced with circumstances in which professionals were actively trying to thwart relationships because it was "generally agreed that mentally defective persons are unfit for the responsibility of marriage and parenthood" (p. 47). When first released, Mattinson's respondents had been forced to adhere to rules that included special precautions to prevent the formation of attachments to members of the opposite sex. "Misbehaviors" resulted in a return to the hospital (p. 46).

A greater percentage of women than men marry; many marry nonretarded men substantially older than themselves (Edgerton, 1967; Floor, Baxter, Rosen, & Zisfein, 1975; Henshel, 1972; Rosen, Clark, & Kivitz, 1977; Scally, 1973). Floor, Baxter, Rosen, and Zisfein (1975) judged that some who married "normals" had "straightened out," whereas others were "overly dependent and regressed to semi-helplessness" (p. 37). Researchers conclude that married individuals are more competent and independent than single cohorts. Of the five never-married women in Edgerton's (1967) study, three appeared afraid of men and sex, and one avoided men because she felt her sterilized condition made her unmarriageable (p. 112). Floor, Baxter, Rosen, and Zisfein (1975) found single individuals had a greater frequency of vocational difficulties, lawbreaking, and drug or drinking incidents than married persons. It is unclear if the marriage/better adjustment correlation results from the selective factor of better-adjusted people finding marriage partners or the positive influence of marital relationships.

In summarizing the quality of marriages addressed in several studies, Haavik and Menninger (1981) conclude that divorce and separation rates are higher and that MR couples require more assistance in maintaining stable and satisfactory marriages than normal couples. Most of Henshel's (1972) married respondents claimed satisfaction with their marriages, but Henshel judged many to have serious relationship and domestic problems. Floor, Baxter, Rosen, and Zisfein (1975) found that although about 50 percent of the marriages were "running smoothly," others were beset with problems, including the chronically poor health of one partner, money management, overindebtedness, erratic employment, legal difficulties, and involvement with difficult or demanding relatives (p. 36). Scally (1973) judged that 40–50 percent of MR adults had "poor" or "bad" relations with their spouses (p. 192).

Although she described problems in the marriages of her previously institutionalized MR people, Mattinson (1971) saw advantages to the marriages. Her observations are insightful and realistic; therefore, it seems appropriate to quote her directly:

It soon became clear that many of them were managing well, maintaining their family life as ordinary citizens, and were not known to the social workers in the area. (p. 20)

Apparently they were quickly able to recognize their need of each other, not only to satisfy their biological instincts and confirm for each other their own heterosexuality, but, recognizing their intellectual limitations, to increase their chances of managing in the community. (p. 131)

They were very much married and very dependent on each other in many areas of their family life. (p. 142)

I was particularly impressed by the mutual help these husbands and wives gave each other and by the complementary nature of the partnerships. Recognizing their own intellectual and emotional limitations, they used their partners for what they could not do or express for themselves. Singly, these people had shown themselves defective in social living; paired, they were much less so. They were very unidealistic and did not set their sights very high, e.g., "I choosed him and his needs so I got to put up with them. I'd be lonely without a man." (pp. 183–184)

They were remarkably honest about their difficulties and realistic in their expectations. The success of many of these marriages seemed to be related to the initial expectation not having been too high. Some failure was not as distressful to them as it might have been to other people whose aims were higher and who might have had a better model in their childhood. Many of them had very few possessions in the earlier part of their lives. (p. 201)

Often with very limited relationships outside the marriage, with few talents to expend in creative pastimes, with the need to prove themselves in this way, the investment in the marriage was enormous. Cocooned and very often unseparated, relying tremendously on each other's abilities, they were able to be surprisingly frank about their difficulties and at the same time to maintain a joint optimism and belief in themselves as a pair. (p. 133)

My ultimate conclusion about these former patients of a hospital for the retarded was that, paired, many of them were able to reinforce each other's strengths and established marriages which, in the light of what had happened to them previously, were no more, no less, foolish than many other in the community, and which gave them considerable satisfaction. (p. 185)

PARENTING

Arguments exist for the advantages of marriage for MR people, but recognizing parenting rights is more controversial. In addition to the general postschool studies, numerous researchers (e.g., Andron & Tymchuk, 1985, 1987; Bakken, Miltenberger, & Schauss, 1993; Bass, 1964; Budd & Greenspan, 1984; Fedje & Holcombe, 1986; Feldman, Case, Rincover, Towns, & Betel, 1989; Madsen, 1979; O'Neill, 1985; Robinson, 1978; Rosenberg & McTate, 1982) have focused primarily or solely on parenting. They address

MR individuals' desire for children, the number of children they typically have, their success at parenting, and the characteristics of the children. Reflecting the heterogeneity of people classified as MR, all studies report a certain percentage of successful parents as well as unsuccessful ones or success in some domains of parenting, but inadequacies in others. Budd and Greenspan (1985) caution that precise patterns of strengths or deficits cannot be predicted on the basis of IQ, noting that three components of intelligence—conceptual, practical self-maintenance, and social—are found in various proportions in MR people and each makes unique contributions to parenting.

Any discussion of parenting for MR individuals must address eugenicists' fear of a national decline in intelligence. Haavik and Menninger (1981) conclude the "data demonstrate that breeding at an inordinate rate appears unsubstantiated" (p. 70). Reed and Reed (1965) found the negative correlation between parental IQ and family size disappeared when childless persons in the parental generation were included in the data: 31 percent of individuals with low IQs had no children in contrast to 10 percent in the middle and 4 percent in the highest range. The Reeds felt that omitting the childless members of the parental generation resulted in biased statistics. It must be cautioned, however, that at the time of the Reeds' study, many MR subjects would have been sterilized. Replicated now, studies would be unlikely to include many sterilized MR individuals. The Reeds found that among individuals having 6 to 10 children, MR people were in the ascendancy. Others (e.g., Heber & Garber, 1975; Henshel, 1972; Mickelson, 1947; Shaw & Wright, 1960) report larger families for MR parents than for the general population.

Three decades after the Reeds' study, Preston and Campbell (1993) point out that population IQ levels have risen, rather than fallen, a fact that they state should curb the common belief and "recurrent fear during the past century" that it would decline because "persons with lower IQs have above-average fertility" (p. 997). Coleman (1993) counters that dismissal of the "common belief" is not well founded because it is based on the implicit assumption that the negative relationship between IQ and fertility has been at least as great in the past as in the present and that evidence points in the opposite direction (p. 1020). Eight years after the original report, Reed and Anderson (1973) cautioned that their findings indicate the importance of accompanying any encouragement of heterosexual activity among MR people with effective contraception. The continuing debates demonstrate the complexity of the problem as well as the lack of consensus among experts about MR people's influence on population trends.

In analyzing within-family trends, Reed and Reed (1965) calculated that the mean IQ of children of two nonretarded parents was 107, those of one MR parent was 90, and those of two MR parents was 74 (p. 115). In Ireland, Scally (1973) found the IQ of offspring to be roughly equivalent to that of the more intelligent parent. In England, Shaw and Wright (1960) found only 12 percent of offspring of MR parents had IQs over 100 and the percentage of children attending special classes and schools was 17 times the national average. In Henshel's (1972) study, 8 (33 percent) of the 24 fertile subjects produced 1 or more disabled children. In contrast, Andron and Tymchuk (1987) found no significant relationship between MR mothers' and offspring's IQs. In examining heritability, the etiology of parental retardation must be considered; if it resulted from prenatal, birth, or postnatal injury or illness, hereditary factors would not be relevant. In Michigan, only 121 out of 727 MR patients (16 percent) screened were assigned specific genetic causes (Thoene, Higgins, Krieger, Schnickel, & Weiss, 1981).

Adult adjustment studies mainly direct attention to men when examining vocational success; the focus is women in discussions of sex, marriage, reproduction, and child rearing. Yet fathers' responsibility for the financial upkeep of offspring is stressed by welfare agencies and supported by courts. Paternity tests, which now are at least 99 percent accurate, enable enforcement of paternal responsibilities. Studies that highlight paternal as well as maternal roles and responsibilities are most appropriate.

Summarizing studies of MR parents, Greenspan and Budd (1986) conclude that, as a group, they are less adequate than nonretarded parents on observed parenting behaviors, children's development, and problems reported to child protective agencies. According to Thurman (1985), children of MR parents have a less-than-average chance of developing into fully competent adults. Robinson's (1978) study found MR mothers more protective, controlling, and punitive toward their children than a control group of college-educated parents. Peterson, Robinson, and Littman (1983) found MR mothers less likely than nondisabled middle- and low-income mothers to display affection, praise, and appropriate discipline. Feldman, Case, Towns, and Betel (1985) found that two-year-old children raised by MR mothers were at risk for language and cognitive delay, although children of mothers who were involved and responsive had higher scores. Schilling, Schinke, Blythe, and Barth (1982) point to a "preponderance of evidence of increased risk of maltreatment and neglect" of children reared by MR parents (p. 206). (Abuse is an act causing injury that can be sexual, physical, or emotional. Neglect is a failure to provide for such needs of the child as food, shelter, and medical care.)

Of the 32 couples with 40 children in Mattinson's (1971) study, two children died (and neglect was queried at the inquest of one of them), six children were removed from their homes, and another three received intensive help from agencies (p. 180). Mattinson concluded that some coped well with one or two children, but "tired" mothers—those with more children—became inadequate, especially when "the wage does not grow with the number of children" (p. 115). Other British studies found that extensive support from social service or health agencies had been required for problems in child rearing for over half of MR parents (Berry & Shapiro, 1975; Craft & Craft, 1979). Scally (1973) judged that 90 percent of MR mothers made "less than adequate contributions to the home and to the welfare of the children" (p. 192).

In the United States, early studies indicated high rates of MR parent involvement with social service agencies and high proportions of children removed from homes because of neglect (Ainsworth, Wagner, & Strauss, 1945; Shaw & Wright, 1960). Mickelson (1947) found that substantial agency support allowed MR people to function better as parents; yet, in cases when support was most needed, it was often rejected by families. All but a few of Edgerton's (1967) participants had been sterilized; two with children (one with three, the other with four) were judged to be good mothers. Both were among the subjects with higher IQs; that is, 73 and 77, whereas the average IQ of the cohort group was 64. Two wives of professional men adopted children, but received support from their mothers-in-law in rearing them.

Henshel (1972) remarked on similarities between her MR subjects' child-rearing practices (relying on corporal punishment as their main disciplinary technique) and those of working-class families described in other studies. Those with MR children were tolerant of them, stating that they would outgrow problems. Nevertheless, concerned about the high proportion of MR offspring and signs of neglect among many, Henshel remarked: "The often erratic childrearing patterns we observed indubitably contributed to the little ones' hyperactivity and unruliness" (p. 225). Some had released children for adoption (usually due to pressure from family), and others had children taken away from them by child protection services. In her conclusion, Henshel stated:

Thus we have two conflicting situations: the individuals sterilized would be very miserable in their childlessness. Still, their yet-unborn offspring could well be a tremendous weight for society to bear. Then there is the added fact that some of these parents could not be entrusted with the care of their own children. More importantly, those little ones, plagued with multiple handicaps, could have only the faintest hope of leading even minimally pleasurable lives. How to solve this dilemma depends to a great extent on the goals and values of society. Obviously, sterilization may be a terrible blow to an individual, especially to a woman who is presently often defined and given a place in society primarily in terms of her maternal role. (p. 244)

Henshel recommends that MR women participate more fully in society at large through meaningful employment outside the home.

MR parents are more likely than others to lose custody of children due to abuse and neglect, but caution must be used in interpreting this finding because high rates of welfare intervention and custody loss may reflect biased perceptions rather than actual parenting attributes (Budd & Greenspan, 1985; Haavik & Menninger, 1981). Judgments of "good mothering" are based on women's social standing, sexual orientation, life style, and disability status (Spallone, 1989, p. 138). Because the danger of misinterpreting "dumb" behaviors (those amenable to change, or at least deserving of compassion) as "bad" behaviors is ever present, there is a need for social service workers to be educated about retardation (Greenspan & Budd, 1986).

Researchers (Abbott & Ladd, 1970; Bass, 1963; Bowden, Spitz, & Winters, 1971; Henshel, 1972; Johnson, 1946; Mattinson, 1971; Peck & Stephens, 1965; Penrose, 1950; Shaw & Wright, 1960) and parents (Fredericks, 1992; Mills, 1977; Wolf & Zarfas, 1982) maintain that parenthood may have a negative impact on MR individuals' adjustment and, in fact, may be an overwhelming experience for some. Neville (1981) believes the definition of retardation indicates that child rearing is beyond MR people's capacities and argues that children not be conceived if there is not reasonable expectation that they will receive minimal care. According to Neville, "For mildly mentally retarded women the physiological and emotional changes that take place during pregnancy and the violence of childbirth are often experienced as disorienting and terrifying traumas. To the extent that a retarded man participates in the birth process, he too can become disoriented and lose his personal equilibrium" (p. 63). Neville argues that paternalism and proxy consent enable MR persons to have human dignity and membership in the moral community by being responsible for their actions.

Others (e.g., Budd & Greenspan, 1984; Zetlin, Weisner, & Gallimore, 1985) contend that normalization principles include the right to take risks and make consequential decisions, so MR parents should be evaluated on the same criteria used with others. Laws that allow termination of child custody solely on the grounds of mental retardation in parents remain on the books (Haavik & Menninger, 1981; Vitello, 1978), and, although there are clear-cut cases in which parenthood is ill-advised, constitutional rights to equal protection disallow treatment of MR people as a class unless it can be demonstrated that restrictions of rights are valid for everyone in that class.

Virtually all studies find a percentage of MR parents to be functioning within, or close to, normal limits, especially when compared to those of similar backgrounds (Greenspan & Budd, 1986). Furthermore, parenting difficulties may stem more from problems in MR individuals' upbringing, lack of education, and current living situations than from intellectual deficits (Rosenberg & McTate, 1982). MR parents have been found capable of benefiting from therapeutic and educational interventions aimed at increasing child-rearing adequacy (Andron & Tymchuk, 1987; Budd & Greenspan, 1985; Rosenberg & McTate, 1982). The trend to work with parents to help them maintain and reobtain custody of children is as much a right of MR parents as of others.

Andron and Tymchuk (1987) note that MR people strive to be good parents and many are self-referred, rather than court-referred, to parenting interventions. They identify factors that influence MR parents' adequacy in providing child care that I have modified, expanded, and clarified in organizing this list:

1. family history (availability of nurturing parental models), personal childhood experiences, and cultural and religious factors conducive to supportive child-rearing practices;

2. independent living skills (not socialized to dependency);

3. adequate income to afford the amenities;

4. access to services from professional agencies;

5. social support, including a positive marital relationship (supportive interaction in relation to the child and each other), extended family involvement, and the availability of support groups;

6. personal strengths such as judgment, health, expressive and literacy skills, and motivation.

In order to establish trust, Andron and Tymchuk have face-to-face contacts with clients and are honest about the legal requirement that any signs of neglect or abuse be reported. They present material in a concrete fashion, make use of peer models similar to parents, and provide in-home training as well as center-based instruction that allows parents respite from full-time child care. MR parents can learn parenting knowledge in group, clinic-based settings (Fantuzzo, Wray, Hall, Goins, & Azar, 1986; Madsen, 1979), but knowledge acquisition alone does not make a significant difference in trainees' parenting (Bakken, Miltenberger, & Schauss, 1993). Applied behavioral home-based skills training in parenting improves performance (Bakken, Miltenberger, & Schauss, 1993; Feldman, Towns, Betel, Case, Rincover, & Rubino, 1986). Most interventions are done on a post hoc basis after MR parents' problems are identified by child protective services. Family-life education is rarely included in schools or teacher education programs (Brantlinger, 1988a, 1988b, 1991, 1992b). In these earlier writings, I recommended that parenting education be part of the secondary school curriculum for MR students.

STERILIZATION

The only quantitative analysis of MR people's reactions to sterilization was done by Sabagh and Edgerton (1962), who report that 44 of the 48 ex-patients had undergone sterilization; of these, 68 percent were disapproving of sterilization, and only 20 percent were totally positive. Henshel (1972) chose not to mention sterilization because of the "painful implications of the topic"; yet many participants reported that sterilizations were done at the insistence of relatives (p. 243). Henshel concluded that people talked into sterilization were unhappy and regretted being unable to have children like everyone else. Those who already had children when they were sterilized were happier than the ones who did not.

Edgerton (1967) provided poignant quotations of fervent desires for children and dismay at infertility. One single woman avoided men because she felt her infertile condition made her unmarriageable. Most were bothered by the dehumanizing stigma of sterilization, which they perceived as an irradicable mark of their institutional past and a permanent source of self-doubt about their mental status that impeded passing as normal. Before laparoscopy, tubal ligations involved abdominal incisions, which left scars that had to be explained in intimate relations. MR people were angry at how sterilization had come about—at not being included in the decision or at the deceit about the nature of the surgery (they often were told it was an appendectomy). In turn, many chose to lie, saying the sterilization scar was from an appendectomy. The reports include a few who were glad that they could not become pregnant or impregnate. In a few of Edgerton's married cases, sterilization was described as a "blessing" by the individual or spouse; a few single men felt it allowed "sexual freedom" (p. 121). Some

of Mattinson's (1971) couples agreed with the reason for the sterilization—
that child rearing would be too difficult for them.

Henshel, Edgerton, and Mattinson were advocates for MR individuals
and spoke respectfully of them. Nevertheless, even as they quoted the outcry
about sterilization, it was striking that all three seemed bothered by participants' desire for children. Intensive contact put them in positions to observe
the immaturity and problematic lives of interviewees. Although they had
compassion for the pain and the sense of loss, none fully endorsed the
respondents' perceptions of themselves as (likely to be) good parents. They
cautioned that sterilization had to be evaluated from many perspectives. In
a statement reminiscent of the eugenicists, Henshel (1972) concludes:
"After studying people whose lives were so often lonely, incomplete, and
full of misery because their handicaps set them apart, we believe that for
those families in which retardation and physical deformities run rampant,
sterilization is strongly indicated" (p. 244).

In terms of access to information and services, Henshel (1972) found that
many women had no idea about sterilization and were confused about birth
control. Mattinson (1971) found the same ignorance. Respondents confided
that not only did they not want more children, but also they had not wanted
some or any of those they had. One woman said: "Well, I didn't really want
this one. I think two's enough!" (J.M.: "Did you try not to have this one?
Did you take any precautions?") "No, I was going to take those birth pills
but a lot of people told me they made them bad and I was a bit frightened
of taking them." (J.M.: "What are you going to do after this baby?")
"There's a place down . . . that if I see the doctor, I can get a cap fitted, but
he said, 'it's only if you've got a big family that you can be sterilized.' I
shall get something done." Another said: "But the trouble is I worries that
the baby's all right. Sometimes you can't feel it and it worries you. I said
to Harry I didn't want this one and that upset 'ee. He said, 'I'll keep it and
look after it.' I didn't want her (other child) either" (p. 106). It was clear
that these individuals had little access to good contraceptive services.

Parenthood, as any parent will admit, can at times be financially, emotionally, and physically draining. For most people, the decision to reproduce
is not a deeply reasoned one. The urge to have children is instinctive, and,
regardless of other considerations, this is often enough to set the process
going (Konstantareas & Homatidis, 1992). Feelings of being bereft, frequently reported by those suffering from infertility, provide powerful evidence of the strength of the urge to have children (A. Smith, 1990). Sherwin
(1992a) theorizes that children are valued as privatized commodities that
reflect the virility and heredity of their parents. She also believes that
because adults are often inhibited from having warm, stable interactions

with the children of others, those who wish to know children well find that they must have their own. Moreover, many women are persuaded that their most important purpose in life is to bear and raise children and that their lives are incomplete and lacking in fulfillment if they do not. For MR women, children may be a hope for real intimacy and for the sense of accomplishment that comes from doing work one judges to be valuable. To combat this nonreason, Sherwin believes that the status of women should be changed from breeder to valued member of a community (p. 135).

7

Sexuality and Parenting among Individuals with Mild Mental Retardation

Sexual expression and birth control are important aspects of most people's lives. For reasons connected with their condition, MR people may have trouble fitting in socially, and they may not have challenging careers and stimulating leisure pursuits. As a result, intimate social and sexual relations may be even more important for them than for others. In spite of their needs and desires, however, before the virginity movement became popular regarding sexual relations for the general public, abstinence had long been recommended and enforced for MR individuals. This chapter includes the results of my own interview studies of adolescents with mild mental retardation and secondary teachers of MR students.

ADOLESCENT STUDY

Seeking evidence about various aspects of sexuality and family living among individuals classified mildly mentally retarded (MiMR), I conducted in-depth interviews with 13 adolescents (5 girls and 8 boys with an age range of 14 to 18 years old). Perhaps the most salient finding of this study was that MiMR adolescents were very ill at ease in hearing or using sexual terminology. For example, Shelly (pseudonym, as are all names in this report) said: "I hate it when boys call me . . . call me . . . it starts with an h . . ." (Ellen: "Whore?") Shelly: "Yeh, I'm not really you know!" Donald admitted: "Talking's hard for me"; Will confessed: "I feel kind of weird saying all those things." At various points in the interview, Terra said: "I feel kind of strange talking"; "Oh, I don't know, I hate to say it"; "I just get nervous about these things"; and "Oh God, I'd never hear the end of it if they found out I was talking about some of these things." It was clear that these students had learned that talking about sex was wrong. By the end of the interviews, most had become remarkably less anxious and much more responsive.

Part of the inability to talk seemed related to negative attitudes toward sex. Most gave the impression that sex was dirty and nasty business—something you did on the sly even though you really should not be doing it or talking about it. Others (e.g., Gollay, Freedman, Wyngaarden, & Kurtz, 1978; Heshusius, 1981; Rosen, Clark, & Kivitz, 1977) note that the lack of knowledge about sex among MR participants was accompanied by the attitude that sexual words and actions are dirty and wrong. These findings emphasize the participants' sense of being controlled by others and of having to please others and not themselves. On the other hand, in my study, when specifically asked why people have sex together, nine responded with some form of "it is pleasurable" ("they enjoy it," "for the thrill," "it feels good," "to have fun"). Three gave social reasons: "when they love each other," "to show you love her," and "to be part of the crowd." A youth who said "to have babies" was the only one to ascribe a reproductive function to sex; yet separating sex from fertility is unwise unless the use of birth control is also assumed.

Two girls had taken fairly comprehensive sexuality courses, and this was obvious in their ease in using sexual terminology and the accuracy and amount of their knowledge. The remaining 11 were judged to be uninformed and misinformed about sex. Four confused the terms "abortion" and "adoption" ("abortion is when the mother don't want the baby and she gives it to the foster people . . . welfare"). Three others said that both were "getting rid of your baby." Rita claimed abortion was "killing the baby after it's been born." Even more off the track, Terra said: "Abortion is if you divorce somebody." After receiving a definition of abortion, 10 claimed to be opposed; 1 said it was okay for others, but she would not do it; and 2 said they would choose to abort if they/their girlfriend were pregnant. Nine felt that giving up a baby for adoption was unacceptable.

Another area of ignorance was the age of onset of female puberty. Four claimed "not to know," six said between 17 and 21 years of age, two said 16, and one (female) said 13 or 14. When an attempt was made to clarify the question by rephrasing ("When is her body first able to have a baby?"), students repeated their original response. Girls were as confused about this as boys.

Regarding the acceptability of sexual relations taking place outside of marriage, eight felt it was permissible ("that's up to them," "it ain't my business," "it's natural," "if they love each other"), two were noncommital, and three stated that premarital sex was unacceptable. Teachers guessed that two who stated their disapproval of premarital sex were sexually active.

When asked about contraception, some named the pill and the condom, but there was considerable confusion and misinformation. In response to the question, "Are there ways to have sex and not have a baby?" Shelly said: "I don't guess not. If you're fixed you're not going to have a baby. You probably won't. Some people has it and some people don't." Will said: "You can wrap a towel around you." Tim responded: "Use petroleum." Later, in response to "What is a rubber?" Tim said: "You wear it on your penis, probably to make her pregnant." The following dialogues illustrate the confusion surrounding fertility and contraception:

Ellen: How does a woman get pregnant?

Seth: Comes natural.

Ellen: Does she have to have a man?

Seth: Yeh, guy helps sometimes [stated in a serious manner].

Ellen: If a woman doesn't want a baby and wants to have sex, is there anything she can do?

Seth: If she don't want a baby, it ain't my reason to say she does.

Ellen: So if you have sex, you're probably going to have a baby?

Seth: Sometimes yes and sometimes never.

Ellen: If they don't want a baby, is there anything a man can do?

Seth: Probably just do it anyway. Take your chances. If they don't want a baby, they could put it up for abortion.

Ellen: What's an abortion?

Seth: To give the baby to another family.

Ellen: Have you heard of birth control?

Seth: Yeh, to have the baby destroyed.

Ellen: What do you think about that?

Seth: It's wrong. I don't think they should do it.

Ellen: What are sperm?

Richard: White stuff that comes out of your penis. It's good for nothing.

Ellen: Do you need it to make a baby?

Richard: No. To have a baby a man has to go real fast. If he wants two kids, he has to go real, real fast.

Ellen: Can twins happen when two eggs from the woman get together with sperm?

Richard: Oh, no. They can't! I found out. The man has to go real fast. How can two eggs come out of the man's john [penis]?

Both Seth and Richard were reputed (by their teachers) to be streetwise and sexually active.

Adolescents were asked how they would feel and what they would do if they got pregnant (or impregnated). Three said they would be shocked, two that they would be happy, and two that they would be unhappy; the remaining six were ambivalent and/or noncommittal. Nine, including all five females, claimed that they would "have the baby" and "keep it." One boy said "get rid of it," but would not say how. One listed abortion as his first choice and another listed it as his second—their other answer was that the baby should be placed for adoption. Two boys asserted that it would not be their responsibility—that it was the girl's concern, whereas the other six boys verbalized that they would take care of the baby or help make decisions about the situation.

Four said their parent(s) would be angry or upset if they (or their girlfriend) got pregnant. One said: "She'd be mad at first but she'd get over it." Five felt their parents would not be upset. As Rita said: "My mom wants me to get pregnant. She wants to be a grandmother. She loves babies. My aunt is only 38 and she has 3 grandbabies and my mother is 41 and doesn't have any." Terra claimed: "My mom already said if I get pregnant before I'm out of school and have a baby, she'll stay home and watch it." (Ellen: "So she wants a grandchild?") "Yeh. She don't mind." Three were unsure of their parents' reactions.

Two males claimed they never would get married. Three (two males, one female) said they were fairly certain they would not want children, reasoning that they were too much responsibility or would require too much care. The most reasonable and stable-seeming of the interviewees, Shelly thought she would remain childless—a choice, she claimed, that was her own. As she said: "I watch little kids at child care [day-care service for students' and teachers' children located in her high school]. I don't know. I'm just afraid and I see other girls pregnant and, you know, it leads them to nowhere. I ain't got nothing against having kids or nothing like that. I love little kids, but I don't think I want to have any." Three (two males, one female) wanted three or more children; five claimed to want one or two. Laura said: "I ain't going to have no dozen—two or three maybe."

Eight students verbalized things to consider before getting married and/or starting a family. Seven mentioned financial stability, six said having a good relationship with the potential spouse, and four named maturity. Donald said: "I'll wait until I get enough money to support my kids and I wouldn't do it until I'm ready." Then he added: "I feel like if you have a kid, you should tell your mom first." When asked about qualities they would like in a spouse, seven wanted someone who "would be faithful," who "would not two-time them" or "run around." One wanted someone "honest." Two girls said a spouse should "be nice," and two males wanted someone who would "take care of" them.

Although I did not ask specific questions about role models during the interviews, 10 students volunteered stories about the relationship or sexual problems of their parents, siblings, friends, or neighbors. One mother was in jail for drug abuse and prostitution, a father had recently "run off" with his wife's sister, several single siblings—mainly adolescents—in their households had children, and four respondents lived with foster parents or grandparents. Only three lived with both biological parents.

Seven, four of whom were girls, claimed their parents (all same-sex parents) had talked to them about sex. When asked who he would go to with questions about sex, Jerry hesitantly replied: "Maybe my mom and dad."

Ellen: Would they give you good answers?

Jerry: No. They don't pay no attention to anything.

Ellen: Would you like to know more about sex?

Jerry: I'll be nowhere if I don't.

When asked if a parent had talked to him about sex, Will said:

Not much. When my dad tries to talk to me, he shakes like a leaf. He just don't know how to explain it to us. He says, "Okay. Now if I can only get up the nerve to tell you part of it." You should know all of it 'cause you might get into trouble, for Heaven's sake! You should know everything, not part of it! You need the whole facts so you won't make no mistakes. Most parents is afraid to tell teenagers but they should so they won't get in deep trouble, you know, like having sex and they didn't know that they was getting her pregnant and then the whole thing would start there. He'd have to get a job and everything. If my parents are afraid to tell me, I'll just have to learn someplace else.

Three girls claimed they had not known about menstruation prior to having their first period. Terra confided: "When I first started, I was afraid. I didn't know I was growing up." Laura said: "I was scared. I didn't know it was going to happen while it was happening." Shelly recalled:

She [her mother] talked to me and stuff like that, I mean, yeh, but I never did really understand it. Like one time when I was 11 years old I started to get my period, you know, I didn't even know it and like I was in the bathroom and I thought, "Oh, my Lord," and I didn't even know what was going on. Mom forgot to tell me. I thought there was something wrong. I thought my insides, or something, was bleeding.

Seven claimed not to have talked about sex with friends or siblings. As Shelly replied: "No. I just feel strange talking about it to other people. I just don't even talk about it, you know." Shelly felt she had learned about sex from "overhearing boys talk." Rita also had learned indirectly by being around two older brothers. Of the six who had shared information with peers, Seth confided: "Mostly from girls, you know, you have to go out and do it yourself, that's where you learn it. I learned from my brother's girlfriends. They do it." (Ellen: "Do you ever talk to them about sex?") "No. Go ahead and get it over with. Girls have to leave their belt buckled unless they want it. I never have taken advantage of a girl." Donald and Will said they learned about sex in drugstores by reading "dirty books" and package labels on hygiene and contraceptive products. Dave asserted that his main source of information was "myself" and "TV." Eight claimed to have had some sexuality education in school, but only two girls were judged to be relatively well informed, and even they had major gaps in their knowledge. These two said they had "enough" information, but others felt they had "very little." Eleven said they would welcome more school-based sexuality education; two were noncommital, but not opposed.

STUDY OF TEACHERS OF SECONDARY MR STUDENTS

A problem with the adolescent study was some students' inability or unwillingness to talk candidly about sex. Believing that teachers would have information about students, I interviewed 22 junior and senior high school special education teachers about their perceptions of MiMR students' sexual behaviors and potential parenting abilities, as well as their own efforts at providing sexuality and family-life education.

All 22 teachers stated that the majority of their pupils had ambitions to establish social intimacy, have sexual relationships, marry, and bear and raise children. A typical response was: "Mine all want to marry and have children and, as far as they're concerned, the sooner the better." A teacher said: "Especially my girls want boyfriends so bad. Having someone to 'go with' makes them feel secure. Most don't have other school interests. Few get involved in sports. They are mainly interested in the social aspects of school."

All felt their pupils generally lacked accurate information about sexual topics. After estimating that 80 percent of her students were sexually active, a teacher said:

My kids are aware of birth control but I'm sure they don't use it regularly. Most of the questions during my sex education course indicated they'd never used it—didn't know how to use it. They were interested in information, particularly the specifics. They had the details mixed up. They didn't know the terminology. They did not know where to get contraceptives and how to use them. There's a lot they don't know.

Many teachers separated their students into two groups: the "streetwise" and the "naive." The bimodal nature of their students' knowledge correlated with socioeconomic status. Low-income MiMR students were judged to be "streetwise" and part of a sexually charged youth subculture. It was surmised that they were sexually active at an earlier age and to a greater extent than either their high-income counterparts or their low-income peers who were more successful in school. As a teacher said: "My students start to hang out at an early age. You can't call it dating, it is more casual than that. I think the kids in regular classes have more formal dates. You know, they call each other up and make plans. My kids just find a place to hang out and they meet there and pair up." Another said: "My special education kids don't play enough. They grow up fast. They're having sexual relationships while they are still watching cartoons."

Teachers felt that the sexual activity rate was higher for some MiMR students because it was one area in which they could compete. A middle school teacher described a student: "She dresses provocatively. Her pants are so tight you wonder how she gets into them. She had a high school boyfriend and talked about him constantly. She's blatant about liking sex—it's an area where she can be successful. She's a dreamer. She thinks a man will fulfill her dreams." Another teacher hypothesized: "My students have encountered so much failure in their lives and there are so many things that they cannot do well. When it comes to sex, once they realize they can do that like anybody else, they think 'I'm good at this.' It's a status symbol to be sought after sexually. Pregnancy is even a status thing. It's seen as sort of an accomplishment, a sign of popularity with boys."

Indications of sexual precociousness and streetwise behaviors have been observed by others. Satterfield and Sugar (1990) found that the majority of prostitutes were sexually abused as children, have serious personality disorders, and are of low intellectual endowment with poor educations. MR girls copy seductive behavior from television, and, hungry for approval and attention, sex may be the most gratifying venture of their lives (Bernstein, 1990). Although these statements could be made for nonretarded adolescents, Bernstein implies that MR girls are unique. Thurer (1991) might counter that the observed behaviors result because MR women are less likely to have paid employment, and the self-esteem that goes with vocational success.

Teachers hypothesized that gender role expectations influenced thoughts and actions. As one 14-year veteran said:

Girls who use birth control are considered "bad girls" because they're preparing for sex. Yet, in spite of thinking that girls should not take precautions against pregnancy, boys turn around and say it is the girl's fault if she should become pregnant. They don't feel they owe the girl and the baby anything if they should father a baby. They act like the pregnancy is the girl's punishment for having had sex. They also think that it is "macho" to father babies and ignore the pregnant girl's situation.

Teachers also thought that girls felt it was wrong to use birth control and plan for sexual encounters; moreover, girls were said "to feel obliged to give in to male demands for sex." Teachers felt many defined "success" as being "popular with the boys" and being "sexually alluring." Teachers complained that girls had narrow sex-role definitions. They felt they could not interest many in jobs or in steps for career advancement because they "only think of themselves as mothers and wives."

Another theory espoused was that the suspected high rate of sexual activity was due to students' low self-esteem and lack of assertiveness. Phrases like "desperate for acceptance," "eager for attention," and "such a need for friends" were frequent. A middle school teacher said: "They're more naive, and less well-informed than their chronological age peers, and they go along with whatever is happpening in their group." Another said: "My students don't seem to think that they have the right to say 'no' to others. They'll go along with anything anybody suggests." A third concurred: "My students have a desire to please others. They are easily led." Still another said: "My students have a serious problem with self-esteem and they become popular, that is boys pay attention to them, when they put out." Another said: "They crave attention. They want to feel loved. They want the status of having a boyfriend. People look up to you when you have a boyfriend. It's the same for boys. Sex is an important part of life. It's the way they earn respect from other guys."

Peer pressure was influential. A teacher said: "They do what their friends do. They want to fit in." Another clarified: "I had a girl who confided all sorts of things to me. I think she really knew she was being taken advantage of and yet she really wanted to be liked and wanted attention from the boys. She would do anything to please if it's put right. She's easily swayed. She wants to be accepted. Many of my kids are real followers." A high school teacher maintained:

Our kids get taken advantage of because regular kids like to get them to do things. We had one boy who was giving blow jobs to a few regular students in the men's room at school. I think he did it because he was used to doing things that other people asked him to do and he didn't discriminate between what is and is not appropriate. He wants regular students' approval and companionship. He seems to drift into things and is not at all active in planning what he'll do. He never questions others' motives.

Lack of evaluative thinking was thought to be critical. A teacher said: "My girls just don't make decisions quick enough. It's hard for them to say no. They talk about not doing certain things but then have a hard time deciding what to do when they are in a situation that calls for a decision." Another said: "I've taught both learning disabled and MiMR students and have found a difference. With the LD there's more boasting and pretending to be cool. They let on that they're sexually active. They're more sophisticated. The MiMR act more according to instincts without thinking of the image or the consequences. They can't discriminate between others' motives and aren't aware they're being taken advantage of."

Vulnerability included not only unequal and humiliating relations with peers, but also more serious, illegal forms of abuse. Twenty (91 percent) had students who had been sexually abused or who were victims of incest; 17 (77 percent) had reported abuse. One said:

Often they get involved with family members or just someone around like a brother's friend. Some don't have friends or events outside the home, so I think they just drift into convenient sexual relationships which often involve family members. Sometimes it happens because someone's taking advantage of them because they are slow and unassertive, but I've had students who have seemed to initiate the sexual interaction. I had a girl a few years ago who miscarried her father's baby. The social worker told us that when she investigated, the father was open about having a severe drinking problem, and he admitted that he had probably had intercourse with his daughter. However, the social worker said that while she was talking to the family, my student was "throwing herself" at her father. Apparently she sat on her father's lap and sat next to him with her arms around him. She did this in front of her mother and other family members, and nobody reacted to her behavior. In that case, the girl was not taken out of the home but the social worker made sure she had birth control. In discussing the situation with the social worker it was difficult for me to decide what the best course of action would be. At first I was mad at the welfare department because they did not take her out of the home, but she loved her family and would have been upset if she had been separated from them.

Some surmised that child protection workers did not intercede because they did not value the low-income MiMR victim of abuse.

In contrast to their low-income counterparts, middle-class MiMR young-sters were described as "naive," "immature," and "out of the mainstream" of secondary school culture in which their chronological age peers were actively pursuing intimate social relationships. Teachers felt that middle-class MiMR students had been prevented from receiving information about sex and from having relationships by protective parents. As one said: "Well-off parents watch their kids closely. They baby them. They are not allowed to hang around the teen hangouts or go on dates. Their parents are very influential in their lives. I had the feeling that mothers pushed their values: 'You can't have children because you're retarded. No kids, no sex!' It was bleak for them—a sad situation. They already seemed depressed, seemed to have given up." Another teacher observed: "More affluent mothers communicate 'No, you can't do it!' Mothers intentionally make their kids look unattractive—their clothes, their haircuts—nothing in style. It is as if they do not want the opposite sex to look at them. On the other hand, low-income parents are tolerant of all their kids' behavior. Their attitude is 'anything goes!' Really, it would be great to compromise the positions."

Naive students' "oddness" was believed due to "inability to distinguish the acceptable from the unacceptable," "not picking up on social cues," "inability to assimilate the adult sexual world," "confusion about how intimacy and affection should be expressed," "impulsivity about things," "lacking awareness of how their behaviors impact on others," and "not having learned to control feelings or appropriately express curiosities."

Eighteen teachers (81 percent) said naive adolescents had trouble distin-quishing whether a peer was interested in them and did not know acceptable ways to approach others. One related: "Like I had one boy who kept touching girls' hair. He was particularly attracted to one girl and wouldn't leave her hair alone. He did it almost unconsciously. She interpreted his touching as sexual and hated it. But I think he really wanted to be her friend, wanted her to know he liked her and thought her hair was pretty. But he went about it all wrong. She wouldn't go near him."

"Immature" pupils were not liked by peers, had limited interaction with others, and often were picked on; hence, they were "withdrawn," "isolates," and "scapegoats." Based on observations in local schools, Evans and Eder (1993) confirmed the fact that special education students, and especially the lower-functioning students, were cruelly teased by regular education schoolmates. Moreover, the teasing tended to have sexual overtones.

Twelve teachers (54 percent) attributed awkward social behaviors to cognitive deficiencies, whereas seven (32 percent) remarked that some socially backward students were academically advanced compared to other members of the MiMR class. They attributed oddness to the way they had been socialized by families—to the result of denial of sexuality or more general overprotection. Three (14 percent) felt students had become "socially peculiar" as a result of having spent many years in self-contained special education classrooms.

Ultimately, in spite of surface behaviors, both streetwise and naive youngsters lacked knowledge about facts, functions, and consequences of sexual behaviors. A teacher said: "My kids act tough—macho! At first I thought that they were well-informed about sex. They treated me as someone who knew nothing about sex. They see teachers as square. But they're not informed. Once you talk to them you realize that they're not as aware as they pretend to be." Another said: "Their only sex education is the media: VCR, and you know how good that is! They are out there doing it—taking their chances—but they don't really know what it is all about."

Twenty (91 percent) felt students thought of sex as a "dirty," "backstreet" "thing to be ashamed of." As one said: "Sex seems tied to recreation and exploitation rather than to a loving relationship." A man voiced a common sentiment:

I was concerned about promiscuous behaviors. They had sex drives. It was natural that they'd want relations, but their framework of thinking of what sex means bothered me. I think they see sexually-oriented magazines, television shows, and movies, and they take it all at face value—quite literally. They take it lightly and don't think of the consequences. I don't think they evaluate the messages that they get through the media. And often they don't imitate the roles very well. They get frustrated and hurt, but they don't know what to do about it.

Pregnancy Rates and Parenting Potential

Nineteen teachers (86 percent), including middle school teachers, had students who had become pregnant. Many estimated that one or two girls got pregnant a year. (For obvious reasons, teachers were less able to judge the rate of impregnation by male students, but guessed a similar rate.) Bothered by their students' lack of control over conception and the randomness of their decisions about when to bear and raise children, teachers believed the early or single pregnancies compounded students' parenting problems. Some MiMR adolescents were described as wanting to have children, regardless of their preparedness for parenting, because they saw pregnancy as a status symbol or sign of being sexually desirable and mature. To others, it meant escape from bad circumstances, from school or families.

MiMR students "romanticized the role of parent" and "were unrealistic about babies." Yet, although they thought some pregnancies were intentional, nineteen (77 percent) felt that the majority of pregnancies resulted from "carelessness and ignorance" or "lack of access to birth control." A teacher said: "They are not knowledgeable about contraception. They leave it up to their partner or chance. They have an attitude that 'what will happen will happen' or 'let nature take its course.' "

It was the teachers' impression that pregnant MiMR girls generally went through with the pregnancies and kept their babies. A middle school teacher recalled:

Over a 3-year-period at that school I taught approximately 40 students, which meant I probably had fewer than 20 girls in all. I had five pregnancies among the girls during those years. The girls stayed in school. One got married. All five were going to keep their babies, but one miscarried. One of the girls told me that she wanted to have an abortion but her mother wouldn't let her. You know, I don't think I have ever heard of an MiMR girl having an abortion. None of my girls' pregnancies were planned. The girls were just ignorant and careless. My impression was that all except the married girl expected to support their babies on AFDC [Aid to Families with Dependent Children] money. You were not allowed to teach about contraception in that school system but the county has the highest teen pregnancy rate in the state. It was very frustrating.

None of the teachers remembered students having placed babies for adoption at birth. Five (23 percent) were aware of ex-students who had voluntarily given up custody of their children at a later date or who had neglected or abused their children, so their rights to custody had been terminated. One claimed an ex-student had lost custody of four children, two at one time and two at a later date.

Eighteen teachers (82 percent) maintained that pregnancy at a young age was not perceived as a great disadvantage. As one said: "My students don't have any postschool plans like going to college and many don't have set career plans. The one thing they look forward to in the future is getting married and having a baby, and it does not necessarily have to be in that order. They don't think that it is any big deal to have a baby without getting married."

When asked if their MiMR students would make good parents, 14 teachers (64 percent) commented immediately: "no way," "probably not," or "no, they'd be very poor parents." Three (14 percent) said they "did not know," and five (23 percent) gave a mixed response, saying "some would, some wouldn't." One predicted: "Some might be okay parents if they had some training, others would be terrible and even with support their having children would be a disaster for everyone involved." Almost all (18, 82 percent)—even those who were initially negative—judged that there were a few who already had skills that would allow them to be good parents or who, with training and support, could learn to be adequate parents.

The major interference with parenting capacity cited by teachers was emotional, not cognitive, inadequacies. One said: "Many of my students are disturbed as well as being retarded. It's the emotional aspects that would cause problems if they were to become parents." They described "quick tempers," "aggressive and violent," "mean and feisty," "selfish," and "egocentric" as negative traits that would be stable over time. Recalling experiences with abused students, 20 (91 percent) mentioned the intergenerational nature of abuse; they felt pupils learned problematic behaviors that would ultimately affect parenting from their own parents. Teachers observed that students projected blame for problems onto others or denied their existence. Thus, those with the most serious emotional problems were judged most unrealistic in assessing their abilities to parent and most likely to get pregnant (or to impregnate).

In opposition to the opinion that gentle, loving, and cooperative MiMR students would automatically be good parents, 20 teachers (91 percent) stated that parenting was complex; hence, it demanded intellectual ability. They reasoned that MiMR students' "general slowness," "retardation," and "cognitive deficiencies" would interfere with competently performing even routine tasks of parenting. One teacher said: "My students lack common sense across the board. All the little decisions that parents have to make would be impossible for many of my kids." They felt neglect due to ignorance would be common. A teacher said: "Most of my students simply do not have the intelligence to be even adequate parents. I am saddened when I hear that one of my ex-students has had a baby. I feel sorry for the baby. I feel sorry for students who have to cope with all the problems that parents are faced with." Yet it was not always high-functioning students who were judged capable of good parenting; 10 (46 percent) emphasized that parenting had more to do with "common sense" than academic skills. A few were bothered that students' negative attitudes toward school would influence the next generation.

Twenty teachers (91 percent) hesitantly expressed concern about a continuation of intergenerational cycles of poverty and special education placement if their students became parents; however, their uneasiness about the potential eugenics interpretations of this opinion was noticeable. Six (27 percent) stated specifically that intelligence was not the most important attribute for potential offspring and perhaps should not be a factor in decisions to parent. Yet 20 (91 percent) also felt that mental retardation in future generations should be prevented.

Teachers suggested that conditions correlated with MiMR status might interfere with adequate parenting. Students were felt to have limited vocational opportunities, and it was assumed that, like many of their parents, they would be poor in adult life. Teachers felt the financial stresses of low-income life would interfere with parental adequacy—that low-income MiMR parents might be depressed or so overwhelmed with demands that they would not be able to provide a calm, optimistic, and supportive environment for children. As one said: "My students are going to have a difficult time providing for their own monetary needs without adding the financial burden of raising children." Another commented: "My students think that what they need to raise a child will simply be there when the baby arrives—that it will all take care of itself. They don't think about the future carefully enough to understand the reality of adult responsibilities." Besides inadequate finances for parenting, teachers worried that students would not be able to maintain a dwelling, get a license to drive and own and maintain a car, recognize their own or their offspring's medical needs, and provide adequate nutrition for a family. Again, they stressed that everyday life in modern times was complex, expensive, and hard.

Four teachers (18 percent) claimed discomfort at blaming students or families for situations they felt resulted from societal conditions and not from inherent traits of MiMR individuals. Their position was that many MiMR people would be good parents if such circumstances as poverty were eliminated. One apologized for "having a biased, middle-class perspective," and wavered:

It's hard to say about parenting. In many ways I did not approve of the way my students were being raised. The parents seemed like they did not care much about school attendance. One of my girls who got pregnant had two sisters living at home with their babies. It bothered me that they were all raising children in that environment. I was upset that my student was going through with the pregnancy. I just could not imagine her as a mother. Parents accept early sexual experience. They don't believe in birth control or abortions. But they all seemed excited about the prospect of a new baby. No one seemed to be ashamed that she wasn't married. In that school there was a 60 percent high school dropout rate and the average student was 4 years behind grade level. I was very confused about my own feelings about the situation. Their values were different than mine, but I'm not really sure that my lifestyle is any more valid than theirs.

Similarly, another related:

I had one extended family with several siblings and cousins, aunts and uncles living together. There were stepbrothers and sisters and half brothers and sisters. It was hard to tell who belonged to whom. Nobody could keep family connections straight. It was the tradition for teenagers in that family to have babies. They kept the babies and did not worry about getting married, though fathers often stayed around. For the most part the babies were well cared for. They looked clean and healthy. They were from low-income, single-parent homes; they had solid family backgrounds.

Yet another said:

Most girls don't marry when they get pregnant and they live with their mothers. The daughters learn how to care for babies from their mothers. I held my confer-ences in my students' homes and I observed that the babies were being well cared for. They were proud of the babies and showed them off. Having babies without being married was an accepted part of their lives. They often have older sisters with kids living at home. I was surprised how well one of my immature girls coped.

Sexuality and Parenting Education

A goal of education is to prepare students for vocational, familial, and citizenship roles in adult life. With MR students—at least in theory—this entails providing a practical daily-living curriculum. Yet the emphasis of functional programming has been almost solely on vocational skills acqui-sition. When domestic skills are included, they tend to be limited to the noncontroversial cooking, cleaning, and personal hygiene. Nevertheless, a normal life includes social and sexual intimacy.

Studies of adults who test in the moderate range of retardation have revealed major deficits in knowledge about sexuality (Edmonson, McCombs, & Wish, 1979; Fischer & Krajicek, 1974), as have studies of those in the mild range (Brantlinger, 1985a, 1988b; Diamond, 1979). Negative consequences result when MR people lack sexuality information and training (Rienzo, 1981; Rosen, 1970). With no preparation for the sexual and intimate social sides of their lives, and with silence or mixed messages from others, MR individuals are often locked into perpetual abstinence or irresponsible adolescence. For MR people—like others—in-timate sexual expression constitutes an important aspect of becoming an adult. Preparation in sexual/social areas should enable students to develop constructive decision-making skills and behave in a fulfilling and respon-sible manner.

Most adolescents do not receive the amount of sexuality education they want or need (Bruess & Greenberg, 1988; Klein, 1992), but the sources of information about sex and models of rational decision making may be even less available for MR individuals. Many adolescents claim peers as a source of information about sex. The peers of MR individuals are likely to be less knowledgeable than average, and they may model problematic behaviors. Because of limited literacy and mobility, MR adolescents may have little access to accurate and informative resources available in libraries or clinics. They are likely to be less capable of sorting through the confusing, disparaging, and dangerous messages about sexuality embedded in the popular media. Lacking funds and communication skills, they may not receive adequate services and advice from medical professionals. Although MiMR secondary students and teachers believe that sexuality and parenting education is needed, it rarely occurs in special classes, and MiMR students are not included in mainstream health programs (Brantlinger, 1985a, 1988a, 1988b, 1992b; Craft, 1987; Fantuzzo, Wray, Hall, Gorns, & Azar, 1986; Haight & Fachting, 1986).

Education reflects providers' perceptions of students. The absence of sexuality education for MR individuals may indicate that others feel their sexual expression is not feasible and desirable; thus, sexuality education is irrelevant or ill-advised. Diamond (1979), a counselor with physical impairments, stresses that adolescents with disabilities have the same physical and emotional needs and the same anxieties about sex-role identification and impulse control as everyone else, but she notes the false belief that the less individuals know about sex, the less likely they will be sexually active. "Invisibility and silence" are barriers to sex equity, but people are "afraid to mention certain ideas in public or to take certain behaviors out of hiding" (Klein, 1992, p. 3). Fine (1988) asks: "How could one continue to believe that naming is dangerous and not naming safe?" (p. 29). Students learn that their sexual participation is to be informed not by openness, enthusiasm, and knowledge, but by fear, furtiveness, and ignorance (Whatley, 1992).

Although sexuality education is integrally related to the topic of this book, it is not feasible to go into sufficient detail to do justice to the topic. Fortunately, fine sexuality programs are available. Among the most comprehensive and practical is Kempton's (1988) multimedia package. Kaeser and O'Neill (1987) address the needs of individuals with severe disabilities, for example, by task analyzing the teaching of masturbation. It is possible, however, to review basic guidelines for sexuality instruction in this book.

Although Diamond (1979) recommends that specially trained personnel are needed to educate and counsel people with disabilities concerning their sexual needs, experts may not be readily available. In the meantime, because it is essential that sexuality education be included in the curriculum on a continual basis, teachers can inform themselves and make attempts at sexuality education even without special training. Preschoolers can begin by learning formal (and neutral) names for body parts. In order that pupils learn about body changes prior to their occurrence, facts about puberty must be taught to third to sixth graders. Because of the finding that girls with Down syndrome are likely to go through menarche 11 months earlier than average (Evans & McKinley, 1988), timeliness is especially important for moderately MR girls. Techniques of contraception should be taught prior to junior high school. To prevent or decrease the pain and cost of failure in parenting by MiMR individuals, it is important to provide instruction during, or prior to, the high school years. (See Table 7.1 for suggested content.)

To enable them to understand themselves and social relations and to make the best decisions, MR students should have access to full information about sexuality. Direct instruction in parenting and exposure to parenting-like experiences have the goal of increasing knowledge, improving skills, and modifying attitudes and behaviors that interfere with competent parenting and successful family relationships.

A contradiction that arose in my study of secondary teachers was that they were not teaching sexuality education even when they said it was extremely important for their students (Brantlinger, 1988a, 1988b, 1991, 1992b). The lack of a sexuality curriculum was explained partly by the fact that teachers had not been prepared to teach about sexuality in either preservice or inservice programs; hence, they avoided a curriculum they were uncomfortable with. Another reason given was the teachers' worry that others would suspect their motives. Women worried they might be typed as permissive about sexual activity, open to a full range of sexual practices, pro-choice, and politically liberal, whereas men were concerned that colleagues and students' parents would suspect ulterior motives related to sexual interests in the children.

An even more important deterrent was the teachers' perception that administrators did not want them to stray from an academic curriculum and would not support them in case of adverse reaction from students, parents, or community members. Principals were said to have a conservative and cautious approach to instruction, avoiding anything that might draw criticism from the community. A teacher confided:

We had the highest pregnancy rate in the state. Still the principal advised teachers not even to counsel students about their sexual problems. He would not allow any sex education without 100 percent parental approval. The health teacher did not really teach sex education. Nobody would touch it! I was afraid of getting into hot water with the principal. But I think most parents would have welcomed it. They felt inadequate themselves.

Table 7.1
Suggested Components of a Parenting Education Course

1. *A general exploration of parenting and alternatives to parenting.*
   - An examination of students' parenting aspirations.
   - An evaluation of common irrational attitudes and myths about parenting.
   - A realistic analysis of parenting skills.
   - A comparison of skills needed for good parenting with personal skills of students.
   - An awareness of the ability to have personal control over parenting.
   - Information about finances involved in childbearing and child rearing.
   - Information about the influence of genetics and the environment on offspring.
   - An exploration of alternatives to (early) parenting.
   - Contact with children of various age levels.
   - A recognition of substitutes for fulfilling maternal/paternal instincts.
   - Practice in making informed decisions about when/whether to become a parent.

2. *Instruction about sexual relations and family planning.*
   - An examination of motives for establishing intimate relationships.
   - An analysis of problematic interactional patterns among adolescents.
   - The development of personal standards for sexual behaviors.
   - An examination of the relationship between behaviors and standards.
   - Practice in making thoughtful decisions about sexual relationships.
   - The development of motivation to be responsible in sexual relationships.
   - The provision of assertiveness training.
   - An examination of double standards related to gender.
   - An exploration of partner selection.
   - Information and practice in initiating and maintaining relationships.
   - Practice in communicating needs and feelings in relationships.
   - Practice in communicating about sexual topics with "helping" individuals and partners.
   - The development of an understanding of the relationship between sexual intercourse and reproduction.
   - Knowledge about safe and effective birth control methods.
   - Information about how to obtain contraceptives.

- The development of an appreciation of the need for consistent use of contraception when engaging in sexual intercourse.

- The development of motivation to prevent unwanted pregnancies.

- An examination of optional resolutions for an unwanted pregnancy for pregnant women, mothers, or families.

3. *Instruction about parenting.*

- Information about the importance of early and continuous prenatal medical care.

- Information about nutrition and safe/unsafe practices during pregnancy.

- Information about birthing.

- Information about child and adolescent development.

- An exploration of parent roles in providing a safe and healthy environment.

- An exploration of parent roles in providing a stimulating cognitive and supportive affective environment for offspring at all stages of development.

- Information about services available to aid in effective parenting.

Another teacher related:

I went ahead and taught sex education anyway, though I knew my principal wouldn't like it. He didn't say much about it, but when I informed him that I had invited someone from Planned Parenthood to talk about birth control, he was not happy. He thought that it was partisan. He told me to invite an antiabortion group to come, too. The person was not even going to mention abortion. She was there to talk about birth control.

Another said:

In my third year I taught in a middle school in an inner-city area. My own perception was that the kids were too young to be sexually active. I was shocked when a 13-year-old got pregnant. I was naive. Sex education did not occur to me as possible curriculum. I remember deliberately trying to avoid sexual topics with the kids. There were four other special education teachers in the school and none of them were doing anything with sex education. Looking back, I don't know who the kids would go to for help or information. Probably the street or some family member. The school sure wasn't providing information.

While I was at that school some regular education teachers developed a sex education curriculum guide but it was not accepted. No administrator ever brought up sex education to me but they were in the teachers' room on many occasions when we discussed the sexual problems that our students were having. Basically I think that there was an underlying fear of irate parents or community kooks who might make an issue out of something that was taught. I think the teachers would have been willing to take risks if we had the administrators' support but their view would have been: "Even if it's good for the kids it is not worth getting into—keep an even keel!"

Vague or ambiguous messages—interpreted as disapproval—were perhaps more anxiety-producing and inhibiting than flat and candid refusals. A teacher confessed: "Sex education would have been a lot more useful than a lot of the things that I did teach. I thought about including it, but I had a sense of foreboding about it—like thinking that it would get out of hand. I knew my kids needed it and wanted it but I was unwilling to take the personal risk."

Due to an improved understanding of human rights in recent years, most would agree that MR individuals have the same right to express themselves sexually as any other citizen. In actuality, however, there are still barriers to sexuality education and sexual expression.

8

Professionals' Attitudes toward the Sterilization of MR Individuals

Social upheavals and legislative trends, such as those pertaining to institutionalization and sterilization, reveal that social constructs and collective attitudes are not static, but shift and evolve with time. In spite of historical trends and patterns in mass sentiments, it is likely that movements and ideologies are never universally endorsed or rejected. Ideas live on in individuals. Attitudes and habits of practice vary according to geographical location, professional role, political affiliation, gender, educational attainment, religion, or any number of idiosyncratic variables such as contact with MR people.

People with disabilities are frequently in the position of having family members and/or professionals make decisions for them. These others, then, have the power to significantly influence MR people's lives. Although family tends to be perceived as subjective, the status of professional connotes an objective and informed expertise. Yet professionals may be equally influenced by perceptions, attitudes, beliefs, and circumstances. Physicians as a group are "generally in favor of sterilizing developmentally disabled individuals" (Haavik & Menninger, 1981, p. 113); that is, they have a bias. The chief argument against medical professionals as principal decision makers is that people overestimate their knowledge of patients' interests and values and they confuse medical judgments with moral decisions for which physicians possess no special credentials (Buchanan & Brock, 1989). The result is that professionals may make decisions for clients that are neither consistent with clients' values nor in their best interests.

This chapter reports a study of the attitudes of people in various professional fields toward sexuality, sterilization, and MR people. The participants were 50 professionals, including family planning clinic employees, social workers, MR agency personnel, educators, gynecologists, judges, lawyers, and Protection and Advocacy and Adult Protective Services workers (see Table 8.1). Participants were intentionally selected (Patton, 1980) to represent populations likely to be involved with sterilization decisions for MR people. All had been employed in south central Indiana for at least one year at the time of the interviews; hence, the study also describes and evaluates present practice regarding sterilization of MR people within a given region.

After a review of the literature on sexuality, parenting, sterilization, and rights, 13 domains were established for investigation (see Table 8.2). Interview and data analysis methods developed by Glaser and Strauss (1965, 1967) and by Strauss and Corbin (1990) included using broadly phrased, open-ended questions likely to encourage disclosure of personal opinions.

Table 8.1
Professional Roles of Participants

```
Legal (N = 14) (6-30 years' experience, mean = 16.9):
     7 judges (5 males, 2 females)
     7 "other" legal:
          3 Protection and Advocacy lawyers (2 males, 1 female)
          2 Adult Protective Services employees (females)
          2 lawyers who served as guardian ad litem (males)

Medical (N = 8) (3-22 years' experience, mean = 12.5):
     6 doctors (all males; 4 obstetricians/gynecologists, 2
          general practitioners)
     2 nurse-practitioners (female)

Family planning agency (N = 4) (3-21 years' experience,
          mean = 14.2):
     2 administrators (female)
     1 nurse-practitioner/clinic director (female)
     1 social worker (female)

Department of Public Welfare (N = 3) (1-16 years' experience,
          mean = 7.3):
     3 social workers (female)

Developmental disabilities agency (N = 13) (2-18 years'
          experience, mean = 11.1):
     4 case conference and community coordinators (1 male, 3
          females)
     2 social workers (female)
     2 agency administrators (male)
     2 residential care administrators (female)
     2 vocational supervisors (female)
     1 nurse (female)

Educators (N = 8) (1-16 years' experience, mean = 10.4)
     6 special education teachers (1 male, 5 females)
     1 special education college professor (male)
     1 principal of a special education school (male)

Total (N = 50) (1-30 years' experience, mean = 12.4)
```

All professionals contacted agreed to be interviewed—a 100 percent response rate. Forty-three interviews were audiotaped and transcribed, but notes were also taken as respondents talked. Two interviews were conducted over the phone. When contacted, a doctor said: "Shoot!" and a judge said: "I have time now so start asking!" Five additional respondents, three of whom were judges, requested that their interviews not be taped. The interviews ranged in length from approximately half an hour to over four hours, with most being between one and two hours.

Table 8.2
Domains and Items Used in Data Analysis

Domain	Item
1. Acquaintance disabled	1. Nuclear family member 2. Friend, neighbor, other relative
2. Professional contact	1. Have had contact 2. Termination of parental rights 3. Commitment to an institution
3. Professional participation	1. Sterilization decision
4. Coursework	1. In disabilities
5. Coursework	1. In sexuality 2. In sterilization
6. Discussion with colleagues	1. Sexuality 2. Sterilization 3. Sexuality/disability 4. Sterilization/disability
7. Awareness of issues	1. Existence of statute 2. Relevant litigation 3. necessity of court permission 4. Equal protection/access to sterilization 5. Interpreting consent 6. Medical implications/contraception 7. Normalization principles 8. Attitude toward people with disabilities
8. Acquaintance with	1. Sterilized individuals
9. Awareness of	1. Performing individuals/agencies 2. Procedures for obtaining
10. Attitudes toward	1. Sterilization
11. Attitudes toward	1. Sterilization of disabled 2. Eugenics position 3. Individual rights position
12. Attitudes toward	1. Parenting among disabled 2. Complexities of parenting decisions 3. Impact of sex/parenting education
13. Concern about involvement	1. Legal ramifications 2. Value conflict or dilemma

The 13 domains specified in Table 8.2 laid the framework for the initial sorting of narrative data. The next step was to find patterns within the domains and subdivide the data according to increasingly more specific criteria (see Table 8.2, Items). When possible, discrete categories were established, and responses were tallied in order to make quantitative comparisons (see Table 8.3). (These numbers or percentages also are referred to in relevant sections of the chapter.) The major findings are presented as summaries of responses, with pertinent arguments or rationales given in direct quotations selected to represent majority, minority, and individual perspectives.

The professionals contacted readily agreed to be interviewed, talked for extended periods of time, showed considerable interest in the topics addressed, and eagerly discussed "controversial issues" with "someone not connected with" their places of employment. Their extensive experience and diverse backgrounds resulted in rich and varied information about sexuality and sterilization issues. For clarity, results are presented in the same order as in Table 8.2. Thirteen respondents claimed to have personal exposure to people with disabilities (Domains 1 and 2). Of these, four were judged to be close contacts: A doctor had a preschool-age grandson with Down syndrome; another had a cousin with cerebral palsy and mental retardation; an agency social worker had a foster child who was emotionally disturbed; a teacher had a sibling with autism and moderate MR. Seven others mentioned more distant contacts (e.g., teenage MR neighbor, colleague's son with autism). All 50 (100 percent) worked with people with disabilities to some extent in fulfilling their professional obligations (Table 8.3, item a). Three common types of involvement provided by respondents are listed in Table 8.3 (i.e., items b, c, and d).

PROFESSIONALS' EXPERIENCE WITH STERILIZATION OF MR INDIVIDUALS

Although 42 professionals had some involvement in cases in which individuals with disabilities had been sterilized (Table 8.3, item b), none had specific statistics on the incidence of such sterilizations in their locale. As the director of the state Protection and Advocacy Commission explained:

I have no idea about the number of sterilizations approved by courts because there is no reporting mechanism. To get that information you would have to talk to each court individually. They don't keep records by context, so you would have to have the names of those involved in the cases and the case numbers. Even then there is no record as to why decisions were made. I suspect there has been a decline in cases since 1975, when the statute was repealed. Courts aren't granting permission without medical reason and doctors aren't doing it without court approval. Superintendents in the state hospitals are not empowered to make decisions on elective surgery—they can only make medical decisions if the situation is life threatening. The state and national trend is for no sterilization. I see law as a pendulum swing—it never stops in the middle.

Professionals at gynecological/obstetrical or family planning clinics and at welfare departments indicated that they dealt with parenting or fertility control of MR persons on a "daily" basis (Domain 3). A social worker estimated: "I have a small percentage of the more severely retarded in my case load—maybe two to three pregnant women a year—but I have a fairly high percentage of LD [learning disabled], slow learners, and school dropouts. I see 20 to 30 unwed pregnancies a month, 15 of whom are young teenagers. A lot of the AFDC mothers are special education."

The welfare department and family planning clinic received money for sterilization surgery, but workers clarified that it could not go to MR women because of guidelines prohibiting the use of federal funds for those with "intellectual disabilities." Both based judgments of "disability" on whether the person attended special education classes when in school. Hence, funds were denied to learning disabled as well as MR individuals.

Judges had responsibility for commitments to institutions, guardianship decisions, competency decisions, custody battles, child abuse charges, truancy cases, and sterilization decisions. A judge in a rural county said:

I do about 60 guardianship cases each year, although most are geriatrics, and 30 to 40 commitments to institutions. They have to be a danger to themselves or others—otherwise you can't take their freedom away. I try to talk them into voluntary commitment and get about 30 percent to agree. I review the cases and go visit each one in the institutions once a year, but from what the wardens tell me, I'm the only judge they see. I couldn't live with myself if I didn't know firsthand what happens to the people I commit.

Judges also said that felony and misdemeanor cases often involved a perpetrator or victim with disabilities.

PROFESSIONALS' PREPARATION FOR WORKING WITH MR INDIVIDUALS

With the exception of educators, who had required coursework for state certification, professionals had little preservice or inservice preparation for working with MR individuals (Table 8.2, Domains 4 and 5; Table 8.3, item e). Of the 13 employees at agencies serving clients with developmental

Table 8.3
Quantitative Results

	Judges (n = 7)	Legal (n = 7)	Medical (n = 8)
a. Dealt professionally with people with disabilities	7 (100%)	7 (100%)	8 (100%)
b. Dealt professionally with sterilization of person with disabilities	5 (71%)	5 (71%)	8 (100%)
c. Dealt professionally with commitment to an institution	7 (100%)	7 (100%)	0
d. Dealt professionally with termination of parental rights	6 (86%)	0	0
e. Had handicapping conditions coursework	0	0	0
f. Had sexuality and/or sterilization issues coursework	0	0	3 (38%)
g. Discussed sterilization with colleagues	1 (14%)	3 (43%)	6 (75%)
h. Aware of legal issues pertaining to sterilization	7 (100%)	4 (57%)	6 (75%)
i. Aware of other issues related to sterilization of disabled	2 (27%)	1 (14%)	3 (38%)
j. Unbiased attitudes toward people with disabilities	2 (27%)	2 (27%)	2 (25%)
k. Believe sterilization a frequent occurrence in general public	7 (100%)	7 (100%)	8 (100%)
l. Aware of acquaintances who selected sterilization	7 (100%)	7 (100%)	8 (100%)
m. Volunteered they had personally been sterilized	0	0	0
n. General attitude toward sterilization positive	6 (86%)	6 (86%)	7 (88%)
o. Attitude toward sterilization of people with disabilities positive	4 (57%)	4 (57%)	7 (88%)
p. Aware of cases of sterilization of individuals with disabilities	7 (100%)	7 (100%)	8 (100%)
q. Believe sterilization of disabled occurs without court consent	4 (57%)	6 (86%)	8 (100%)
r. Concerned about parenting skills of disabled	7 (100%)	6 (86%)	8 (100%)
s. Concerned about personal involvement with sterilization cases	2 (29%)	0	8 (100%)

124

Family planning (n = 4)	Welfare (n = 3)	DD agency (n = 13)	Educators (n = 8)	Total (n = 50)
4 (100%)	3 (100%)	13 (100%)	8 (100%)	50 (100%)
4 (100%)	3 (100%)	12 (92%)	5 (71%)	42 (84%)
0	3 (100%)	11 (85%)	4 (50%)	32 (64%)
0	3 (100%)	8 (62%)	1 (12%)	18 (36%)
1 (25%)	1 (33%)	4 (31%)	8 (100%)	14 (28%)
4 (100%)	1 (33%)	2 (15%)	3 (38%)	13 (26%)
4 (100%)	2 (66%)	6 (46%)	5 (71%)	27 (54%)
4 (100%)	0	1 (7%)	1 (12%)	23 (46%)
4 (100%)	3 (100%)	4 (31%)	4 (50%)	21 (42%)
2 (50%)	3 (100%)	7 (54%)	7 (88%)	25 (50%)
4 (100%)	3 (100%)	13 (100%)	8 (100%)	50 (100%)
4 (100%)	3 (100%)	13 (100%)	8 (100%)	50 (100%)
3 (75%)	0	7 (54%)	2 (25%)	12 (24%)
4 (100%)	3 (100%)	11 (84%)	8 (100%)	45 (90%)
4 (100%)	3 (100%)	7 (54%)	6 (75%)	35 (70%)
4 (100%)	3 (100%)	13 (100%)	8 (100%)	50 (100%)
4 (100%)	3 (100%)	9 (69%)	8 (100%)	42 (84%)
3 (75%)	3 (100%)	13 (100%)	7 (88%)	47 (94%)
4 (100%)	3 (100%)	8 (62%)	4 (50%)	29 (58%)

disabilities (DD), 5 had unrelated degrees (psychology, sociology, religion, history, business). Even nurses and social workers at DD agencies had little coursework specifically on working with MR clients.

Professionals in leadership positions in organizations whose primary function is serving MR people (Protection and Advocacy, Adult Protective Services) claimed little preparation for their professional roles. One, a lawyer, assumed he had received his political appointment because he had successfully prevented his suburban community from having to take part in the capital city's racial desegregation plan. An Adult Protective Services manager, who worked with MR people "on a daily basis," had been promoted from a secretarial position. She admitted: "I was not remotely trained to deal with the handicapped."

Medical professionals recalled learning about genetic syndromes and/or brain injuries, but not the "human side" of MR individuals. A doctor said: "Aside from learning the names and symptoms of syndromes, I don't think the word 'handicapped' was mentioned—but I've had plenty of exposure through my practice." Another said: "The closest my training came was a course in genetics but on my internship rotations I dealt with handicapped patients; I had spina bifida, geriatrics, alcoholics, cerebral palsy, and drew blood from an autistic." Legal professionals mainly recalled covering specific litigation pertaining to people with disabilities in case law courses.

PROFESSIONALS' TRAINING IN SEXUALITY AND CONTRACEPTION ISSUES

Neither university nor subsequent inservice preparation of 37 respondents included sterilization content (Table 8.3, item f). As a notable exception, personnel at family planning clinics claimed ongoing staff development on sterilization, sexuality, and serving clients with special needs. Five teachers and DD employees had attended workshops on sexuality but, as one said: "I've been to workshops on sexuality but sterilization has seldom been mentioned. I feel discouraged from dabbling in that area—it's such a difficult issue. Workshop leaders avoid controversy and our staff doesn't discuss it. It's almost as if it's taboo to touch on the topic."

Twenty-seven (54 percent) had talked about sterilization of MR people with co-workers (Table 8.2, Domain 6; Table 8.3, item g). Four family planning clinic workers, two social workers, and two doctors said their discussions resulted in formal decisions about dealing with sterilizations; others claimed "brief," "casual," "unfocused and unproductive" conversations. As a teacher said: "We see problems among our students all the time and, although we gossip about them, we do nothing to help students understand their sexual feelings or drives. Really, we avoid getting involved. It's easier for us that way." Later, she said: "Sterilization's been mentioned but not loudly!" A social worker at a DD agency said: "Sex is really invisible in this place. It simply does not exist."

Seven of the 23 who had not discussed sterilization of MR people with colleagues admitted to deliberately avoiding such subjects because, as a social worker said: "They are too controversial and feelings about them are too intense." In addition to those who had discussed sterilization of MR people, 10 recalled general discussions about sexuality, 2 recalled general discussions about sterilization, and 7 (DD agency staff and educators) recalled conversations about the sexuality of MR people.

AWARENESS OF STERILIZATION ISSUES

Respondents were evaluated as informed/aware of legal issues pertaining to MR sterilization if they discussed at least one of the first four items in Domain 7 (Table 8.2) with some accuracy. According to this criterion, 23 (46 percent) were at least minimally informed (Table 8.3, item h). In spite of working with adults and adolescents, educators and DD employees were surprisingly uninformed and misinformed. Two knew of the absence of a state law, and four vaguely recollected court cases. An administrator said: "I know there was some brouhaha in the South; the state overstepped legal boundaries and sterilized people without consent." A vocational counselor conjectured: "I don't recall specific laws or cases. I know the law has not protected the mentally retarded—that's a court tradition. Maybe there is a law concerning sterilization—either that or a bunch of judges are cheating." An educator wavered: "There's a conflict between parents, child, and state, but I don't know anything for sure. My impression is that laws and legislation for the handicapped are archaic." These professionals might advise clients, parents, or guardians, but had little accurate information to share.

All judges knew the law regulating sterilization had been repealed, and all brought up *Stump v. Sparkman* (1978). Although they were aware that the case involved the sterilization of an adolescent presumed to be MiMR, *Stump* was meaningful to them because it established legal immunity. A judge said, "What *Stump* means to me is that as a judge I can do anything and suffer no legal consequences. Judge Stump was careless, sloppy, biased—but the Supreme Court did not penalize him for his errors on the bench."

Two doctors admitted total ignorance of litigation and legislation. Others implied they were knowledgeable when, in fact, the information they had was not accurate (thought there was enabling legislation; thought they needed court permission to do sterilization surgery on anyone with disabilities). Family planning personnel had specific and accurate information about legal ramifications of sterilization. An administrator said: "We make it our business to keep informed. There could be serious repercussions for our clinic if we were to become embroiled in a court case. We are funded through United Way and we receive federal funds. Both funding sources could be cut off if we violated a legal code or federal guideline."

Knowledgeably discussing one of three nonlegal issues in Domain 7 (Table 8.2, items 5 through 7), 21 professionals (42 percent) were judged "aware" (Table 8.3, item i). Confused about parents' and guardians' roles, respondents assigned them more authority than they technically have. If they mentioned consent, they focused on verbal, rather than nonverbal, consent modes. Twelve thought sterilization was inappropriate for people who could not give informed consent, but did not bring up discrimination in denying sterilization to nonverbal or cognitively limited people. Two judges did use equal protection arguments. One said: "Well, if the normal public can get sterilized then there ought to be opportunity for the disabled to get sterilized too. That is why we have to look at this one case at a time and decide what is in each person's best interest."

Forty-one did not differentiate between clients' present information and their potential to gain from training. Few discussed the ramifications of different types of sterilization surgery, such as their invasiveness, the chances of reversing infertility, and their likelihood of causing problematic side effects or influencing sexual development or sexual response. They also did not offer arguments about the availability, safety, convenience, and effectiveness of other contraceptive methods.

STEREOTYPED ATTITUDES

The total narrative response of each participant was scanned for evidence of stereotyped and prejudiced views of MR people and for use of derogatory terminology (Table 8.2, Domain 7, item 8); half were judged as unbiased (Table 8.3, item j). Disparaging terms (animals, vegetables, children) for MR people were rare except among doctors and judges (five of each used at least one of those terms). A doctor declared: "With semi-vegetables there's not much chance of pregnancy." A gynecologist said: "I have a 12-year-old MR neighbor and I worry what will happen when his hormones get loose. I worry about neighborhood girls and that he will drive his mother frantic." Another doctor said: "I've been told the autistic don't have sex drives." A judge stated, "Most retarded people are not interested in sex."

Twelve DD employees and teachers were concerned about bias. A conference coordinator said: "The public views the handicapped in a collective sense—based on stereotypes. It has a drooling image of retarded people." A teacher said: "The public at large don't see them as human—it is easy to deny their humanity—even for those of us that work with them. We have to realize they have human feelings and adult rights." Nine specified that MR people's sexuality was particularly distorted. One asserted: "The public needs a good education. They see males as oversexed and females as alluring, seductive, and passively willing. I see nice young ladies with strong moral convictions."

Fourteen teachers and employees at DD agencies accused co-workers and administrators of discrimination, particularly of finding it convenient to avoid situations that might be frowned upon by relatives of clients or other members of the community. One complained: "Our knee-jerk response to anything that verges on being sexual is 'no.'" A vocational programmer elaborated: "The classic word around here is 'redirect'—interpreted as 'you can't do it here' or 'that is not appropriate.' The problem is there is nowhere where sex is appropriate. 'Redirect' sounds objective but it is really oppressive. Administrators talk out of both sides of their mouths. They sound like they are for normalization but, in truth, they're not—at least when it comes to sex."

The four administrators spent considerable time explaining their worries about reactions of clients' relatives or about a sexual incident being turned into a scandal by the press. They worried about reconciling supervision codes and practical constraints with normalization and human rights principles. Some advised that the best course was to keep clients involved in nonsexual pursuits and separate individuals who began to show signs of sexual attraction. Some maintained birth control was unnecessary when clients were "appropriately supervised," by which they meant prevented from having sexual relations. Their narratives revealed a cautious and conservative approach to sexual matters.

PERSONAL EXPERIENCE WITH STERILIZATION

Professionals knew that tubal ligations and vasectomies were frequent among the general public (Table 8.3, item k). All knew such surgery was performed at local hospitals and in doctors' offices. All were acquainted with people who had been sterilized (Table 8.3, item l), and 12 (24 percent) volunteered that they or their spouses had vasectomies or tubal ligations (Table 8.3, item m). Five said they would not select sterilization themselves. One said: "It's a fairly terminal step. I wouldn't take that route personally."

A judge wavered: "Sterilization is a reasonable option but even at 39 I'm not willing to be sterilized, though I don't want more children. It is convenient birth control but I'm reluctant to do it myself or tell others what to do."

Attitudes toward sterilization were generally positive (Table 8.3, item n), but ranged from 21 who were emphatically positive to 24 who were indifferent or ambivalent to 5 who were opposed. Of the opposition, two (doctor, judge) were categorized "pragmatically opposed"; they thought people might regret being infertile at some later point. The doctor contended:

I used to recommend sterilization to patients who wanted 100 percent birth control, but I've seen so many people change their minds after they did it that now I am reluctant to do it. You also can have some pretty negative problems: scarring, people claiming it's diminished their sexual feeling. I don't need that business. I generally recommend against unless there are medical reasons why someone should not become pregnant.

The most intense opposition came from three who were philosophically against sterilization. A Protection and Advocacy administrator said: "I have a bias against sterilization—it seems like maiming a normal function of a human being." The most vociferous, a residential supervisor at a DD agency, expounded:

I have strong feelings against it. I've almost come to blows with others about sterilization. I feel that fertility is a natural biological process. I would only intervene with natural processes in extreme cases for life preservation reasons. It may be a convenience for other people, but it is radical and needs justification for people who can't make choices. It's a violation of civil rights. Sterilization is a radical solution for anybody. I think it should be a last resort for fertile people who want to control reproduction. There are lots of other alternatives. When an acquaintance chooses sterilization I am sad. Most people do not have strong feelings. Most are ambivalent. I feel that they hold their positions because they haven't thought about it as much as I have. I don't know of any colleague who feels as strongly as I do. I feel I have a mission. I want to influence others—to change minds. I try to present my position reasonably and objectively in the framework of human rights. I've done a lot of pro-life work. I'm opposed to abortion and do not feel knowing that the baby will be handicapped is a reason for abortion. The public at large tends to be passive. I've thought about the issues more philosophically, medically, ethically than most.

In contrast, among the most positive, an administrator at a family planning clinic stated: "Sterilization is fantastic! When you don't want children, it's a for-sure method. I like things black and white." A social worker said: "Sterilization is a convenient and reliable birth control choice." Respondents mentioned such advantages as "long term," "reliable," "relatively risk-free," "few side effects," and "comparatively cheap." More ambivalent, a social worker said: "It's a serious decision that no one should make lightly. I wouldn't rush into it. You never can tell the blows life will deal you. I mean, maybe something will happen to your family or you will sometime marry someone who wants children. But, on the other hand, there are real advantages. It is the most convenient and safe method of birth control." A social worker at an adult day-care center said: "I used to think 'barren' about sterilization and associated it with animals, criminals, or DD people. Now I'm positive. I think 'lucky people who are sterile.' With age I'm less appalled by sterility. I see it as a blessing."

Just as opinions about general sterilization varied, so did views about sterilization for MR people (Table 8.3, item o). As a supervisor for a residential DD agency observed: "On my staff philosophies on sterilization vary from mandatory to choice to never." Ten (20 percent) disapproved of sterilization for MR people. The rationale for the discrepancy between their feelings about sterilization for nondisabled and disabled persons tended to be that it should not be done to someone incapable of choosing. Five disapproved only when the person involved was cognitively unable to grasp its significance. Three were opposed in all circumstances in which mental impairment or emotional disturbance was involved because they believed that, by definition, such persons would be unable to fully understand and make sound choices. A principal of a special school said:

I see it as a violation of personal civil rights. There is nothing more personal than your own body. It's an extreme, irreversible act. All it prevents is pregnancy, not promiscuity. I have friends who have been sterilized and it doesn't bother me but the difference is informed consent. Many retarded people can't make the decision to be sterilized. The word "sterilized" implies that it is being done against their will.

Those opposed to sterilization also believed that sexual relationships were inappropriate for MR people. An administrator of a DD agency, who had been sterilized himself, said: "I guess I'm opposed to sterilization for them. I worry that others think sterilization is protecting clients who are vulnerable. It only protects them from the physical impact of pregnancy, but not the emotional impact of exploitation." A judge who allowed sterilizations of MR people because he was "inclined to side with the family" added: "Sterilization is not an issue with the severely handicapped. They have no opportunity for intercourse—not unless it's inappropriate. Not unless they're taken advantage of by others. The client doesn't want sexual intercourse in those cases."

Two judges worried about complications; as one said: "Professionals would be taking risks if they got involved with sterilization given the current political climate. I worry about the strength of the right-to-life movement." The other stated:

I have nothing against sterilization, in general, but I hate to make irreversible decisions. It is a grave decision, so strict legal procedures must be followed. I would be inclined to turn down a sterilization appeal, especially if it involved someone who is emotionally unstable. I know *Stump v. Sparkman* signified judicial immunity, but I don't need the publicity of somebody who later changes their mind and decides to implicate me.

Another judge said: "I have a tendency to deny sterilization if there is no life-threatening reason for it. I know a state hospital superintendent who puts the women on the pill. It is pretty easy to keep them on the pill in those circumstances." He appeared unconcerned about long-term side effects of the pill.

Of the five generally against sterilization, four also disapproved of sterilization for MR people. The other, the doctor "pragmatically opposed" to sterilization, responded:

I wouldn't want to advertise this but I think it should be routinely done with people who are retarded or disturbed. These people don't have the good sense to know that they won't be good parents. They are better off without kids. Some of the ones I see are really children themselves. They are also very careless in using conventional birth control. I have one patient who lost two kids to welfare and here she is pregnant again. She doesn't want another baby but she's too far along in her pregnancy to have an abortion. My partner has her convinced that she should be sterilized. That's a good thing in her case.

All respondents were aware of cases involving sterilization of an MR person (Table 8.3, item p). Nineteen approved of the decisions, 23 had mixed feelings, and 8 were upset—even indignant—about them. An ambivalent workshop supervisor said:

I knew clients in the workshop had been sterilized. With some of the higher functioning ones I felt badly that control had been taken away from them. One married and wanted a child. She did not talk much about having been sterilized and did not seem generally depressed about it. Life went on. She was reconciled to the fact. She did get sad when she talked about it. With training she could have been a good mother. She had good self-help skills and was emotionally stable. I felt a moment of anger that she had so little control. No one had even asked for her opinion. But pragmatism reared its head. I concerned myself with how to help her get through it—to get on with life. It seemed important not to overreact. It had happened. It would not change. Dwelling on it would not help.

An Adult Protective Services employee complained: "I heard the judge say 'sterilization prevents a female handicapped person from being a victim.' He implied that pregnancy would victimize a woman. Now, I'm not in a position to render an opinion on sterilization but it does not prevent abuse, only pregnancy. Sterilization is ancillary to the problem. There is no need to sterilize someone who does not wish to be sexually active."

Seven educators and agency personnel disagreed with decisions about sterilization. A workshop supervisor recalled: "I knew of a 28-year-old who was capable of understanding and making decisions. Her mother forcibly got her sterilized. She lied to her daughter—never told her what was happening. We are wary of parents and reluctant to oppose them, so I just observed the whole thing and stewed. I was annoyed at how dominating and sure of herself that mother was. I didn't oppose the sterilization but how it came about."

Twelve professionals were aware of situations in which families had trouble getting court or medical cooperation in what they thought were justifiable sterilization decisions. A case conference coordinator for an adult DD agency said: "I've had three parents in the last year who said they were pursuing sterilization. They went to local doctors and hit a brick wall—they wouldn't perform them without a court order. One doctor said he would do it, then he checked into it and changed his mind. He was worried about liability." Similarly, a nurse at a DD agency complained:

Doctors are shirking their responsibility. The average doctor prefers to ignore the handicapped. I know they're afraid of lawsuits and have terrible insurance problems, but, still. . . . A mother talked to me about her sexually promiscuous daughter. She's had four abortions but the mother can't find a doctor who will do a sterilization. The mother is hysterical. We take our clients to Planned Parenthood even for general physicals because the staff is nice. Doctors don't want to bother with the handicapped.

A social worker hypothesized: "The parents of many of our clients are rather ignorant, nonassertive people. All you have to do is mention the word 'court' to them and they drop the idea of sterilization. They are easily intimidated by authority and have pretty negative feelings about sterilization anyway. One called it 'getting neutered.' I've also heard 'getting fixed.'" A social worker with a residential program related:

I went through court for one case. The girl was in her mid-20s, sexually active, and was adamant that she didn't want kids. The guardian ad litem they appointed was a zealot. He interviewed several staff members several times. He went to the files, ordered new IQ tests. He talked to the woman's boyfriend. I suppose I should be impressed with how seriously he took it, but he was coming from a certain position and I believe he had made his mind up before he ever got involved in the case. In spite of the guardian ad litem's opposition, the sterilization was finally granted but it was a long drawn-out thing. In another case the mom mentioned going to court but she was not persistent. You have to be persistent to make things fly.

A residential administrator said: "At one time they were doing steriliza-tions wholesale. Now, it seems, our clients can't get them without a real hassle. I don't think sterilizations should be easy decisions but they have so many advantages they shouldn't be impossible either. If the man on the street can get one, then why can't the retarded person?" Similarly, a vocational supervisor said: "I'm annoyed at the difficulty the handicapped have getting sterilized. It's harder than heck to get sterilizations for the handicapped now—not for anyone else though. Everyone I know is steril-ized."

In contrast, 14 believed sterilizations were being approved routinely. A woman in charge of group homes related:

I was in the position of being primary information-giver for an 18- to 19-year-old girl whose guardianship was held by the welfare department. I knew the case was proceeding and I kept waiting for them to come to me for information. They made no effort to declare her incompetent—it seemed like they were only interested in her IQ level. I was only contacted for the record. I felt mildly negative—I could see the benefits of sterilization—I was mainly upset about the way they went about the whole thing. The judge said, "Let it be," and so it was.

Forty-two (84 percent), including all doctors, family planning clinic workers, social workers, and educators, believed that sterilization opera-tions were performed on MR persons without court approval (Table 8.3, item q), but felt that only a few doctors were willing to do such surgery and they were doing it surreptitiously. A small town judge said: "I don't like to see parents spend money on court costs, so in clear-cut cases I recommend a local pediatrician who does sterilizations without court orders. I can't tell you his name or he'd flip!" Of all the professionals, judges were least likely (four of seven) to believe that sterilizations occurred without court approval.

Six (two doctors, two family planning clinic employees, two DD agency members) mentioned a doctor who, as one doctor said, "did wholesale sterilization—anybody handicapped or poor—if a patient couldn't pay he'd do it for free. He was doing the right thing for the wrong reason. His motives were all wrong. I'm not big on the master race idea—that less than perfect should be eliminated." A family planning clinic administrator recalled the same doctor:

It was wonderful for us because we could refer to him. He would sterilize anybody, anytime, no questions asked. He had problems with a patient and got sued. I haven't heard about him for many years. Now I only know a couple of doctors who will do disabled sterilizations and they are about to retire. Doctors have pressures—malpractice suits are increasing tremendously. You have to find a doctor who practices old-fashioned medicine; who believes in serving, in taking risks. It has to be someone who's established, gutsy. Doctors are right to refuse services in some cases.

CONCERN ABOUT PARENTING ABILITIES OF MR INDIVIDUALS

Participants believed MR individuals wanted children, yet 47 (94 percent) worried about clients' parenting competencies (Table 8.3, item r). A social worker at a DD agency estimated: "Of those I see at my agency I'd say 5 percent would make decent parents and perhaps an additional 5 to 10 percent could with training." A doctor said: "Some parents are abusive, and the reason for the abuse is that they're retarded." An Adult Protective Services employee said: "The MR/DD I see should not have children."

Concerning parenting decisions, opinions ranged from belief in allowing complete freedom of choice for MR people (3, 6 percent) to belief in not allowing MR people any role in decisions (13, 26 percent). The majority (34, 68 percent) felt parenting decisions should be made on a case-by-case basis, with most indicating they would tend to discourage or educate against parenting, but that it was ultimately the right of MR individuals to decide. A family planning administrator said:

I saw a television program about two people who had been stuck in institutions all their lives. They met and fell in love. They had menial jobs in sheltered environments. Someone helped with shopping and cooking. They wanted to have a baby but understood that they had to save money and be on their own. Why shouldn't they have a family? Why deny them the joy of having a child? As long as someone could provide support I don't see a problem. The kid might not be retarded. Anyhow it's their choice. Even if they're pretty sure they would have a handicapped child, it's their decision. I wish them luck. Society has a tendency not to want to see DD. They have feelings. We all do. They are still people and should have a normal life. Human rights should not be denied. We should stretch their lives.

Taking an opposing view, a judge complained: "I'm appalled that some people think that dependent handicapped should have children. I read an article by a person who said that handicapped have a right to have children, that they need someone to love. I believe you need intelligence to raise a child."

Discussions centering around who should parent and how to decide who should parent were plentiful, with most acknowledging the complexity of issues. One said: "I know my feelings are embedded in middle-class values." A doctor stated: "I would be skeptical about MRs being parents. To have a kid dependent on you is a big responsibility. Parents of an MR person have to worry about who will take care of their grandchild." Some felt that multiple perspectives should be addressed in decisions about parenting—fulfilling one party's desire to parent might have a negative impact on offspring, guardians, and taxpayers. They felt fair resolution would be a compromise of prerogatives.

The dilemma of "preferences" and "best interests" was also discussed. A secondary teacher argued:

I can't picture my students going through pregnancy, labor, and the birth process. Raising children is a financial and emotional burden. My students are all different. Some might be loving and caring but still would be unable to handle all aspects of parenting. Students talk about marriage, kids, cars, house but they still see themselves as kids. They don't have realistic plans for getting those things. I have real reservations about childbearing and rearing for the population I work with. They are not mature enough to handle another life. But very few girls would know or admit that they wouldn't be good mothers. They all want babies. You have to protect them from the trauma of their own inability to cope.

Respondents opposed people who were obviously mentally ill having children, referring to an inherent contradiction in facilitating parenting aspirations when there were indications that they could not meet even minimum standards of parenting. They stated the need to be pragmatic and balance a convenient (and perhaps realistic) approach to people with restricted competencies with idealistic goals for expanding their lives in accordance with normalization principles.

Respondents thought the lack of match between parenting aspirations and skills was confounded by the scarcity of good parenting education for MR people. A vocational supervisor said: "About 40 to 50 percent could be trained to be good mothers, about 5 to 10 percent are already capable, about 40 percent I couldn't perceive as parents even with a lot of work. Most are unable to care for themselves. They need a lot of supervision and they even view themselves as dependent children—it's difficult to change that role." They complained that it was difficult to evaluate potential for parenting success on the basis of present skills because MR people had not been educated to parent. The need for education for both personnel and MR individuals was a central theme verbalized by welfare, family planning, school, and DD agency personnel. As a social worker said:

My retarded clients seem so ignorant and apathetic. They don't mean to get pregnant but they make no effort not to. They act as if they've caught a cold—that it's just one of those things that happen—as if there is nothing they could have done to prevent it; that it's beyond their control. The slow are not well informed about sex. They don't make connections. I guess the kids are loved and as parents they try their best but they have a lot of problems. Sex education and parenting education are definitely needed. A lot of times I don't like to see them become parents. Working with Child Protective Services has made me biased against parenting for many. But I don't like to be negative in dealing with them. I wish that I had received more training about sexuality. We all shuffle our feet around here and hope for the best.

PERSONAL ROLE IN STERILIZATION DECISIONS

Twenty-nine professionals (58 percent) were apprehensive about personal or agency liability when participating in sterilization decisions (Table 8.2, Domain 13; Table 8.3, item s). Doctors were anxious about potential malpractice lawsuits. Four of the six said they would not risk performing sterilization surgery on someone they knew was retarded or disturbed. Welfare department and family planning clinic employees worried about giving advice about sterilization to clients because they feared losing funding or receiving damaging publicity. A county welfare worker said: "I don't have to judge competency. Thank goodness! If they say they want their tubes tied, I give them Medicaid forms and send them to the doctor. I can't suggest a ligation. It's against the law. Sometimes I bite my tongue."

Judges did not worry about the legal ramifications of sterilization decisions; as a judge clarified: "I knew the *Stump* case related to sterilization of an incompetent but the case is important to me from another perspective; to judges it indicates that we can get away with anything. The case was handled horribly, yet judicial immunity was secured." Two judges anguished about the human impact of sterilization decisions. A juvenile judge said: "I have not dealt directly with a sterilization case since I've been on the bench. I cross my fingers that I won't get one. For me, sterilization would be the worst case to deal with."

Removed from personal involvement in granting permission, performing surgery, or providing funds, employees at DD agencies and teachers were still wary of taking part in decisions or expressing opinions to others. A social worker said:

> I've been involved in custody of children cases. They're very messy. I had to testify to character, work potential. The baby's grandmother got custody, but she was almost as retarded as her daughter and she lost custody because of neglect charges. It was an ordeal for me watching the tension and anguish. Getting the baby back was the grandmother's reason for being—she was in turmoil over losing the baby. The attorney did well but the women ruined their own case by causing a spectacle. I tried to calm them down. With training they probably could have made it as parents. I was sorry to see them lose the baby.

Others claimed to be unprepared to deal with certain people with cognitive or emotional impairments. Medical professionals worried that instructions for treatment would not be understood or that prescribed medication would be misused. A family planning clinic nurse practitioner said:

> Our philosophy is to treat all people alike. We're required by the government to be barrier-free. I'm glad to serve them but I'm always frustrated dealing with retarded people, especially if they are unable to communicate verbally. I can't get a history of menstruation, they can't discuss ramifications of pregnancy, their support system. I have trouble explaining what I am doing in the exam. Then, with the handicapped, I worry about incest, medications that they might be on, eating habits, congenital abnormalities. . . . They seem so vulnerable and I am so powerless.

A nurse practitioner in a obstetrical clinic related:

> The retarded usually come in with their mothers or with staff from their group homes. We don't take risks with pregnancy for handicapped women. Others can bear children and live with it but for them it's a tragedy. I try to explain things so they feel like they're making an informed choice. Working with LD [learning disabled]—those that don't catch on real quick—is also problematic for us. Our visits are geared for minimal time with patients—15 minutes average. Our reduced funding makes us short-staffed. For persons with LD it takes an hour. We can't say, "Here, read this." We have to use films, brochures; even then we worry that the person may not understand. We try to include a friend or relative. Most of them opt for the pill but they don't use it consistently. They tend to need birth control for a long time because men in those circles don't opt for vasectomies. We have a high failure rate with that group.

Doctors also had stories of difficult cases. One recalled: "I had a patient who was 35 years old—obviously mentally retarded. She had already had four or five pregnancies and one baby had ended up in the commode. She was upset at being pregnant. She did not want children and was not able to care for them. It was a sad situation. I would not have wanted to adopt her baby. That was one situation where I brought up sterilization." In describing a patient with autism, a doctor said: "It's difficult to give a physical. I have to follow her as she walks around the room. She's known to scratch and bite so I'm very apprehensive dealing with her." A gynecologist said: "I have trouble keeping this one young retarded lady on my examining table. I live in fear that she'll fall off and get injured." Doctors who advocated sterilization, but would not do such surgery themselves, seemed most problematic. "It's not worth the effort or the risk" echoed through their responses. Conscience statutes permit doctors to refuse to participate in sterilization on moral or ethical grounds (Sloan, 1988, p. 41), but that should not extend to the rationale of avoiding responsibility and risk.

IMPLICATIONS OF STUDY OF PROFESSIONALS

Because sterilization laws are nonexistent or outdated, advocates for MR people have explored guidelines to ensure that practices relating to sterilization, sexuality, partnerships, and parenting are sound (Irvine, 1988). Yet, in recognition that laws are made and enforced by people who may not be objective and well informed, persons must cautiously pursue such goals. The motility of ideologies impacts on real-world politics; sensible positions are not always popular, and good intentions do not always result in desired outcomes. As a judge said: "I would like to have legislation about sterilization on which to base my decisions but taking a bill to the present legislative bodies would be opening a real can of worms. Any bill I proposed would be so radically transformed before it was enacted that it would end up being worse than what we have now. I would leave things alone given the present political climate in this state."

The results of this study indicate that professional values and practices are as diverse as those of the lay public and families of MR individuals. Attitudes toward sterilization of MR people are likely to be dependent on values related to sex as well as perceptions of disability. Opinions are conflicted; on one level, it is believed that MR people should not have children, but it does not follow that sterilization or any other birth control is endorsed. Some imply that sexual expression is not appropriate. Because of the force of their feelings, neither professionals nor parents can necessarily be counted on to make decisions that are consistent with MR individuals' own values or interests. As parents and social service agencies search for scarce resources to manage often overwhelming demands of MR individuals, they both may consider what is personally convenient or satisfying rather than what is best for an MR person. Perhaps through the interface of formal and informal care—through a critical juncture of family relationships, health care, and social policies, boundaries can be defined for obligations of each (Zarit & Pearlin, 1993).

Sterilization is complicated by the fact that it is rarely addressed in professional training or literature and is infrequently discussed among colleagues. Because of its unmentionable status, professionals lack opportunity to critically examine their views and develop more enlightened ones. Best practice is more likely to result from a thorough understanding of circumstances and issues than from ignorance and avoidance (Ducharme & Gill, 1991). MR people rely on professionals to help them make decisions; therefore, it is essential that they be prepared to deal with sexual, intimate social, and contraceptive needs of MR clients.

Part III

STERILIZATION CASES

9

Individuals with Mild Mental Retardation

During the early part of this century, anyone with mental retardation, including those in the mild range, was subject to compulsory sterilization laws. This chapter includes five very different individuals' experiences with sterilization. Pseudonyms are used and facts are altered to protect anonymity. The cases are presented as they occurred; hence, they do not reflect my own attitudes about what should have happened. It is hoped that previous chapters have prepared readers to form their own opinions about the appropriateness of each sterilization decision.

TAMARA

Michelle was doing a three-week, end-of-the-year practicum with junior high students classified mildly mentally disabled. After consulting with Katherine, her supervising teacher, she decided to teach a family life unit that she had developed in a methods class. Older than most undergraduates, Michelle had married and become a mother shortly after high school. After working as an aide in special education classrooms for many years, she started college. At 31, Michelle was one semester away from her undergraduate degree. Her own two children were in sixth and eighth grade.

Permission slips for participation in the sexuality unit were sent home with students. The students groaned and giggled, "Oh, no. Do we have to?" when the unit was announced. Katherine warned Michelle, "It's like pulling teeth to get anything from home." Eagerness to start the unit was revealed by the presence of 14 permission slips the next morning. One student, Tamara, had not returned the slip. When Michelle quietly reminded the 14-year-old to bring it soon so she could be part of the unit, to her astonishment, the usually polite and timid Tamara glared and snarled: "I don't need no sex ed., I'm not going to have no babies." Michelle informed Tamara that they would be discussing other interesting and useful things besides having children and assured her that she would enjoy the unit. Tamara promptly retorted: "It's my own business to take the class and I don't want to. Just leave me alone!" and rushed out of the room. Tamara's friend and neighbor, Tracy, tattled that Tamara had thrown the permission slip in the waste basket the day she received it. Tracy ventured: "Maybe she thinks her grandma would be mad." Tamara soon returned to the room, slammed herself down in her seat, and did not say anything the rest of the morning.

Before Michelle introduced the first lesson, she gave Tamara a pass to the library. Again, uncharacteristically, Tamara bolted from the room without a word to anyone. Moreover, when Michelle went to retrieve her from the library at the end of the period, Tamara was nowhere in sight, and the librarian could not recall her having been there. A search of the restrooms revealed a familiar pair of shoes in one of the stalls. After Michelle said "Tamara?" with no response, she questioned the person in the stall if she had seen Tamara. Again, no answer. Michelle waited a few minutes and then, convinced it was Tamara, said: "Are you alright? Is something wrong? I wish you would tell me what the problem is." Tamara's response was smothered sobs and a "go away!" Michelle offered: "Let's go to the conference room and talk about this." When Tamara slinked out of the stall, Michelle put her arm around the frail teenager and whisked her off to prevent the embarrassment of being seen in her puffy-eyed state.

They had barely entered the room when Tamara blurted out: "My grandma got me fixed so I can't have no babies, so I don't need your stupid sex ed." Michelle paused, waiting for the first round of sobs to subside. Then she quietly said: "Would you like to talk about it?" With anger addressed at anyone in her range, the usually quiet Tamara shouted: "Nothing to tell. She thinks I'm too dumb to have babies so she made me have an operation." Michelle said: "When did that happen?" Tamara replied: "I don't know. Two years ago, maybe. Dr. H. did it at the hospital."

Michelle: "Did he ask you if you wanted the operation?"

Tamara: "No. He only asked me what class I was in."

Michelle: "What did you tell him?"

Tamara: "I didn't talk to him. I wouldn't say. Grandma told him I was in special ed.—in a class for mentally retarded."

Another outpouring of tears. Michelle put her arm around Tamara, and this time her attentions were not rejected. After 10 minutes of sitting quietly together, Michelle asked Tamara if the operation had hurt. Tamara replied: "Yes, they said it wouldn't, but it did. They are big liars. Grandma didn't tell me what the operation was for, and the doctor told me it was 'just to help with a little problem you have.'"

Michelle: "Then how do you know that you are 'fixed'?"

Tamara: "Grandma caught me and my boyfriend and said that she was glad she got me fixed 'cause I was a slut. She says I'm 'man-crazy' like Mom and she 'ain't going to raise any more kids.'"

Michelle: "Where is your mother?"

Tamara: "I don't know. Maybe Texas. Grandma doesn't know. I saw her when I was 10. She came back and took Grandma's money. She took her car. Grandma had to call the police."

Michelle: "How do you feel about that?"

Tamara: "I hate my Mom. She's mean to me and my brother. She's mean to Grandma. I hate her."

Michelle: "Do you like living with your grandmother?"

Tamara: "Most of the time. But I don't like her to lie to me. She shouldn't have got me fixed. I'm not a slut."

Michelle announced that it was about time for the dismissal bell to ring and that Tamara would have to hurry to make her bus. Anger returned to Tamara's voice as she threatened: "You better not tell. Grandma said if I blabbered about it, it would just prove that I'm really retarded. I don't want anyone to know." Michelle said that she would like to talk about it with Ms. S. (Katherine) and added: "Ms. S. is worried about you. She didn't like to see you upset. I think it is important for her to know what's bothering you." Tamara replied: "I don't care if you tell her, but you guys better not say anything to my Grandma and I don't want the kids to know."

The next day, Michelle confidentially whispered to Tamara: "We're going to talk about puberty in my class this afternoon. I'd like you to be there. Why don't you stay?" Tamara promptly retorted: "But I don't have no permission and I'm not going to ask Grandma to sign." Michelle assured her that it was okay for her to be there, adding: "We just get those as a precaution, so families know. They're not required." As other students entered hearing range, their conversation halted, with no commitment from Tamara about her plans. But Tamara stayed in her seat for the film about puberty in boys and was still there during the discussion, although she did not enter into it and did not laugh with the others at the humor they saw.

When Michelle introduced contraception on the tenth day, she started with hormonal and barricade methods, then permanent surgical techniques. Although wary of looking in Tamara's direction, when Michelle glanced her way she saw the same nonexpressive face that Tamara had held since the beginning. She did not call on Tamara, but included her in the activities and Tamara dutifully participated. In fact, Tamara's behavior was not atypical—she was always passive and compliant. But she usually smiled and sat close to others. This time she sat apart, and her peers kindly gave her space. Michelle was pleased with Tamara's classmates' reactions. They witnessed her outburst and knew she had been dismissed the first day; nevertheless, nobody mentioned her presence or nonparticipation. Katherine remarked: "These kids have been together since first or second grade and are more like siblings than classmates. They squabble, but are kind to each other at difficult times. It's not easy being in a class for retarded students, and they give each other a lot of support."

Perhaps another reason the students ignored Tamara was that they all were absorbed in the unit. As Katherine noted: "It sure is easy to get their attention when you talk about sex. They act like they know it all ahead of time, but they start getting a little more humble as time goes on. Then you notice what they don't know. Most are naive about sex, even though I'm sure at least half of them are already sexually active."

Because they had the rare luxury of two adults in the classroom, Katherine suggested that Michelle spend more time with Tamara. As Katherine said: "This situation is clearly something she needs to talk about. The counselors are too busy this time of year, plus I think she is comfortable with you." So on the pretense of helping Michelle get Katherine's things packed for a move to a new building, Michelle and Tamara spent a couple more hours together working and talking in a small conference room adjacent to Katherine's classroom. This arrangement seemed natural to everyone because Tamara was a conscientious student who had finished much of the work while her classmates were still procrastinating or fooling around.

During their time together, neither Michelle nor Tamara brought up the topic of the sterilization. Michelle saw no need to pry. She was not a trained counselor and did not want to get in over her head. They mainly talked about each other's summer plans, Tamara's feelings about going on to the high school, and Michelle's plans for student teaching in the fall. Michelle did give Tamara her phone number and said: "It would be nice to hear from you this summer. Give me a call. I'll miss you." Tamara did not call. It was not until her second student teaching placement, which was at the high school, that she ran into Tamara. She felt a presence at her side and turned to see Tamara with a shy smile. Michelle was delighted to see her. She had worried about her since their conversation. In fact, Michelle was a Catholic and was tempted by the "Right to Life" movement on purely philosophical grounds. Nevertheless, in a conversation with her younger classmates in the teacher education program, she was overheard to say: "I've known too many people who really would have been messed up if they hadn't had an abortion to deny anyone that choice. You guys are too idealistic. Wait until you've been around awhile." Michelle confided that she thought she was against sterilization, but was "so happy" that her husband decided to get a vasectomy a few years earlier. Nevertheless, Tamara's sterilization bothered her: "Of the 15 kids in that class, Tamara would probably make the best parent. Some were aggressive, and others had no common sense. Tamara was kind and gentle and got along well with others. I felt sorry for her. Oh, well. What's done is done."

Michelle's interaction with Tamara was limited. Her student teaching placement was in a multicategorical resource room with mainly students with learning disabilities. Michelle smiled at Tamara when she saw her in the corridors and always got a timid smile back. A week before she was to finish her student teaching placement, Tamara appeared at her classroom door and announced in an embarrassed manner that she had been thinking about something that Michelle had said in "that class last year." Then Tamara queried: "Why did you say that sometimes people need to use a condom even if they've been fixed?" Surprised at her recall, Michelle responded: "If you have more than one sexual partner or if that partner has sex with someone else, then you need to worry about sexually transmitted disease. Remember we talked about the dangerous diseases that spread when you have sex with someone who has a disease." Tamara said: "That's what I thought. That's what I told my boyfriend." Michelle added: "It is always good to use a condom. Better safe than sorry" and thought to herself, "Tamara had been listening—that really makes my day."

RHONDA SUE

Dr. Michael was a senior member of an OB/GYN group of five doctors. He had been employed at the clinic since he completed his residency 19 years earlier. His practice was in a university town, and the majority of his patients were connected to the university; the minority were rural folk and local townspeople. Unlike his colleagues, he came from a rural town within the state and almost preferred serving "locals." Perhaps sensing this, they requested him. His partners fondly referred to him as "hick doctor." In turn, he called them "snobs." He and his wife, a guidance counselor, often discussed the elitist attitudes of those affiliated with the university or "from the suburbs," although they were now suburbanites themselves. They felt educated people underestimated the local people's intelligence and ethics. Other doctors made fun of the hoards of kin who accompanied pregnant women. Dr. Michael loved to see families involved, so he welcomed them when they accompanied patients.

Dr. Michael prefaced his remarks by expressing admiration for rural culture and by categorizing Rhonda Sue as an exception to other country people he served. He first met Rhonda Sue when she was a pregnant 13-year-old. He remembers it was his tenth year in practice because his partners and office staff had thrown a surprise luncheon in his honor. As Dr. Michael was locking the door to the clinic at a little past 6 P.M., Harvey, who he assumed was Rhonda Sue's father, drove his truck so close to the entryway that he blocked the stairs. Dr. Michael was on his way home, and it was not his turn on call that evening, but before he could collect his thoughts, Harvey had bundled Rhonda Sue out of the truck and up the stairs. Dr. Michael was so intrigued with the size of Rhonda Sue's belly that, without thinking, he reopened the clinic door and helped her through.

He had never seen Rhonda Sue before; nevertheless, it soon became clear that she was in labor. Apparently, Harvey and Rhonda Sue had intended for her to have the baby at home, but after many hours of labor with no sign of the baby, Harvey got alarmed enough to pack her into the truck and drive the 30 miles to the clinic. Harvey, a burly man of indistinguishable age, announced that Rhonda Sue would have the baby "right here" (in the clinic waiting room). Dr. Michael protested: "That's impossible. We have no delivery room. We'll have to go to the hospital." Harvey flatly replied: "We ain't goin' to no hospital." Dr. Michael pointed at the hospital in clear view across the street. Harvey stared at Dr. Michael, spit a thug of chewing tobacco out the door, and restated: "We ain't goin' to no hospital!" His bulky body blocked the door. At that point, Rhonda Sue, who was sprawled across the couch in the waiting room, groaned. A quick examination indicated the baby was in position for delivery. The baby made the decision by pushing his head through. He was a hefty eight-pounder. Because both baby and mother seemed healthy, but also because Harvey insisted on "no hospital" and there was nowhere else to go, after about an hour of medical care and filling out the paperwork that he had a clerk at the hospital bring across the street, Dr. Michael said it was all right for them to go home. Looking back, he felt Harvey and Rhonda Sue would have left his office regardless of what he said. He never billed them, and they never left an address where they might be reached. Rhonda Sue had not spoken a word. She also had not seemed interested in the baby, but dutifully wrapped him up and carried him out when Harvey told her to.

One afternoon many years later, when Dr. Michael was seeing his usual round of patients, the receptionist poked her head in his door and nervously whispered that a woman had arrived wanting to see "the baby doctor." The receptionist added: "She doesn't have an appointment and she is not listed as a patient, but she is *very* pregnant. A few minutes later the receptionist ushered a sullen woman into his office. He would not have recognized Rhonda Sue—she looked to be 40 years old—except he did remember the name. On questioning, it turned out that she, indeed, was the same Rhonda Sue that had delivered in his office almost a decade earlier. She gave monosyllabic or no replies to his inquiries, but he eventually discerned that this was her fifth pregnancy. In response to questions about her other children, Rhonda Sue said: "Welfare's got 'em, except Junior, he's gone." In reply to Dr. Michael's inquiry about what "gone" meant, Rhonda Sue said: "Shot dead. Brother shot him. Welfare got the rest." Dr. Michael vaguely remembered reading about the case in the paper a few months earlier. Nine-year-old Harvey ("Junior") had apparently died of a gunshot wound inflicted by his eight-year-old brother, who the family referred to as "Brother." Besides Junior, the other children had been born at home. Further questioning revealed that the Harvey who had come with her when Junior was born was also "gone." At the time they removed the children, "welfare" moved Rhonda Sue to a subsidized housing complex when they learned she was pregnant.

Rhonda Sue had no idea about what month of the pregnancy she was in, but Dr. Michael evaluated her as fairly close to term. During the examination, he asked whether she wanted a boy or a girl—she did not care. He then asked what she planned to name the child—she did not know. Dr. Michael noted: "I get a number of quiet patients who are scared or embarrassed. I try to chat with them to calm them down. Most patients are enthusiastic talking about possible names and, particularly, about whether it will be a boy or a girl. Even those who give babies up for adoption often volunteer what they would have named the baby if they had been able to keep it." It was Dr. Michael's judgment that Rhonda Sue was not interested in the baby. He recalled: "I finally asked her right out: 'Rhonda, do you want this baby?' I got a solid 'no' from her. The first sign of emotion I had seen. I asked how the baby's father felt about her having the baby. She responded that she did not know and did not care. I then asked if she was going to give it up for adoption. Again, I got a negative response. I usually don't ask these questions—finding out the mother's plans is up to the welfare department.

But I had a sinking feeling when I thought about sending this woman home from the hospital with a child. On the other hand, I did not know who would adopt her child. I know I wouldn't."

Dr. Michael continued: "I knew I was opening a can of worms when I asked her if she wanted any more babies after this one. I got a decided 'no' from her. I told her that when I delivered her baby, I could make it so that she would have no more children. I asked her if she wanted me to do that surgery. She said 'yes'. I rarely initiate talks about sterilization. I let the patients bring it up. We keep signs posted in the office and there are brochures about birth control, and sterilization is described, but I was pretty sure that Rhonda Sue could not read. I got the permission forms for sterilization. Sure enough, Rhonda Sue could not read. She could sign her name. Turns out her last name was Harvey. I couldn't figure that one out. I had a nurse come in and read the statement on the permission slip a second time—I also made her sign her name as witness."

After Rhonda Sue left, with her permission, because she said welfare would pay the costs of the delivery, Dr. Michael called the Welfare Department. Rhonda Sue Harvey was a client, and the social worker was familiar enough with her that she did not have to get out her records. Rhonda Sue had very willingly signed the papers releasing custody of her three children and said she did not want them because they were "bad kids." The only one she appeared to care about was Brother—the one who shot Junior. During the investigation of the shooting, Rhonda Sue told the police: "Junior got it comin'. He wouldn't leave Brother be."

The social worker informed Dr. Michael that Rhonda Sue had never asked about the children during the five months since they had been taken away. She added: "They were terribly neglected. The house was a pigsty—that sounds awful to say, but it's true. They had no indoor plumbing and only a space heater. I guess their electricity got turned off, so most of the time they had no heat. She was living with a man called 'Herve,' who claimed to be Rhonda Sue's uncle." After he shot and killed his brother, Herbie (Brother) had been sent to a residential school for seriously emotionally disabled children. Rhonda Sue's two daughters (aged six and four) were in a foster home in Vandalia (the neighboring) County. The Welfare Department there was trying to place the girls for adoption. Rhonda Sue had recently moved to the local county because welfare workers had encouraged her to move into public housing when they learned she was pregnant. Herve stayed in the house in the country.

Dr. Michael told the social worker that Rhonda Sue had readily consented to a tubal ligation, and, even though she was only 22 years old, he believed sterilization would be a good idea. The social worker immediately agreed.

They discussed the funding, since regulations required that Rhonda Sue sign the papers giving consent for sterilization a month prior to surgery. Dr. Michael predicted that the baby was likely to arrive much sooner. It was convenient to do the sterilization surgery immediately following the birth, especially since he felt that someone like Rhonda Sue would not return for surgery later. The social worker added: "There's another hitch. We can't use the sterilization money for anyone with a mental disability. It is obvious that she is mentally retarded. We don't have anything in our records that states her disability but that is because she just entered our case load. If we go back to the old records, I'm sure we'll find that she was in special education. That's the criterion we use. I'll check it out."

The social worker called back later in the day to say: "We are in luck. Vandalia County School Corporation has no record of her attending school. We do not have to classify her retarded—there is no evidence. The main problem is she is only 22 years old. In my opinion, the fact that she has had five children and totally lacks interest in them justifies sterilization. Plus, she neglected and abused the ones she had. The girls had bruises on their bottoms and Junior had black and blue marks on his upper arms. During the investigation, the girls said their mother, father, and brothers often hurt them and threatened to kill them. Vandalia County could back us up with pages of data verifying the horrendous condition of her home and kids. The *Vandalia Times* has condemning pictures in their account of Junior's shooting."

Rhonda Sue's fifth baby was born exactly 20 working days after she signed the permission forms at the Welfare Department, so the sterilization could be done at the time of the birth. In spite of earlier protestations about "giving up" the baby, Rhonda Sue suggested this solution to her case worker, and custody was signed over shortly after the birth. Apparently, the case worker had visited her apartment and had informed her that it would have to be cleaner for her to keep the baby. Her response was: "Okay, you can have it. I don't want no more kids." The case worker told Dr. Michael: "We usually help mothers keep their children. Our department's philosophy is that birth mothers have the right to their children. We do everything in our power to help them be good mothers. I was pretty fatalistic about Rhonda Sue. She made it clear that she did not want the baby. She is so sullen and lethargic. I just do not think she could change—maybe with intensive therapy but where's she going to get that? I knew if she took that child home, even if we visited daily, it would suffer. Babies placed for adoption immediately after birth stand the best chance of getting a good home and a good start. I sometimes have second thoughts in custody termination cases. I watch the mother's pain—even if they were rotten mothers, they show regret about losing children. Rhonda Sue showed no signs of caring. She is signed up with Adult Basic Education and Vocational Rehabilitation will try to place her in a job."

Dr. Michael usually discussed tough cases with his partners. In fact, they had an informal pact that touchy decisions would be made jointly. They knew the clinic's insurance would go up with a malpractice suit against any one of them. On this occasion, with the exception of talking to the case worker from Welfare and the pediatrician in the delivery room, Dr. Michael kept Rhonda Sue's situation to himself.

LEEANN

LeeAnn Barrow was born seven years after Roberta, her half sister, to a man in his mid-forties and a 17-year-old woman who had been deaf since birth. A spunky, energetic child, LeeAnn's own opinion was that she had "run circles around Mom and Dad—been in trouble all my life." On her sixteenth birthday, unemployed and living in a public housing project with her six-month-old daughter, McKella, and her widowed mother, LeeAnn survived with help from Aid to Families with Dependent Children. Also unemployed, Mrs. Barrow received a disability pension. Tears came to LeeAnn's eyes when she told of her father's death from a heart attack two months earlier: "I really miss that man. He was everything to me. Mom's a retard. She's no help at all."

LeeAnn made this speech as her mother was by her side holding McKella, who was named after a favorite soap opera star. Both grandmother and baby beamed at each other with delight. Neither understood what LeeAnn was saying. About every fifth sentence, LeeAnn said something negative about her mother. Mrs. Barrow, on the other hand, was eager to please. She brought LeeAnn soft drinks and, without being asked, brought more ice when the first round melted. She changed McKella's diapers and amused the baby for hours. Mrs. Barrow smiled lovingly at LeeAnn and nodded at me to show her approval of my conversation with her daughter. She could not hear the soaps, as one program after another boomed out at top volume. LeeAnn periodically turned aside from talking to say: "Just a minute! I've got to see this."

LeeAnn's past year had been eventful. First, the school had taken her to court on truancy charges. She would have been sent to a juvenile correction center, but when it was discovered that she was pregnant and nearing the age of 16, the school dropped charges. About the same time, Roberta separated from her husband, and she and her three preschoolers moved in with the Barrows. Four adults and three children lived in the two-bedroom apartment for three months. Then McKella was born. Four months later,

LeeAnn's father died suddenly from a heart attack. Next, Child Protective Services threatened to take McKella on neglect charges.

McKella was not a neglected child in the traditional sense—LeeAnn and Mrs. Barrow competed constantly for McKella's affection and attention. The problem was that the house was filthy. Mr. Barrow had organized cleanups. He shut off the television until the apartment was clean. Within a month of Mr. Barrow's death, the apartment manager tried to evict them because of the foul condition of the apartment. When they refused to leave, the manager reported them to Child Protective Services.

Although the Barrow family had been known to the Welfare Department for a long time, Kim, employed by Child Protective Services, first met LeeAnn after the neglect charge. When she heard about the charge, LeeAnn cursed out the housing manager; however, when Kim warned of the possibility of losing McKella, the two women rallied to do a better job with housekeeping. Perhaps it had improved, but it was still littered with dirty disposable diapers, half-eaten TV dinners, and pop cans. In broad daylight, cockroaches skirted around the edges of the room.

Four months after Kim met them, Mrs. Barrow died. Then, LeeAnn's care of the baby, her housekeeping, and her relationship with Kim rapidly deteriorated. Her attitude toward Kim was erratic: One day she would be glad to see her, the next time rude. She became obstinate and uncooperative. Kim felt that LeeAnn manipulated her by saying that she was sick or that she had sprained her ankle so that Kim would do the housework. With her mother's support gone, the reality of being stuck with a child hit her. Although McKella was cute, she was energetic—a handful. She made typical toddler messes, and LeeAnn did not feel that she should be the one to clean up after her. She treated McKella more like a sibling than a daughter. Eventually, Kim started visiting daily to monitor McKella's care.

Within three months, LeeAnn had once again been cited for child neglect. The neighbors called police about incessant crying. The police arrived at about 10 P.M. to find the door unlocked, McKella crying in her crib, and LeeAnn nowhere in the vicinity. They called Child Protective Services, and Josephine, its head, came immediately. Within an hour, McKella was in a temporary boarding home. When LeeAnn arrived home shortly after midnight, she was arrested. She argued that the baby had been fast asleep when she left and that she had not intended to stay away so long, but "something had come up" to detain her. Although LeeAnn was arraigned, she was not tried because this was her first offense. She was allowed biweekly visits to McKella at her foster home.

Kim had driven LeeAnn to Planned Parenthood, where she was given a supply of birth control pills. Because LeeAnn was so heavy, it was not until she was several months pregnant that Kim became suspicious about her condition. When asked about it, and LeeAnn said, "I guess so," Kim asked what had happened with taking the pill. LeeAnn laughed and said she had thrown them away. Kim reminded LeeAnn that she had said she did not want another baby. LeeAnn's reply was: "I don't." "Well, why didn't you keep taking the pill then?" Kim asked. LeeAnn snapped: "I got tired of taking them." This conversation happened after McKella had been put in foster care. Kim asked what she was going to do about the baby. LeeAnn said: "Keep it." Kim said: "Why? You said you didn't want it." LeeAnn's response: "Shit. Do you think I'm going to be a bad mother and give a baby up for abortion?" Kim said: "It's too late for that anyway, but you can put it up for adoption. There are many people who would love to have a baby and they can't." LeeAnn glared at Kim and said: "I ain't giving up no baby!" End of conversation. Kim said: "We aren't supposed to impose our values on clients, but, boy, did I have to bite my tongue."

Because of loneliness and depression, the pregnant LeeAnn went to live with Roberta in a housing complex on the north side of town. That arrangement lasted four months. Shortly after Lauren's birth, LeeAnn said, "My sister kicked me out. Her boyfriend did not like to hear Lauren fussing." LeeAnn got an apartment in the same housing project. Kim was curious to see how LeeAnn would react to Lauren. At first, she did better. She kept Lauren fairly clean, and, as far as Kim knew, LeeAnn did not leave her home alone. She mainly did not pay much attention to Lauren. Unlike McKella, Lauren seemed content to just lie there. When Lauren was two months old, LeeAnn convinced Josephine, the department head, to let McKella live with them. By the time Lauren was four months old, LeeAnn seemed to give up on her. When Kim visited, she always found Lauren's diapers full, and she had terrible diaper rashes. LeeAnn yelled a lot, but there were never bruises on either McKella or Lauren.

Kim took a two-week vacation. When she returned, not only was the apartment in disarray, but also McKella and four-month-old Lauren were dirty and undernourished. LeeAnn, who had probably been 50 pounds overweight the previous year, had put on at least another 25. A soap opera was on full-blast, and when Kim asked LeeAnn why she had not done the housework before turning on the television, as they had agreed, LeeAnn retorted: "Just fuck off! Mind your own business." Kim reminded LeeAnn that she could not keep the children unless things changed. To that, LeeAnn responded: "Who cares! Get off my back!" Kim switched off the television and said: "You need to find the list we made of the things you have to do." LeeAnn shoved past Kim and, as she turned the television on, said: "I ate it, okay?" Then she plunked herself down in the chair with her arms stubbornly folded across her chest. At that point, McKella appeared in the kitchen doorway with a large knife with which she was trying to open a can of pop. Lauren was discovered on the floor in the kitchen, wide awake, but seemingly unaware of the ruckus going on around her.

Kim went next door to use the telephone to call Josephine at Child Protective Services. Within 10 minutes, Josephine appeared, and they took the two girls. McKella was welcomed back to the foster home where she had spent most of the past year. Because they had other children, the couple was reluctant to take Lauren. Lauren went to live at a temporary boarding home, where she was able to stay on because "she was so good—so little trouble."

Two years later, LeeAnn was in another subsidized housing complex, but a newer housing project. This time the apartment was more sparsely furnished and much neater. LeeAnn, again, had an infant, Jared. She had recently signed papers relinquishing custody of McKella and Lauren. Jared was dressed in hand-me-downs, but they were clean and fit him well. They were also appropriate for the weather. LeeAnn bragged: "I'm keeping my house clean and I'm not going out on him. I'm going to hang onto this one. I've always wanted a boy."

Because she had been accused of neglect and not abuse, LeeAnn had been allowed to visit her daughters frequently while they were in foster homes. At first, she did visit, but her visits decreased in frequency, especially after Jared's birth. Even though both girls lived within three miles, transportation was difficult. LeeAnn did not have a car, nor did she drive. Nevertheless, Kim was willing to drive her during her weekly half-day visits. But, when given a choice, LeeAnn preferred shopping or visiting Roberta. After a visit to McKella, LeeAnn complained: "McKella acted like I wasn't there. She calls that foster lady 'Mom.'" Her lack of interest in the girls and their clear preference for their foster parents, as well as their improved appearance and behavior since being removed from LeeAnn's care, had precipitated the initiation of permanent removal. Kim expressed surprise at how readily LeeAnn had agreed to losing custody and at how little concern she had shown about the girls since. It was also interesting that she was so attentive to Jared. Kim conjectured that her mother's death had made LeeAnn "the person in charge." But LeeAnn had also just turned 19 and seemed generally more mature and less frustrated.

McKella was adopted by her foster parents. At the age of three, her development was pretty much on target. She had been hyperactive and aggressive when she first arrived at her foster home, but had calmed down and was well behaved after a few months. Lauren had not fared as well. She was a year and a half old before she walked, and, at two, she still had few words. Her foster mother had enrolled her in a preschool for children with disabilities. Although loving and caring, the foster mother, a widow, felt she was too old to take another baby on a permanent basis. She had grandchildren older than Lauren. Because Lauren was not an infant and was developmentally delayed, she was placed on a national list for hard-to-place children.

Like McKella, Jared was alert and responsive. Unlike the girls' situation (LeeAnn claimed not to know their fathers), Jared's 17-year-old father, J.R., was interested in him and remained in contact with LeeAnn. J.R. was a dropout from a program for seriously emotionally disabled youths. He did not have a full-time job, but was cooperating with Vocational Rehabilitation to get more preparation. Although they did not always get along, LeeAnn and J.R. had some good times. Because he had access to his parents' car, he was a help to LeeAnn in getting groceries and taking Jared to the doctor. He lived with his parents in the same housing complex as LeeAnn, and his parents were pleased to have a grandchild. Their willingness to take care of Jared probably prevented the neglect situations that LeeAnn was charged with when McKella and Lauren were at home.

The next conversation about birth control was right after Kim found out LeeAnn was pregnant with Jared after she had lost custody of both girls. Out of the blue, LeeAnn announced: "I am getting my tubes tied. Roberta got it done. She says it's great. She doesn't have to worry about more kids. She said I should ask the doctor to do it when I have this one." Kim recalled: "I almost jumped up and down with joy. It is so tragic for her to keep having kids that she doesn't want. To her, getting pregnant is like catching a cold—it just happens." A frustration of Kim's interaction with LeeAnn was her repeated pregnancies. At 40, Kim and her husband had finally resigned themselves to being childless. As Kim said: "I marvel at LeeAnn's fertility. As far as I know she wasn't even having sex all that much."

Kim was delighted that LeeAnn brought up the tubal ligation. The Welfare Department gets funds for sterilization surgery, but has a waiting list of women who want it. Kim tried to get LeeAnn on the list and was disappointed when Josephine told her LeeAnn was ineligible. Federal regulations do not allow the use of funds for people with intellectual disabilities. Their way of complying with the regulation was to disqualify anyone who had been in special education. LeeAnn had been in classes for the mildly retarded as well as for the emotionally disturbed.

Kim had promised LeeAnn that she would look into funding for the tubal ligation and had to tell her the bad news. As usual, LeeAnn just shrugged. Kim cynically thought: "More babies, more jobs for social workers!" After LeeAnn had Jared, Josephine, who does the books, saw an unexpected tubal ligation charge. She could not wait to tell Kim. When Kim saw LeeAnn, she asked her about the delivery. LeeAnn did not say anything about a tubal. Kim's first thought was that the doctor was padding the bill, but when she came out and asked, LeeAnn said: "Oh, yeh. I had that done. I just told him that you guys would pay." Kim said: "Usually there is elaborate paperwork. We have to make anybody wait a month after they've signed the papers in case they change their mind. There wasn't any paperwork. We are afraid to ask Dr. —. We don't want to make him nervous. But we're real curious. Believe me! LeeAnn is not yet 20 years old. Maybe she'll change her mind and decide she wants another kid. But she has one baby. I mean, right now she is raising Jared. She's lucky. And she never mentions the girls. If I happen to see them, I report how they're doing and she doesn't even seem interested." When Josephine mentioned the sterilization to the doctor, he said: "Oh, that was medically indicated because she has diabetes. Her mother died of complications from diabetes, you know."

After Jared's birth, Kim got LeeAnn connected with Vocational Rehabilitation services. They helped her get work in a restaurant that was on a bus route from her home. LeeAnn's sense of humor and extroverted behaviors were appealing to most of her co-workers, but she often irritated her boss. He had several MR employees and worked well with them. After LeeAnn was almost fired for her disrespectful reaction to his criticism, her boss learned that LeeAnn responded well to subtle suggestions, and he subsequently used that approach.

LeeAnn got two meals a day at the restaurant, and Jared got the same at day care. LeeAnn lost some of the weight that she needed to lose because of her diabetic condition, and Jared was robust and healthy. Kim judged that LeeAnn was "doing okay with Jared. Not great, but better than with the girls. I think it helps for her to be working and out of the house. It keeps her from messing it up so much." By the time Jared was a year old, J.R. had another girlfriend, but J.R.'s mother continued to be good to LeeAnn and Jared. Public transit had a convenient route to Roberta's house, and LeeAnn's bus pass got her there free of charge. Roberta was more stable than LeeAnn and was family.

LINDSAY

Lindsay, a bright-eyed, red-headed four-year-old, drove her nursery school teacher crazy. She could not sit through a story, never played with a toy for more than about 30 seconds, never followed—in fact, seemed not to hear—directions, and begged her classmates to join in their play without knowing how to be part of their play. Yet Lindsay was cheerful and eager to please.

Thinking that Lindsay might have a hearing problem, the teacher referred her to a speech and hearing clinic. They found no hearing loss, but the therapist noticed that, although she chattered incessantly, Lindsay's sentences were no more complex than a two-year-old's and her vocabulary was limited. Because of her language delay, a twice-a-week speech therapy routine was initiated that was to continue for eight years.

Meanwhile, a few of the parents at the cooperative nursery approached the board to "discuss the appropriateness of this preschool for Lindsay." They quoted their children's complaints that Lindsay bothered them and interfered with their activities. The teacher suspected that these parents were mainly reacting to their own observations of Lindsay. In spite of her pestering, the other children were fond of Lindsay and liked to help her do the things expected of nursery school children. Although Lindsay was a challenge, the teacher opposed her dismissal and got the support of other parents to block such action. In response to parents' concerns, she started a program to include Lindsay in positive social interactions with peers and to increase her individualized interaction with adults in order to promote her language development and improve her readiness skills and attention span. With deliberate efforts to include and engage her, Lindsay's negative behaviors subsided, and time spent in constructive activities and cooperative play increased.

In contrast to the patience and flexibility of preschool staff, Lindsay's kindergarten teacher was neither tolerant nor resourceful. Within two days of the start of school, the special education director received a report of the "inappropriateness of the kindergarten placement" that stressed the urgency of making other educational arrangements for Lindsay. Her parents were called to a conference. Mrs. Steppenbach was well aware of her daughter's problems. Involved in the cooperative nursery on a biweekly basis, her efforts and honesty, in fact, had bolstered the preschool teacher's determination to keep Lindsay in school.

The Steppenbachs had three children: Alice, aged 11, who was in a gifted and talented middle school program; David, aged 9 and a straight A+ fourth grader; and Lindsay. Mr. Steppenbach had started a computer business about the time Lindsay entered preschool, and his attention had been devoted almost solely to that thriving business. He proudly monitored the report cards of his two older children, although in other ways he had not been a very active parent. His wife loved children, and he left family and home responsibilities to her. He had not wanted their "accidental" third child. Mr. Steppenbach was often irritated by Lindsay and was happy that their home was big enough that he could "get away from her antics." In fact, he was at his computer business at least 10 hours a day, 7 days a week. He had mentally noted that Lindsay was not like his other two children, but he attributed this to his wife's not being sufficiently strict with her; as he called it, "spoiling her rotten." After such accusations, Mrs. Steppenbach kept Lindsay out of her husband's way as much as possible. Anticipating that she would be blamed, Mrs. Steppenbach rarely passed information about Lindsay's school problems on to her husband.

It was Mr. Steppenbach who received the official call about Lindsay at his computer store. The principal tactfully informed him of "some problems," and then was taken aback by the animosity of Steppenbach's reply. Steppenbach demanded to know exactly what Lindsay had done and then interrupted the principal's account with an accusation of the teacher's mismanagement. When her husband notified her about the call, Mrs. Steppenbach was not surprised. Every day when she met Lindsay at the kindergarten door, the teacher had reeled off her daughter's wrongdoings.

The conference, which began right after school the following day, was a nightmare for Mrs. Steppenbach. Her husband was rude, his voice was at a volume that could be "heard all over school," and he denied the accuracy of the teacher's evidence about Lindsay. He literally told his wife to "shut up" when she tried to confirm the validity of the teacher's observations. What puzzled her was that the teacher was not saying anything that Mr. Steppenbach had not himself said about Lindsay over the past three years. The conference ended 10 minutes after it started with Mr. Steppenbach's demand that Lindsay be transferred to the other kindergarten room immediately. Mr. Steppenbach announced that he was "going back to work" and stomped out of the office. As his wife followed, he turned and yelled: "You go back in there and make sure they switch that kid today." She reluctantly walked back into the school in time to overhear the second kindergarten teacher protest the decision to the principal. She had 31 students (3 more than the other teacher) and had observed Lindsay on the playground enough to know what she was in for.

Lindsay soon was enrolled in a "developmental kindergarten"—an all-day arrangement mainly comprised of children who had not fared well in their first year of kindergarten. Shortly after that, Mr. Steppenbach filed for a divorce. By the end of the year, Lindsay had tested "educable mentally retarded." After a second year in the developmental kindergarten, Lindsay was placed in a class with nine other children similarly labeled—a placement that was to mark the beginning of her school career in self-contained special education classrooms.

Shortly after the separation, Mrs. Steppenbach "lucked into" a job that suited her well—a salesperson in a fancy household goods store. She got along well with her boss and was soon promoted to assistant manager. Her request for custody of the children went undisputed. Mr. Steppenbach sent a monthly check that, combined with her own salary, allowed her to keep the family home and continue the family's predivorce life style. In spite of her successful career, Mrs. Steppenbach's family came first, and all three children could be seen helping around the store or sitting in the back storeroom doing homework after school. Her boss, a grandmother whose children lived far away, loved the Steppenbach children, especially Lindsay.

Mr. Steppenbach took Alice and David on weekly outings, but Lindsay was never included. This arrangement went unchallenged, until Alice's sixteenth birthday. As Alice told it 10 years later: "Dad—who was rolling in money—drove me to the car dealer's. He told to me to 'pick one out, honey.' He and his wife were standing there grinning. I just suddenly got furious. It seemed so unfair that he should be acting like Santa Claus after being so mean to Lindsay. I couldn't stand it. All I said was 'Take me home!' He hasn't talked to me much since then, but he put the money for a car in my bank account—it's still there. During my sophomore year of college, Mom helped me buy a car anyway." Alice's and David's relationships with Lindsay reflected that of their mother. They helped her cope with frustrating tasks, they were affectionate friends, and, when they were older, they drove her to movies or school events.

Lindsay received 12 years of education in self-contained classrooms for students with mild mental handicaps (previously educable mental retardation). Her years of speech therapy had resulted in fairly good communication skills. She had learned to focus on what was said in conversation and to express herself simply and slowly, and her pronunciation was clear enough that she could be understood by most people. By the time she reached high school, she read at a third-grade level, could handle small sums of money, and was able to get around the community using public transportation. The schools' focus on social skills had somewhat checked her pestering. She was mainly cheerful and cooperative, but even in secondary school, she still had almost daily outbursts of anger when she was unable to do a task or when plans did not go as she had hoped or expected. She also stomped out of the room at least once a week because she was "mad at" someone.

In terms of a social life, Lindsay was more fortunate than many others with her label. During her first year in the primary special education class, she met Carrie and Melanie, who both were within six months of her age. At the first parents' meeting, their mothers brought up their concern about the social isolation of their daughters because of rejection by neighborhood peers. From then on, these mothers faithfully drove the girls across town to each other's house and arranged weekend events. They also provided occasional respite when one of them had weekend plans. During their many years in the program, these three grew to be like siblings. As with siblings, there was a good deal of jealousy and competition between them, but, in the end, they enjoyed each other's company and support.

From an early age, Lindsay had been obvious about her "crushes." In kindergarten, she was enthralled with the principal and rushed up to hug him or wrap her legs around his. High-school-aged neighbors were also the embarrassed recipients of her affection. Up until about fourth grade, she was tiny and cute, and these behaviors were tolerated with some humor and even affectionate reciprocation. By fourth grade, puberty had set in and with it a rapid weight gain. Suddenly, the "cute" behaviors became repugnant to others, and she was chided or teased. Mrs. Steppenbach expected each new teacher to recite tales of Lindsay's romantic transgressions. By the time Lindsay was in high school, the most popular football and basketball players were selected as "boyfriends." She never was attracted to the boys in her classes—they were "just friends" and convenient, or accessible prom partners. Lindsay followed her current crush around school corridors and giggled when he looked her way. Sometimes she would stuff love notes in his locker or write her name and his within arrowed hearts on school supplies. Most of the youths ignored her and tried to escape her attentions. Some of them—or their friends—made a joke of the situation and sent notes back or pointed her out to others as "the girlfriend." Her feelings were hurt when she realized she was the butt of jokes, but this consequence did little to deter her blatant crushes.

During her last two years of high school, Lindsay took part in a transition-to-adulthood program through which she was placed at a variety of job sites. She tended to start out well at the tasks involved (e.g., filing or duplicating materials, preparing or serving food, cleaning), but after a couple of weeks, she lost interest and skipped work, argued with co-workers, or talked back to employers. Her aggressive crushes, now directed at men at work or customers, also interfered with her work performance. Family and teachers worried about postschool arrangements.

Although her two best friends had obtained permanent jobs in competitive employment—Melanie in the library and Carrie in the cafeteria of the local junior college—Lindsay had not been kept on at her last job as a motel room cleaner. Everyone planned on this job turning into permanent employment. The teachers were frustrated that she was engaging in the same kinds of disruptive and nonproductive behaviors time after time. They worked

with Vocational Rehabilitation staff to find full-time work for their graduates as they exited from school but, as with Lindsay, clients sometimes
thwarted their plans.

A discussion with Mrs. Steppenbach ended with a decision to let Lindsay
face the reality of pounding the pavement in search of a job. Mrs. Steppenbach, along with Alice, who now had a master's degree in social work and
had always been generous with her sister, agreed that they would not give
Lindsay any money besides a small allowance. Lindsay had plans to get an
apartment with her long-term friends, but was informed that she would have
to live at home unless she earned the money for rent. Lindsay was impressed
with Alice's apartment in the capital city and talked constantly about the
kind of apartment she would get when she graduated from high school. She
was upset when her relatives broke the news of the conditions for her move
because she assumed the money would be there to do what she wanted.

Because Carrie and Melanie were counting on Lindsay to pay a third of
the rent for the apartment, they asked about jobs for Lindsay and got one
for her at the cafeteria where Carrie worked. Lindsay had worked at busing
and dishwashing and had not wanted that kind of work, but she had few
options and was desperate to earn the money needed for the apartment. She
took the job. She and Carrie had the same hours. Carrie made sure Lindsay
got to work on time. She also reminded Lindsay to get back to work or to
calm down when it was necessary. Lindsay's success in keeping the job
could certainly be credited to Carrie. But, in the end, friction with Carrie
resulted in Lindsay's suspension.

Of the three women, Carrie was the "most normal" socially, in spite of
the fact that she had the hardest time academically. As a senior in high
school, she was still reading at a second-grade level, and her math skills
were equally poor. She was pretty and neat in appearance, and her cooperative attitude and smiling response to others had resulted in her being a
favorite at school and now on her job.

Melanie was the opposite of Carrie. She rarely smiled, and her knitted
brow and tendency to stay on the fringes of social action meant she was
often left alone and ignored. She did not seem to mind. Teachers described
her as a social isolate and immature. Of the three friends, she was the most
advanced in reading and math. Melanie had been at the top of her special
education class. She received excellent evaluations at her library job. The
job suited her, and she was conscientious in fulfilling responsibilities. Her
vocational success was partly a result of what teachers felt were problematic
behaviors. She was vehement about tidiness and order. As a youngster, she
got upset about any change in routine. She still liked routines, and the
operation of the library depended on efficiency in routine tasks. She wanted

the books to be in their proper places and worked hard to make sure this was the case. She liked being by herself and did not bother librarians or students who used the facilities.

For two years after high school graduation, the three women lived together fairly peaceably. Lindsay liked to cook and, when reminded by the others, did her share of cleaning. Although she was emotional and erratic, she was the leader with ideas about what to buy, what to cook, how to decorate the apartment, and what to do for entertainment. In fact, because the other two were passive and insecure, Lindsay's initiative was essential to their living independently. The others' temperance, however, kept Lindsay out of the trouble she would have gotten into on her own. When Carrie turned 18, her father promised her the old family car if she got her license. With enthusiastic coaching from Melanie and Lindsay, Carrie managed to pass the written part of the driving test, and, in spite of her extreme timidity, she was eventually convinced to do the road test. She failed the first time, but made it the second time around. The three friends took advantage of Carrie's "wheels" and had fun going to restaurants and shopping for clothes or things for their apartment.

Just at the start of their third year as roommates, Carrie started to date Lee, the dishwasher at work, and they were soon making their own plans. This left Lindsay and Melanie with no car. They had depended on Carrie and were out of the habit of taking public transportation. Both were very upset at this turn of events. Moreover, Lindsay was upset for other reasons. She had always considered herself to be favored by the boys—and was genuinely unaware of evidence that most boys preferred Carrie. Lindsay had been the one to talk about "boyfriends." Carrie had nervously avoided men's advances. Lee, who was as shy as Carrie, was slow to ask Carrie out, but, after a year and a half working together, their attraction to each other was obvious to everyone except Lindsay. To make matters worse, Lindsay had counted Lee as one of the young men who liked her, and when she finally was apprised of the relationship between the two, she accused Carrie of stealing her boyfriend. Melanie had never shown any interest in men. Her main concern was the loss of transportation, and she was very upset about Lindsay's intense reaction.

Lindsay was extremely jealous of Carrie's relationship. She stormed around at work and criticized Carrie to anyone within earshot. After two years of fairly successful employment, she got several warnings about inappropriate work behavior. The cafeteria workers were patient with Lindsay and sincerely wanted her to do well. Several of her co-workers had taken her aside and tried to get her to be reasonable about Carrie and Lee. Instead of getting over the blow, her anger got worse during the next few weeks. Not only did she complain about Carrie to employees, but also she began to call her names and berate her in front of customers. When a supervisor told her to stop, Lindsay walked out of work two hours before quitting time, announcing she was "not going to work with that bitch." After Lindsay walked out the first time, the manager telephoned her to remind her that when she was scheduled to work, she was expected to be there working appropriately. She also warned Lindsay that if she left work again, she would be suspended. When Lindsay marched out the second time, she was suspended from her job for the week.

Mrs. Steppenbach had been delighted with her daughter's living arrangement and was relieved that she had kept the same job for so long. She was grateful to Carrie for her important role in those successes. Although it was not Carrie's fault, her new relationship with Lee had changed everything. In spite of Lindsay's ugly treatment of her, Carrie had first tried to appease her and, when that failed, to keep out of her way. Nevertheless, Lindsay was on the rampage. Lindsay demanded to move home and was shocked when her mother refused to let her. Furthermore, after listening to Lindsay's endless harangues against Carrie, the exasperated Mrs. Steppenbach announced that she did "not want to hear anymore nonsense" and accused her of "acting like a 10-year-old!" She knew that Lindsay had also tried to get Melanie to side with her in kicking Carrie out of their apartment, but Melanie was loyal to Carrie and would not take sides. Mrs. Steppenbach felt that Lindsay would eventually adjust to the disappointment and get over her jealousy and that this would happen more quickly if she did not intervene. Quite frankly, on a personal level, Mrs. Steppenbach had no desire to share her space on anything more than a temporary basis with the demanding Lindsay. She had sold her home in the past year and had bought a two-bedroom condominium. She loved the quiet neatness of her new home. This was the first time she had a place of her own. Both Alice and David had jobs in other states, and both had recently married. Perhaps it was not a coincidence, but about the time of Lindsay's problems with men when she was in high school, Mrs. Steppenbach had become depressed enough to see a counselor. The three years of therapy had helped her deal with the guilt and anxiety she felt about Lindsay. She was feeling happier and more relaxed than she had ever felt before. When she hung up the telephone after refusing Lindsay's demand to move in with her, she first felt the old tensions and pangs of guilt returning, but then recovered and laughed to herself about Lindsay's expressions of disbelief at her mother's reaction.

As a child, Lindsay's crushes and her blatantly sexual behaviors had embarrassed her mother and siblings. Several times neighbors or relatives had complained that Lindsay had fondled a cousin or a neighborhood child.

She had also been caught in various stages of undress with other children numerous times. Usually the other children were confused onlookers. David, who was four years older than Lindsay, was particularly upset at her behavior around his friends. Mrs. Steppenbach tried to keep Lindsay engaged in other things and out of David's way when his friends were around.

During most of high school, as far as Mrs. Steppenbach knew, Lindsay's relationships with men had mainly been fantasies and flirtations. In spite of her many crushes, Lindsay had never had a real boyfriend who returned her affections. The boys in her special education class were friends, but she was not interested in them. During her senior year of high school, when Lindsay was 19 years old, there were several occasions when she was not at home when Mrs. Steppenbach returned from work. A few times she did not return until late at night. When questioned about it, Lindsay was evasive, except to say she had been "on dates." Lindsay had always been impressed with Alice's and David's "dates." Shortly after that, Lindsay complained of vaginal irritation. A visit to Planned Parenthood revealed that she had gonorrhea. What most troubled Mrs. Steppenbach was hearing from Carrie's mother that Carrie had observed Lindsay asking men—mostly strangers—for rides. In consultation with Planned Parenthood staff, it was decided that Lindsay should start taking birth control pills. A counselor at the clinic also volunteered to work with Lindsay to help her understand the dangers of having sexual relations with strangers and to convince her of the importance of getting her partners to use condoms even when she was on the pill. The counselor reported that Lindsay was responsive during these sessions and appeared to "catch on."

Perhaps the excitement of living in an apartment had kept Lindsay entertained and away from men for the first two years. Carrie and Melanie were disgusted at Lindsay's heavy-handed flirting with men they encountered in various settings, and they shamed her about what they considered to be social and moral transgressions. Her peers' admonitions influenced Lindsay. They were a threesome who did things together, and Lindsay had not gone off to her old haunts. Things quickly changed after Carrie started dating Lee. The marriages of David and Alice and David's wife's pregnancy added to Lindsay's frustrations. Torn between the thrill of weddings and excitement of becoming an aunt and the envious bitterness about others doing the things she would like to do, Lindsay's mindset became that she was going to "show them."

The manager of the cafeteria had fully expected Lindsay to "pull herself together" and was prepared to welcome her back. Although Lindsay was not the best worker, she did fairly well when she was in a good mood. The manager was proud of employing MR workers, and Lindsay's failure made her sad. But stubborn Lindsay made no effort to return to work. Two weeks after her suspension, Lindsay received a letter terminating her employment. Unemployed, Lindsay had time on her hands and began to hang out at the mall and downtown. With no transportation, she begged for rides. She was open about her determination to find a boyfriend.

About a month after Lindsay had been fired, Mrs. Steppenbach was awakened in the middle of the night by the telephone. A policewoman identified herself and said that Lindsay had been admitted to the hospital. She asked Mrs. Steppenbach to meet them there. Lindsay said that she had been raped by three men and had been left out on a country road. She had gone to the first house on the road. The residents would not let her in, but offered to call the police. A medical examination revealed evidence of sexual intercourse. Lindsay's story about what happened that night varied with each telling. At some points, she said that she did not know any of the men, but then said that someone named Jimmy was there. Later, she told police that Jimmy had raped her before, but then changed the story to say that he had been her boyfriend two years earlier. She first could not remember his last name, but then remembered it was Jones.

When the police arrested Jimmy Jones, he first denied knowing either Lindsay or anything about the rape. Later, he confessed that he and his friends had sex with Lindsay, but that she was a voluntary participant. In fact, he said that Lindsay had run into them at a discount store and had begged for a ride. When they agreed to drive her home, she asked instead for them to take her with them. At that point, she initiated sex with Jimmy in front of his friends. They drove to the country road, and all three had intercourse with Lindsay. Apparently, at first she agreed to have intercourse with Jimmy's friends, but changed her mind when they called her "retard." One of the men recognized her as having been in "that retard class" and taunted her with the fact. Lindsay had, in fact, known Jimmy since elementary school. He had been bused in from a rural town to the same developmental kindergarten. After that, he had attended classes for students with learning disabilities until he quit school at 16. He had attended the transitional program with Lindsay for a few months before he quit school. Jimmy also confessed that he had slept with Lindsay several times "a couple of years ago," but insisted that she had initiated sex and he was not her boyfriend. For a number of reasons, the case did not go to court. The gynecological examination of Lindsay revealed not only her recent intercourse, but also the fact that she was about two months' pregnant. Lindsay named several men as possible fathers. To her mother's relief, Lindsay fairly readily agreed to have an abortion.

Carrie's relationship with Lee blossomed into an engagement, and she decided to live with her parents until their wedding. Melanie was going to move into a supervised apartment arrangement at the end of the month (when their present lease was up). Although she was capable of living independently, her parents knew she would become a hermit if not encouraged to socialize with others. Lindsay was in a position of having no job and no place to live. She could not live in the supervised apartments because they were only available to employed people. She did not want to live with the "retards" in a group home that she visited. Personnel from mental health, who became involved with Lindsay because of the rape incident, suggested that she live in the temporary shelter for abused women. She would become part of their group therapy sessions. In the meantime, they insisted that Lindsay be on some form of reliable birth control.

Mrs. Steppenbach's boss and long-term friend encouraged her to look into sterilization for Lindsay. Both groaned at the idea of Lindsay getting pregnant and deciding to keep a baby. Lindsay was now 22 and could make her own decisions. Mrs. Steppenbach and Lindsay went to Planned Parenthood. The nurse practitioner reviewed her birth control options. When she mentioned a tubal ligation, Mrs. Steppenbach asked Lindsay what she thought about that. Lindsay's response was: "But, Mom, I want to get married and have a baby." Mrs. Steppenbach was actually relieved at this response because she worried that sterilization was too major a decision for them at this time. After all, Lindsay had worked and lived independently for two years and perhaps would mature in the future. She also conveyed her worry that Lindsay would not be reliable about taking the pill or using a barrier method. Eventually, they settled on Norplant, which could be inserted into her arm surgically and would be an effective contraceptive device for five years. The nurse warned Lindsay that she should insist on partners using a condom. She did not dwell on this message because she did group sessions for residents at the women's shelter and knew Lindsay was scheduled to live there for a while.

STEVEN

Steven Brytcha was removed from the care of his unmarried teenaged mother for the first time when he was a 17-pound two-year-old. Police reported Sandra, his mother, to Child Protective Services when they found the malnourished Steven asleep on a couch in the middle of a party during a drug bust. Over the next three years, Child Protective Services worked cooperatively with Mental Health Services to try to get Sandra off drugs and to get mother and son reunited. During the time Steven remained in

foster homes, Sandra visited regularly and sometimes took him for weekends. Then, Sandra was arrested on drug and prostitution charges, found
guilty, and imprisoned. Sandra refused to give up custody of Steven, and he
was moved to a foster home in the area of the correctional facility so that
he could visit Sandra twice a week. When Sandra got out of prison, the
nine-year-old Steven went to live with her for the first time in seven years.
Within the year, Sandra was murdered by an ex-boyfriend, and Steven was
again placed in a foster home.

When Child Protective Services first took custody of two-year-old
Steven, they found him to be a poorly coordinated little boy whose body
was covered with scrapes and bruises. A physical examination confirmed
the hunch that the injuries probably resulted from falls rather than beatings.
In the years that Sandra visited Steven while he was in foster care, foster
parents claimed that Sandra was casual, inattentive, permissive, and ne-
glectful, but not violent. Steven did not appear to understand others or did
not pay attention. He was continuously and randomly active, and this
behavior was the reason ("he wore them out") foster parents gave for
discontinuing his care. Another problem in foster care was that he did not
bond with others, rarely gave them eye contact, and did not like to be held
or cuddled. His reactions to Sandra were about the same as to anyone else.
One foster mother described mother and son as having "parallel relations,
they're with each other but don't notice each other."

The first social worker assigned to the case suggested that Steven enter
a preschool for children with disabilities because of various developmental
delays. Moreover, because Steven was hyperactive and not responsive to
foster parents, she felt he would be tolerated longer in the foster homes if
he were not there on a full-time basis. Nevertheless, the first foster mother
terminated his care after seven months, giving a pending lengthy family
vacation as the reason. She also refused to have him back when they
returned from their trip. Steven then was taken on by a woman who had
previously worked well with MR children. Within a month, she asked to
have Steven placed elsewhere, stating: "I just can't learn to like him." He
stayed in the third foster home for a year, until he followed Sandra to the
location of her correctional institution. When he left, the foster mother said
she was relieved and complained that Steven "did not seem to like anything
or anybody."

At five, Steven generally complied with commands, but never stayed
with an activity for more than a minute or two. He rarely smiled and never
laughed. Not only did he not bond with adults, but also he was indifferent
to children. Within a week of entering kindergarten, Steven was referred for
special education services and was placed in a primary class for mildly

mentally retarded students. During the four years his mother was in prison, Steven moved to nine different foster homes. When Sandra got out of prison, Steven's case worker said: "It's a good thing; we've run out of foster homes for him." After Sandra's death, Steven's maternal grandfather was contacted, and he agreed to "look out for Steven," but could not take care of him at his home. Steven was sent to his tenth foster home, where he lasted one week.

Steven had been sent back and forth between classes for the emotionally disturbed and classes for the mildly mentally retarded during his first five years in school. He spent his eleventh year at a short-term residential treatment center for children with emotional handicaps. When he was twelve, Steven was placed in a children's group home. Within the month, he was transferred to the adolescent home because "he was initiating sexual interaction with other children" (both males and females).

Steven's grandfather visited him once a month in each of these settings. After a couple of holiday visits, however, Mr. Brytcha refused to take Steven home because he was unable to handle him; as he said: "Steve does not mind me, he gets away from me." When Steven was 14, his grandfather married a woman who was proud of her ability to deal with children and who expressed an interest in "taking care of Steven." She was a "take charge" type of person and felt that she could "turn that boy around." Steven was a challenge for Mrs. Brytcha. She tried to keep him clean and neat, but by the time Steven got to school, he was disheveled. The teachers noticed bruises, which they assumed were from his being hit, since Mrs. Brytcha had advised them that they should control Steven with "smacks." Although Steven flinched when she was around, he was also much more responsive to her than to anyone else. His skinny frame filled out some. When she told him to sit, Steven did just as she said.

Steven fascinated his middle school teachers. He was a short, slender 15-year-old with light brown straight hair. Basically handsome, his expressionless face communicated little. He was neither popular nor unpopular—asocial, he was just there. He fidgeted as he worked at academics, achieving close to a second-grade level. He never contributed to discussions, nor would he write anything other than short routine sentences. He showed no emotions, and attempts by psychologists to discuss his feelings about his traumatic and disrupted early years drew no reactions. He would flatly answer yes and no to earlier events that they asked him about, but would offer no further information and showed no sign of emotion even about his mother's death, which he had witnessed. At the moment, their biggest concern with Steven was that he was rarely in school. He had missed 35 out of the 47 school days that year. He would ride the school bus to school and either take off without coming in or sneak out at lunchtime. Attempts to prevent truancy had not been successful. When asked what he did, he said: "Hang around." Those who had seen him said he would go in and out of stores and fast-food restaurants. Workers at those places said he went through trash and picked cigarette butts out of ashtrays.

After Steven had lived with his grandparents for two years, shortly before his sixteenth birthday, Mrs. Brytcha came to an annual case conference. The teachers were floored when Mrs. Brytcha announced that she "was trying to get Steven sterilized" and asked for their opinions. When asked why, with Mr. Brytcha sitting silently by her side looking at the floor, Mrs. Brytcha said: "He gets at girls—that's all he wants to do." She added: "You heard what that bus driver said about him. If I let him out of my sight, he is off with girls." Mrs. Brytcha said she had talked about "gettin' him fixed" with their doctor, who said "it was a good idea," but that a "judge would have to sign the papers." Mrs. Brytcha said her reason for telling them was that the school would have to "sign that he was retarded and crazy." The school psychologist offered to send Steven's papers to the judge, if Mr. Brytcha gave permission, which he did.

During the two months before his sixteenth birthday, Steven was at school a total of two days. Nobody saw Steven after his sixteenth birthday. About a year later, curious about what happened to Steven, the school psychologist called Mr. Brytcha. Mr. Brytcha reported that "Steve took off. We don't know where he is." When asked about the results of the attempts to have Steven sterilized, Mr. Brytcha said: "Judge wouldn't sign. Said he wasn't retarded enough."

10

Individuals with Moderate and Severe Retardation

This chapter details the cases of five individuals who test in the moderate to severe range of mental retardation. "Darrell," "Colleen," and "Roger" are well adjusted, perform everyday life functions fairly competently, and are integrated into family and community. "Trish" and "Penny" are severely retarded, and both have autism. A frequent assumption about individuals who are moderately and severely retarded is that they are not interested in sexual interactions with others. Some of these cases reveal the fallacy of that assumption.

DARRELL

Darrell went into a severe depression when his 80-year-old mother suffered a stroke. His mother's stroke occurred two days before Darrell's fifty-second birthday, so his immediate disappointment was that his birthday celebration, which also served as an annual Fourth of July reunion for a large extended family, had to be cancelled. Darrell did not want to be alone in the mobile home where he and his mother had lived since his father died in a farm accident two decades earlier. At that time, Darrell's sister, Sonia, and her husband, John, took over the management of the family orchard and moved into the large house with their four children. Darrell and Mrs. Gintel were happy to live in a mobile home on the property.

Diagnosed as retarded when he was four, Darrell had gone to school at the ARC Opportunity Center in the basement of a church from the time he was 8 until he was 17. Even as a preschooler, Darrell had been his father's "little helper" and had trailed Mr. Gintel as he worked in the orchard and produce garden. Mr. Gintel had enjoyed Darrell's company and was patient in teaching him chores. Darrell was a strong and willing worker and was good at the routine tasks. After his father's death, Darrell did some work with his brother-in-law, but John had new ways of doing things and was annoyed at Darrell's resistance to change. Darrell could tell that John resented his presence, which added to his stubborn response. John was used to working alone and did not like the constant company of his retarded brother-in-law, so he gradually eased Darrell out of orchard tasks. Darrell continued to mow the lawns and worked in his mother's garden.

Darrell and his mother enjoyed each other's company and had been best friends. Except for his experience with John, Darrell never felt unwanted or a burden. Included in family gatherings, he had lots of friends in his parents' generation. In the past few years, his nurturing aunts and uncles had died. He had been independent around the house, doing most of the cleaning and cooking as their mother weakened. In the four months between their mother's stroke and her death, Sonia and Darrell had gone to the nursing home daily even though Mrs. Gintel did not appear to recognize them. During his mother's illness, Darrell sat in the trailer and rocked—a way he had dealt with stress since he was a child. Sonia brought him food, but returned to find most of it uneaten. After Mrs. Gintel died, Darrell sat on the steps to the trailer and refused to go into "Mom's house." Sonia insisted he move to their house. Sonia was a teacher and did not have much time to spend with Darrell. Her children had always had fun with Darrell, but they no longer lived at home. John made no effort to conceal his annoyance at having Darrell in the house. He accused Sonia of babying Darrell and asked her to make him move back to the trailer. The sensitive Darrell was aware of John's feelings and would not come to the dinner table or family room to watch television, but broke into tears at the idea of going to the trailer. Sonia felt "terribly in the middle."

Nobody had talked about what should happen if Mrs. Gintel died before Darrell. Her mother was so positive about things that Sonia rarely broached "depressing subjects" in her presence. Sonia knew her mother expected her to take over. Sonia's older brother had moved to California 35 years earlier and was nearing retirement himself. Telephone conversations revealed that he, too, assumed Darrell was Sonia's responsibility.

Over the next few months, Darrell became more sullen and withdrawn, and he was losing weight at a great rate. Although Darrell and John scrupulously avoided each other, Darrell's presence in the house put "a strain on their marriage." In spite of tremendous guilt feelings, she eventually called a cousin who was a social worker at an institution. Arrangements were made for Sonia to visit, although her cousin warned that "because of deinstitutionalization we rarely admit new clients" and Darrell was "too high-functioning to fit in." Sonia took the day off, and her cousin showed her around the wards. Sonia quickly realized that most patients, though Darrell's age, were "much worse off" and concluded, "I couldn't live with myself if I sent him here." Her cousin gave her information about ARC residential care.

Sonia was impressed with her tour of ARC group homes, but remarked to John that "the staff are all hippies." Many of the staff were college students, as ARC was located in the same town as the state university. Sonia did not have a "big thing" about hippies; her youngest son wore his hair in a ponytail and had a pierced ear. Darrell was tearful when Sonia told him about the possibility of "a new place to live." This reaction was new; Darrell always had been docile in complying with her requests and usually looked forward to new adventures. Sonia was uneasy when they took Darrell on a separate tour and thought they were unrealistic in expecting him to make up his mind about things, but added, "He's obviously flattered by all the attention." Since they were children, Sonia had expected to answer for him. Sonia told John: "I must admit, those kids were great with him. He's been acting like the end of the world since Mom's stroke, but I believe he took some interest in that place."

Sonia told the staff they wanted to move quickly to relocate Darrell. The residential manager felt a supervised apartment was most suitable because Darrell was high-functioning. It was Sonia's least favorite place. Clients lived with roommates of the same sex, but the apartments were clustered together, and it was clear to Sonia that there was "a lot of back and forth between men and women." She told John: "I made it clear to them that Darrell had no interest in women." John joked: "Oh, I wouldn't be so sure!" but quickly added: "Just kidding!" John was in a better mood since plans were under way for Darrell to move. Darrell made John uneasy, although he was ashamed of his reaction because "everyone else in this family thinks Darrell is Mr. Nice Guy." About 10 minutes later, John heard Sonia talking to herself as she cleaned up after dinner: "I think it best that Darrell live with just men, really. Mother would have been horrified to see those posters in the apartment."

It was agreed that Darrell would try the adult group home with three men: one 19, one 27, and one 39. Although younger than Darrell, Sonia thought they "seem older anyway, and Darrell won't know the difference." The next time Sonia told Darrell "they were going to see the people at the group home," he went without grousing. She was pleased that things were "falling into place so nicely." Her mother's illness had "worn her out," and she was looking forward to Darrell and John being in better moods.

A month after their first visit, Darrell had his boxes packed and was eager to move. During the first weeks, Doug, the director of Darrell's home, called Sonia about twice a week to ask questions or report Darrell's adjustment. Darrell was evaluated by Vocational Rehabilitation—all residential clients had jobs, worked in sheltered employment, or went to adult day care. They had to be out of the residence at least six hours a day. Doug reported that Darrell would start in a job enclave arrangement doing such outdoor maintenance as mowing, raking, shoveling snow, and cleaning parking lots. Doug added: "We like having Darrell here. He's a nice guy and a good housekeeper. But he is really ready for the supervised apartment." That made Sonia uneasy, and she defensively said: "We prefer the group home."

Sonia made arrangements for Darrell to visit every third weekend. The first two visits went well, but Darrell kept asking if it was "time to go back." On the third visit, he mentioned "Marty." Sonia assumed Marty was someone from his work. The fourth visit was cancelled at the last minute. The ARC homes had scheduled camping at a state park, and when Darrell placed his suitcase by the door and was informed that he was not going because it was his weekend to go home, he sulked to his room and shut the door. Doug assured Darrell that it was "his choice" and he could call his sister to rearrange his home weekend. The next weekend, Darrell announced proudly that he "danced with Marty at the camping." In response to Sonia's "Who's Marty?" Darrell said: "My girlfriend." Sonia's youngest son, who had always been "pals" with his uncle, said, "Cool." This son was a senior in college in the town where the group home was located and had been driving Darrell the 60 miles each way for his home visits. Sonia bit her lip. Darrell was two years her senior, but she thought of him as her "kid brother" with an emphasis on "kid."

Sonia decided to drive Darrell back herself, and John, who had yet to see the group home, was convinced to accompany them. They were greeted by Mark, rather than Doug, and were told that Doug did not work weekends, but maybe could be reached if it was an emergency. Mark later said he could tell she was "uptight about something." Sonia said: "It's not quite an emergency, but I need to talk with him" and went in to use the phone. John sat uncomfortably watching television with the men.

When Doug answered the phone, Sonia went straight to the point: "Darrell says he has a 'girlfriend.' What does he mean by 'girlfriend'?" Sonia noticed the hesitation on the other end of the line. Doug slowly answered: "Was her name Marty?" To her affirmative, Doug clarified: "Marty attends afternoon classes at the ARC Center with Darrell. She was on the camping trip last weekend. They seem interested in each other." This report confirmed Sonia's fears. She tried not to sound accusing, but she could not help but say: "I thought we talked about 'not being with girls.' He couldn't handle something like that, you know. He is *very* retarded. He can't even read or write. He has no business having a girlfriend." Again, silence. Then Doug said: "The men and women frequently are in programs together. We do not prevent contact. It is normal for relationships to form. We find they are good for clients—healthy psychologically. I noticed that Marty seemed attracted to Darrell and he was happy to dance with her." They were both quiet on the phone, and then Sonia said: "Well, thanks, bye." On the way home, she could not keep off the subject. John finally said: "Calm down. It's probably nothing." He asked what Marty was like, and Sonia admitted she had not asked. But she said: "She has to be retarded since they're in the same program."

At their weekly staffing, Doug discussed his conversation with Sonia and asked the residential staff to help him "think this thing through." His undergraduate degree was in psychology, and he was doing graduate work in psychiatric social work. This was not the first time someone had expressed an opinion about the way things should be for their retarded relative, but he could tell by Sonia's voice that the idea of her brother being sexual was very threatening. Yet in just three months he had watched a depressed Darrell start to enjoy life. Staff were pleased with Darrell's adjustment at work, home, and social settings. Doug knew he would be an advocate for Darrell's right to intimate relationships, but he wanted to proceed in a manner that would not alienate Sonia. He was not sure that anything would come of the attraction to Marty, but he could tell that Darrell was interested in women, in spite of his sister's censure. Staff decided to "wait it out" and let Sonia adjust to the "new Darrell."

Darrell came to an Easter celebration that included three of Sonia's grown children, two spouses, and two grandchildren. They all remarked on how great Uncle Darrell looked. The whole family had worried about what would happen to him after Mrs. Gintel died. Sonia confided Darrell's "romantic attachment" to her two oldest daughters. One laughed and said: "You mean he's having sex? Good for Uncle Darrell!" The other, always more sensitive to her mother's feelings, said: "Oh dear, that could be a problem." Word of the girlfriend got around. One son-in-law came right out at the dinner table and said: "So, Darrell, I hear you have a girlfriend. What's her name?" Darrell blushed and said: "Marty." The next question was: "What's she like?" Darrell said: "She's real nice. She likes me a lot." John asked: "How old is she?" Darrell did not know. At that point, Darrell got up from the table. He got nervous when people asked him things that he did not know. He also could sense that he was being teased.

It was the end of May before Darrell visited Sonia and John again. Either they had weekend plans, or there was some outing or occasion at the group home that Darrell did not want to miss. Besides, whenever he visited, he was ready to go back as soon as he entered the door. A little jealous that she was not needed, Sonia was also relieved. Not only had Darrell improved, but also Sonia was feeling better than she had in years. She had not realized the strain of mothering four teenagers and managing her mother and Darrell. Although mostly independent, neither drove, so Sonia had taken them shopping and to church for 23 years. Plus, she felt obliged to look in on them once or twice a day even when she wanted to "lie down and put her feet up after teaching all day." John was grateful to her family for the opportunity to run the orchard—he was an efficient manager, and the business was thriving, but Sonia knew that on some level he resented obligations to Darrell and Mrs. Gintel. Now that their youngest was finishing college, they had the money and the freedom to travel. They were eagerly planning a Christmas trip to the Caribbean, and both felt better about their marriage than they had in years.

Darrell's relationship with Marty was also thriving. When Sonia asked about Marty, Darrell "dropped the bomb" that "Marty and me are getting married." Sonia got on the phone to Doug, who replied: "That's news to me. I never see them together. They see each other at the Center and at weekend social functions. I usually have the weekend off. I'll check it out if you want me to. It might just be talk." Sonia got the distinct impression from his tone that Doug thought it was none of her business.

After school was out in June, Sonia decided to visit the ARC Center. Darrell was proud to introduce his friends (staff and clients). He introduced Marty with no special fanfare. Sonia had not been around many MR adults and found herself somewhat repelled by their appearance, although they were neatly dressed and seemed clean. Marty, for example, had missing teeth and was considerably overweight. She had a high-pitched, nervous laugh that was disconcerting to Sonia. Sonia stayed for their health class, in which they were learning to recognize the signs of fever, how to read a thermometer, and what do to in case of a temperature. Again, she observed little interaction between Marty and Darrell and was becoming relieved that the "marriage thing was a false alarm." After class, she accompanied Darrell to the Rural Transit van that transported them to their respective homes. No sooner were they out the door of the Center when Marty came up and took Darrell's hand and he turned and gave her a kiss on the cheek. The kiss made Marty dissolve into her irritating (to Sonia) giggle. Darrell was "clearly happy as a lark." As they were waiting for the van, Darrell recited: "No hanky panky at work. Only kiss on cheek and handholding in public."

Again, Marty and Darrell laughed joyfully. Sonia said goodbye and pondered the situation on her drive home. She reported to John: "They look like the 'Jack Spratt' couple: Marty is short and round and Darrell tall and thin as a scarecrow." For the first time she laughed about it.

Sonia did not think much about Darrell over the summer. Her second oldest daughter had her first baby, and Sonia flew out West to help and ended up staying three weeks. Then, she had to plan for her youngest daughter's August wedding. Sonia had just started back teaching when Doug called. He had frequently mentioned that supervised apartment living would be more appropriate for Darrell because of his housekeeping skills and independence. She had remained firm on her preference for the group home. Doug indicated that it was illegal to keep Darrell in a setting that was "too restrictive" and reiterated that they were obliged to push clients toward independence. He also said there was a waiting list for the adult men's home. They had accepted two new clients since Darrell arrived, and there was another client who needed to move from the children's home because he had turned 18. Doug pointed out that Darrell was 20 years older than the next oldest client and people in the supervised apartment setting were more like Darrell—he would have more in common with them.

Darrell graduated from enclave to semi-independent work in maintenance at the mall. He took the city bus to and from his job and worked independently, although a Vocational Rehabilitation counselor checked periodically. Darrell's main problem was his confusion about money. He was careful with cash, but could not tell the difference between a ten-dollar bill and a one-dollar bill and could not make change or write checks. In the supervised apartment, he would get help with shopping and managing his wages. Sonia felt pressured to agree with the move. Darrell was delighted about it. Marty lived in an apartment. Although Sonia raised her eyebrows and shook her head when she reported this to John, again, the report ended in their both laughing. Sonia realized she was putting "some distance" between herself and Darrell, and she was pleased at herself for "not worrying all the time."

The next shock came when Doug called about the possibility of Darrell's having a vasectomy. He said Marty "was on the pill," but because she was only 37, it might be some time until her menopause, and it would be safer if Darrell had a vasectomy. Sonia later admitted that she was surprised at her "naivety"—she had assumed that kisses on the cheek and handholding were the extent of the relationship—but she was "taken aback that a young man like Doug could talk about these things so easily." Her first reaction was an angry "Why didn't you tell me they were having sex? I told you we did not like the idea of women. He's too immature." Again, Doug's characteristic silence. Then, he said: "Darrell is an adult. Our clients make up their own minds about relationships. We help them protect themselves from pregnancy and disease. We don't know for sure if they are having sexual intercourse. Darrell and Marty are embarrassed talking about sex. We do know they are intimate. In these situations, we assume they are having sex." He added: "I know you are not Darrell's official guardian but we try to involve next of kin in medical decisions. Vasectomy is relatively safe and easy—much easier for males than the tubal is for women. That's why we think Darrell should be the one to get it done, not Marty. Marty has medical problems anyway." Sonia said: "I'll call you back."

She repeated the conversation to John, who nonchalantly said: "Seems reasonable to me." It was a couple of days before she was calm enough to call Doug and "give him the go-ahead." Doug seemed relieved and said: "Darrell wants this operation. He is very protective of Marty and says he 'wants what's best for her.' I don't think he'll have a problem getting it done. He is 53 and he can verbalize that he wants the vasectomy and why." The vasectomy was done within a month of this conversation.

When they called to invite Darrell for Thanksgiving, with some mixed feelings, Sonia asked if "Marty would like to come too." Darrell said he would ask and yelled to Marty, who was obviously in his apartment. Sonia could hear that high shrill giggle, and she cringed. "Yes, she would like to come." At dinner, Darrell and Marty sat next to each other, smiled at each other, and patted each other continuously—something Mrs. Gintel had always done to Darrell. Darrell also announced to the whole family that "Marty wants to be my wife." Again, the giggles. Neither could answer the "So when's the big day?" questions.

Darrell's visits were now limited to the major holidays, and Marty always accompanied him. They remained affectionate, but Marty's excited giggling diminished considerably. Doug's next call was to inform Sonia that Darrell and Marty wanted to move out of the supervised appartment into their own apartment in the same complex. Sonia was happy that her mother was not around "to witness all this. She'd be horrified." But the call was not unexpected. Sonia avoided the subject of "marriage," although her children seemed determined to bring it up at their family gatherings. For the most part, Darrell and Marty were out of her mind. She was more and more grateful that Darrell "had his own life." At the same time, she felt less responsible for him.

When Darrell was 55 and Marty 40, they got married in a church they had been attending close to their apartment. They had the reception at the ARC Center cafeteria, which had been decorated for the occasion. Sonia and John were amazed to see how many friends the couple had. Vocational

Rehabilitation, residential, and ARC staff were there, as well as about 30 clients. Marty had no relatives. She had gone from foster care to an institution as a pregnant 16-year-old. Her baby was placed for adoption; Marty stayed there 15 years. She reentered the community with the deinstitutionalization movement when she was in her early thirties.

Marty worked at the sheltered workshop—her social behaviors interfered with community work. Sonia was not the only one to find Marty's mannerisms irritating. Marty had trouble with roommates, and staff said she got on their nerves. Darrell took pride in his ability to "calm her down." Darrell continued to work at the mall, but supervision had been discontinued because it was not needed. Darrell did most of the cooking and cleaning. Marty could read at a third-grade level and could handle money they needed for shopping. Residential staff helped deposit Darrell's checks and budget for expenses. Marty read the bus schedule, so they were mobile in the community. As with many retarded couples, they pooled their competencies and functioned better together than either could alone. Marty and Darrell were an affectionate couple and enjoyed each other's company.

COLLEEN

One morning I received a call from a woman who practiced law in a nearby county. Sarah Jones clarified: "You don't know me. My sister attended your sexuality workshop and suggested I call." Sarah had been appointed guardian ad litem for Colleen, a 12-year-old with Down syndrome. Mrs. C., Colleen's mother, and Dr. K., the family doctor, had petitioned the court for Colleen to have a hysterectomy, which "was advisable to prevent pregnancy and for personal hygiene." Dr. K. said he routinely did hysterectomies in such cases. The case made Judge D. nervous. He had recently been assigned this court, and his predecessor had presided over it for 30 years. Dr. K. had confided that he and the previous judge had been "very good friends." This announcement made Judge D. uncomfortable—he felt it implied that the previous judge had always sided with the doctor. A perusal of the petition made it clear that this was not an open-and-shut case. Well aware that the infamous *Stump* case also involved sterilization of an MR minor, Judge D. was determined to avoid the pitfalls of that case. He asked Sarah to check the accuracy of the diagnosis of retardation and the desirability of sterilization. Judge D. also informed Mrs. C. that she would have to get a second medical opinion about the advisability of surgical sterilization.

The next day, a letter from a second doctor, Dr. Q., appeared on Judge D's desk. The letter stated that Colleen was "severely retarded and could not cope with the problems of menstruation personally nor from a standpoint of hygiene." He stated that, "for her own protection, hysterectomy is indicated." When Judge D. discovered that the address on the letter matched that of Dr. K., he insisted Mrs. C. obtain a medical judgment of someone further removed from the case. Within a week, a letter arrived with the postmark of the large city on the other side of the river. The letterhead indicated that Dr. P. was the Director of the Division of Maternal/Fetal Medicine at—University. Dr. P. recommended hysterectomy on the following grounds: "The likelihood for offspring to be genetically normal is extremely small and the likelihood that she can satisfactorily take care of herself is extremely small. In my own experience, for individuals with this condition who reach maturity, hygiene poses a significant problem to their own health and well being as well as general appearance and comfort. It also offers significant stress, particularly with diminished intellectual function, to be faced with hidden and unexplained bleeding." From the wording of the letter, Judge D. suspected the doctor had not seen Colleen. A follow-up call confirmed his suspicion. Because he had not specified a personal examination, he resigned himself to accept this "second opinion."

The scheduled surgery was pending, and Mrs. C. and Dr. K. stressed the urgency of the decision. When Judge D. mentioned the case to his wife, a nurse, she asked if a hysterectomy or a hysterectomy/oophorectomy was intended. Judge D. had not known there was a difference, so he had not asked. After clarifying that a hysterectomy/oophorectomy would halt hormone production, thus affecting the development of secondary sexual characteristics such as breast growth, pubic hair, and body shape, Mrs. C. said her intention was for Colleen to have only the uterus removed. This confusion made Judge D. even more uneasy. He called Sarah and told her to check everything about the case very thoroughly.

Sarah took her role as guardian seriously and was frustrated at being uninformed about sterilization and disability. When alerted to the fact that Down syndrome was not synonymous with "severe disability," Sarah checked a psychological evaluation that had been done seven months earlier. Colleen's score on the Stanford-Binet was 51 (borderline between mild and moderate MR), which "was consistent with scores from previous testings" and "was better than normally seen in children with Down syndrome." She scored in "kindergarten to first grade range academically, expected for a child with her mental age." Although Colleen was eligible for classes for "educable mentally retarded" persons, the psychologist recommended that she "continue in the trainable class" because "the curriculum was more appropriate for her." He noted that Colleen had "a speech dysfluency and severe articulation problem which made her hard to understand and presented difficulty in communicating"; however, her receptive language was quite good. The psychologist maintained, "There is no evidence of mental health or behavioral problems, Colleen is easy to work with, a well-adjusted child who presents no problems in the testing situation." "Well adjusted," "cooperative," "congenial," and "cheerful" were terms used by her two teachers, her mother, and Sarah. Friendly with classmates of both genders, unlike some 12-year-olds, Colleen had shown no signs of romantic interest in boys. Her mother predicted that "because of her immaturity, I don't think that she'll be interested in boys for awhile."

The rationale given for a hysterectomy, rather than a tubal ligation, was hygiene. Yet she had already had three periods. At her first menses, Colleen said to her mother that there was "catsup" on her panties, but she was not upset about the bleeding. Colleen's two sisters were a year or two older, so perhaps she was more aware of menstruation than she was given credit for in the doctors' letters. With reminding, Colleen changed the sanitary pads by herself. The teacher said, "Students less able than Colleen care for their menstruation. Colleen will be independent because she wants to keep herself clean." Hygiene is a usual part of the curriculum for moderate MR children. A previous teacher who taught Colleen for six years said, "Colleen handled the physical parts of taking care of herself very well. Even in preschool, she had "few accidents with urine or bowels."

Mrs. C. said her decision to seek sterilization for Colleen was motivated by fear of pregnancy. She worried that, if Colleen got pregnant, the family would face a difficult decision about abortion or about what to do with a child, especially if the child were handicapped. Not opposed to abortion herself, she worried what others would think if she was forced to seek an abortion for Colleen. Although Colleen was not interested in boys or sex and was always in supervised settings, Mrs. C. worried about her "vulnerability to rape while at the sitter's house or on the bus. Even at home, someone could break through the screen and rape her." She felt because of her reticence: "Colleen would not tell me if she were raped. She would suffer in silence. That's her usual reaction to stress or problems."

Mrs. C.'s second concern was that Colleen might "have an accident with her periods at school and [nonhandicapped] kids would notice," which would result in "ridicule and embarrassment" not only for Colleen, but also for her sisters. Mrs. C. had not been in favor of moving the moderate class from a special school to the new middle school because she worried about teasing and because Lisa, her middle daughter, had been very upset when she learned that she and Colleen would be in the same school.

A third concern was that others would have to help Colleen with her periods. Involving others in unpleasant duties would reflect negatively on the family, and they would spread rumors and shun them. She worried that Colleen's stepfather and stepbrothers might witness "disgusting things." Mrs. C. did not want her husband to "take care of Colleen's mess. I leave for work an hour earlier than everybody else and they're responsible for getting Colleen off to school." At the same time, Mrs. C. said her daughter "was very independent in getting dressed and eating breakfast but had a couple of accidents [blood on her sheets]."

Mrs. C.'s first husband left when her daughters were four, two, and one. She felt the birth of a Down syndrome child was mainly responsible for the breakup. Previously a housewife, she was forced to make day-care arrangements when she went to work in the medical records department at the local hospital—a job she had held for 11 years. Her first husband did not stay in contact with his daughters, nor was he consistent in support payments. In fact, she had received no support for seven years. Mrs. C. tearfully told of the lonely, worrisome years as a single mother. A year earlier, Mrs. C. married a man with two sons the same ages of her older daughters. Although his ex-wife had custody of the boys, they were increasingly at Mr. and Mrs. C.'s house because of conflicts with their stepfather. Alluding to problems of blended families and stressing the importance of making this marriage work, Mrs. C. was obsessed with not burdening her husband with unpleasant duties. A conscientious mother and wife, Mrs. C. felt the hysterectomy would simplify things and diminish anxieties.

Sarah took a keen interest in Colleen, particularly after Colleen had taken the "visitor" on a tour of the school. Hard to understand at first, Sarah found within minutes she adjusted to Colleen's "accent." At one point, Sarah observed Colleen give a quick wave to a girl in a cheerleader's outfit who looked like her. After they passed, Colleen proudly whispered the girl was her sister Lisa. Sarah's impression was that Colleen had been coached not to make their association known. Sarah called Colleen "a dignified little lady who is a pleasure to be around."

In preparing for the case, Sarah addressed these questions: Will Colleen want to be a mother, and would she be an adequate mother? Will she want to have sexual intercourse? Is she at risk of sexual abuse and pregnancy? Is she capable, or will she be capable at some later date, of making her own decision about contraception? What kind of birth control method is best for her? Is she able to take care of the personal hygiene connected with having a period? In collecting responses, she realized there were no absolute answers for many of her questions.

The psychologist who tested Colleen declined to answer many questions: "I do not know Colleen all that well, and many of your questions rely on issues I'm not sure about, like who should become a parent and who should make that decision." He did create a scenario that he imagined for Colleen: "She might live in a group home or somewhere she could receive supervision if she leaves home. A statistical leveling off in IQ means she is unlikely to advance mentally more than a couple of years by adulthood and I suspect that she will not be able to understand the abstract concept of sterilization. I do not believe she could adequately care for a child at any time in the future."

Colleen's teachers drew up "probabilities," projecting that "Colleen will want to participate in caring for children—like being an involved aunt—but having full responsibility will be too hard for her and she will get frustrated. She will want to be part of a family—she is affectionate and loyal—but she will not want to head a family. It is reasonable to assume that she has sexual drive and will want the intimacy and closeness of a sexual relationship; because of immaturity, she will probably be older than many girls when an interest in sex first develops. Concerning vulnerability, because Colleen is always supervised, her risk of abuse from strangers is remote. She likes her space, asserts her preferences, and would reject sexual advances unless they were from someone she trusted or to whom she felt beholden. She will probably tell if abuse occurs unless she feels like it is her fault or fears the perpetrator. Colleen is able to state that her body is her own and that others need her permission before they touch her. She has learned to say "no" very loudly and ask for help when someone does something she does not like. We have done abuse protection training with our students. With information and education, she will understand birth control options and, with support, she can decide which technique is best for her if she becomes sexually active. Because she is unlikely to want to become pregnant, a tubal ligation might be the safest, most convenient method in the long run. She is conscientious so any short-term method would work as well for her as for any other woman. Regarding personal hygiene, Colleen discreetly carries a little brown bag with her sanitary pads to the restroom. We have reminded her because Mrs. C. said she would need reminding, but we will work with her on being aware of the need to change pads." When asked about the consequence of having blood show through her clothing, they said: "Children in the moderate class would not notice. Others might notice and snicker but would not make a big deal of it. We have witnessed no teasing of our kids—they are more likely to tease each other. They are kind to—even protective of—our students."

In my discussion with Sarah, we examined how normalization principles might figure in the case. Hysterectomies are not normally done to 12-year-old girls. Regardless of how the surgery is explained to Colleen or others, they will associate it with her retarded condition—a time in the hospital or a scar would further stigmatize her. Although menstruation is rarely valued—on the contrary, it is something women complain about—it is a common experience that serves to bind women together and signify womanhood and adulthood. If Colleen does not menstruate, she will be excluded from the rituals that surround it. In Colleen's case, a hysterectomy will add to the stigma of her condition and further distance her from others.

Sarah talked to her own gynecologist about the medical effects of a hysterectomy on a 12-year-old with Down syndrome. These are the facts that she presented in a brief to the court:

1. A hysterectomy is major surgery; therefore, Colleen would be subject to all the risks of major surgery. Because of Down syndrome, she might have abnormalities that would complicate surgical procedures. (The National Down Syndrome Society includes "dysplastic pelvis," an abnormal development of the pelvis, as a "common characteristic" used for diagnosis of Down syndrome.)

2. A healthy uterus is an organ that plays a role in the body in relation to other organs or systems. It is inadvisable to upset this balance without sound medical reason.

3. The rate of major and minor complications is very high (estimated at between 20 and 45%) for a hysterectomy. Adhesions, in which bodily tissue abnormally grows together causing pain or interfering with other organs, frequently result from surgery.

4. Menstruation is one of the few outward signs of healthy (or problematic) functioning of other (e.g., hormonal) systems. By removing the uterus, signs of dysfunction may go undetected.

5. Major surgery is painful and frightening for anyone, but even more so for a child with cognitive limitations who may not fully understand what is happening to her and why it is being done.

Library research pointed to evidence of diminished sexual response after hysterectomy (Kolodny, 1979; Morgan, 1982; Zussman, Zussman, Sunley, & Bjornson, 1981):

1. During the excitement phase in sexual arousal, blood rushes to the entire pelvic area causing vasocongestion and a feeling of arousal. After the removal of the uterus, there is less tissue in the area to engorge, which may lessen sensation.

2. During sexual excitement, the uterus is elevated into the pelvic cavity. After a hysterectomy, the scar tissue replacing the cervix is inelastic, so it may prevent full ballooning of the vagina.

3. The vagina may be shorter following surgery, or the vaginal stitches may be positioned so that sexual intercourse is painful.

4. During orgasm, the uterus contracts rhythymically; the more severe the contractions and the longer they continue before tapering off, the more intense the woman perceives orgasm. Uterine contractions seem to add to the orgasmic experience.

5. During the postorgasm phase, sexual tension and engorgement of blood gradually recede, and additional orgasms can follow the first one. After a hysterectomy, multiple orgasms are less likely.

Judge D. told Sarah that the evidence on sexual response was "irrelevant" and "far-fetched" and he did not intend to have it introduced in court. Based on the other evidence, he decided that a hysterectomy was counterindicated and that his court would not hear the case again until Colleen was at least 18. Sarah kept her mouth shut, but she had concluded that the quality of MR individuals' sexual response should enter into decision making.

In most respects, Mrs. C. was reasonable and realistic about Colleen, yet she desperately wanted her sterilized. In an irrational way, Mrs. C. repeated her fear that someone would "break through the screen and rape Colleen." She perseverated on the "accident" of blood getting on sheets or clothes. When asked if the same things might happen to her other daughters, she answered affirmatively, but returned to her conviction that a hysterectomy was in Colleen's best interest. There appeared to be hidden motives for the hysterectomy. Mrs. C. may have suspected, or even known, that Colleen was being sexually molested by either her husband or her teenaged stepsons. This would explain why she felt compelled to stress how difficult it was to raise children alone and to justify her desire to stay married, although these seemed to have no bearing on the court case. This possibility also explained her obsessive desire to have nobody in the family get close to Colleen to help with personal functions, her impatience in getting the sterilization done, and her reluctance to put it off until Colleen was older and sexually active. When informed that most sexual abuse was done by someone known to the victim and that mental health services were available for families with such problems, she hesitantly replied: "I know. I work at the hospital and check people into the Mental Health Center" and promptly changed the subject. Perhaps she, her friends, and her co-workers all lived too close together in this small town to make channels of support feasible. Mrs. C. was silent about the possibility of within-family sexual abuse.

ROGER

Roger was a "surprise" child born 15 years after David, his only sibling. Within his first year, Roger was diagnosed as having a mild case of cerebral palsy, which affected the left side of his body, leaving his arm and leg clumsy and limp. At the end of his second year, his parents were not surprised to learn he had developmental delays, although they hated to hear "mentally retarded." Speech therapy was added to the physical therapy he received twice a week at the local hospital. When Roger was four years old, he started at a preschool sponsored by United Cerebral Palsy located in a church on the other side of town. Roger was thrilled to ride in the van and loved his teachers and peers. In spite of speech impediments, Mrs. Peterson wrote in Roger's babybook that her four-year-old was an "expressive and social child, who loves attention and affection." Roger attended the half-day preschool until, at seven, he went to a school sponsored by the ARC that was in a somewhat restored, ancient four-room schoolhouse. Although he liked school, Mrs. Peterson worried about Roger being in the same building with the "big kids" and felt justified in keeping Roger home frequently.

Mrs. Peterson taught elementary school prior to David's birth and since then had done substitute teaching. Mr. Peterson was a pharmacist. By the time Roger was born, David was in high school and was an outstanding student, active in many activities. David was excited about Roger's arrival and was an affectionate older brother. Although the Petersons did not go out much, David took care of his younger brother when they did. The brothers enjoyed each other, and as Mrs. Peterson said: "Roger worships David."

When Roger was nine, his ARC school closed, and students were dispersed throughout the district to "educable," "trainable," or "custodial" classes. Roger was sent to a trainable class in a town about 10 miles from his home. Besides disliking the fact that he would be farther away from home than before, his parents worried that he would "be teased by regular kids." As Mrs. Peterson said: "I've taught in all the schools and I know how cruel kids can be—not all of them, but it only takes one to cause a problem." After some "fierce battles with the school administration that got us nowhere," they resigned themselves to what Mr. Peterson sarcastically called "the improvement." To their relief, Roger preferred the new school— the longer van ride was seen as a plus. The Petersons admitted that Roger "probably was bored seeing the same faces every day at the ARC school."

When he was 13, Roger went to junior high school. He had the option of riding the regular bus or the special education bus. Without hesitation, his parents selected the special bus. At some point, they told David about their choice. David had finished graduate school and was working as an engineer in a city about 60 miles from his parents' home. He had married a woman he met in graduate school, also an engineer, and they were expecting their first child. David asked if it was Roger's choice that he ride the special education bus. The Petersons admitted that they had not asked him. David asked Roger about the two buses. Roger had always loved vehicles, especially buses. They teased him about being "a bus driver" when he grew up. Roger told David that he would like to ride the "big bus with Charlie." The Petersons were not happy with David's interference, but asked school officials if they could change their minds. In the third week of school, their eighth-grade neighbor, Charlie, arrived at their door to accompany Roger to the bus stop. Roger was delighted; his parents were nervous. Within a couple of weeks, Roger was getting to and from the bus stop, which was three blocks away, on his own. Perhaps because the popular Charlie accompanied him the first few days, schoolmates greeted Roger as a "buddy," but never included him in their social events.

By the time Roger was in high school, the Petersons were concerned about his "taking off on his own." Sometimes he walked down to the store from the bus stop after school. Occasionally he ended up at somebody's house. He knew how to call home, but usually forgot. He was in work-study classes, so he had job experiences at various locations in the city and had learned to ride the city bus. He became more and more venture-some, often heading off on foot for fast-food shops several miles from home. His parents punished him when he did this, and although he was apologetic, before long he was missing again. In spite of his limp, he moved at a fast pace and had a surprisingly good sense of direction. He had never gotten lost. In fact, he often corrected his parents when they were confused about a location.

By the time Roger received his certificate of attendance (an alternative to a diploma for students who had been in moderate-level special education classes) at age 19, he had a "survival vocabulary" that allowed him to function in the community fairly well. He recognized common things on menus and knew warning and direction signs. He was careless with money, but could make change for a dollar accurately when he took his time. He had a good sense of the price of things that he was likely to buy, but these were mainly items under five dollars. His math and writing skills were not good enough to successfully use a checkbook.

Roger had mixed reviews on his work-study assignments. He had high self-esteem and did not seem bothered by occasional teasing. In spite of years of speech therapy, Roger was still difficult to understand. This did not stop him from talking. His cheerful personality made him popular with teachers and peers in special and regular education classes, and these social graces continued to serve him well in out-of-school settings. On the other hand, his poor coordination and careless "let's get this work over with and go attitude" (as described by one of his employers) interfered with job success. During his last year in high school, in planning for the transition from school to work, special education and Vocational Rehabilitation personnel decided to start Roger out in a job enclave arrangement at a motel with four other MR workers. Roger had to get soiled linen from the room cleaners (three of the four were MR workers), take it to the laundry room, put it in the washers and driers, fold the linen, and put it back in the carts correctly. Roger was responsible for keeping the laundry room tidy and for stocking the cleaners' carts with toilet articles. Roger seemed to like this work, but his usual casualness and lack of perfectionism meant the job coach had to get after him about being neat and sticking to tasks through completion. In spite of constructive feedback, he got even sloppier. And Roger was paying too much attention to the room cleaners and hotel receptionists. He hung around and talked when he was supposed to be in the laundry room. Roger's job coach felt he was bored with the work. Roger was transferred to a carwash. When that closed down, he bused in a cafeteria. He typically worked four to six hours a day and had classes at the local adult ARC Center for two to three hours in the afternoon.

Roger lived at home and rode public transit buses to work and the ARC Center. In the evening, Roger and his parents did things together. Roger gave them the excuse to go for ice cream, to movies, to the park—to "stay young," as Mr. Peterson said. Mr. Peterson turned 70 the same year Roger finished high school and was gradually turning his pharmacy over to a nephew who had worked with him for several years. When he was 71, Mr. Peterson had a stroke and spent several months in a convalescent center. About the time he was to come home, Mrs. Peterson was diagnosed with cancer and was hospitalized. Although there was a waiting list for the group homes, David convinced the managers of the urgency of the situation and got Roger placed on what was to be a temporary basis. The death of both parents within the year made him a permanent resident at the adult men's home.

In contrast to David's fears, Roger adjusted well to the group home, but suddenly his interest in sexual intimacy with women became apparent. When Roger lived at home, David had seen few signs of interest in sex, with the exception of occasional public masturbation when he was younger. Roger quickly stopped touching his genitals when his parents reminded him that it was "not nice." Suddenly, David noticed that Roger was staring at his own wife and giggling. He was also giggling in a prepubescent way at girls and women in restaurants or places they took him on weekend visits.

Perhaps the sudden severing of home ties had triggered this seemingly urgent interest in women and sex.

Roger had not been at the group home long when David was contacted about a concern on the part of both residential and vocational staff. Roger had a number of freedoms at the home because it was for high-functioning clients; however, he was disappearing for hours at a time. When he returned, he was vague about where he had been. On the last occasion, they got a call from the manager of a restaurant where Roger had once worked, who said he had been found having sexual relations with one of their MR employees in a supply room. Staff reported that on three occasions he had been found having sexual relations with women (twice with one and once with another) at the ARC Center. They had not brought this to David's attention because they felt that the interactions had been initiated by the women and both were using birth control. Roger's engaging in sexual relations with women in the community caused them to worry about the possibility of impregnation and sexually transmitted disease.

Roger had sexuality education at the ARC Center as well as at the group home. He knew how to use a condom and knew that he was to use a condom during sexual intercourse. Nevertheless, on each occasion that he had engaged in intercourse, the condom was squared away in his wallet. He verbalized responsibilities, but failed to use a condom when it was needed. David shared the worries of group home staff. He knew of laws about paternal responsibility and the accuracy of paternity tests. David felt that, if Roger made someone pregnant, as next of kin he would be responsible for financial repercussions. Besides, he thought it would be irresponsible for Roger to father a child. After he and his wife had two children, David had a vasectomy. He made an appointment with the same urologist who had done his vasectomy the year before.

On the way to the doctor, David explained what was to happen and the rationale for surgery. Roger treated the whole thing like a nice outing with his beloved older brother. David filled out the form for Roger as they chatted in the waiting room. When they were called into the examining room and David introduced Roger, he noted a nervous look come over the doctor's face. David apprised him of his brother's recent sexual behaviors and his own concerns. The doctor turned to Roger and asked if he knew what a vasectomy was. Roger had learned it was easiest to answer "no" to such questions. If you answered "yes," teachers often asked you to explain. The doctor described the nature and purpose of the surgery. He mentioned there would be some pain, but a shot would prevent pain. Roger perseverated on the pain and the shot. He had always fussed about shots. When the doctor asked if he wanted to have the vasectomy, Roger said "no." As David tried to reason with Roger, the doctor excused himself and left the room. In about five minutes, he was back. He asked Roger if he knew that the operation would prevent him from having children. Roger answered "no." He then asked Roger if he wanted to be a father some day. Roger responded "yes." Roger typically mirrored the emotions of those around him and sensed that the doctor was ill at ease and his brother was mad at him. David assumed the doctor would perceive the childishness of Roger's behavior and this would convince him of the importance of surgery, but, instead, the doctor asked David to step outside, adding: "Is he alright in here by himself?" David said: "Sure. I'll be right back, Roger." At that point, Roger started to cry. David had not seen Roger cry in about 15 years. The doctor announced that David should call him and left the room.

When David called, the doctor informed him that he had consulted his partner and lawyer and both advised against the vasectomy. David's protest caused the doctor to impatiently say: "There are too many risks. I am not going to do it unless you get a court order." David was a busy man. He had been promoted in his job, he had a young family, and he and his wife were restoring an older home. He had taken time off "to get this thing done" and was frustrated that he would have to spend more time making sure that Roger would not by chance end up a father. He knew he could draw from Roger's inheritance for court costs if he had to go that route, but he could not pay himself back for the time. Besides, he did not like the idea of court. He might look bad if he ended up with the wrong judge. On the other hand, Roger was a willing participant in sexual affairs, and he would continue to be erratic about condom use. When he was not apologizing "for doing bad things," he was bragging about who "loved him."

When they were in the doctor's office, it was the first time David had thought that Roger might want to be a father. Roger always presented himself as a child. On family occasions, even now, Roger expected to be with the children. David criticized his mother for being overprotective and wondered if Roger would act like an adult if he had been treated more like one. Roger showed little comprehension of conversation between David and his wife. To include him, they talked about television kid shows, his work, or the group home. Conversations were stilted. Roger had shown little interest in David's children; he mainly seemed jealous of the attention shown them. David had seen no evidence of parenting behaviors or desires in Roger.

After an initial outburst at Roger in the car on the way home from the doctor's office, David tried to put the whole thing out of his mind. Saturday was his wedding anniversary, and he did not want to spoil the weekend by dwelling on this matter. They always had Roger one weekend a month, and this happened to be the designated weekend. David realized he was starting to resent Roger. He and his wife would have celebrated by going out to dinner and the theater, but they could not leave the girls alone with Roger, and they knew that any of their usual teenaged sitters would be uncomfortable having Roger around.

As Roger was delivered on Sunday night, Greg, the group home manager, greeted the brothers with a "Well how did it go?" Roger was silent as David explained what had happened. David crossly said: "I think Roger should be grounded until he can show that he is responsible enough to use a condom. If he is not going to have a vasectomy, he is going to have to use something else." Bothered by his brother's anger, Roger assured David and Greg: "I will. I will next time," to which David's disgusted response was "When have we heard that before?" Greg walked David to the car and encouraged him to call other physicians and volunteered to work on a plan to better prepare Roger for consenting to surgery.

Greg discussed the situation with group home staff. Because Roger was sexually active with willing partners and had not used condoms during intercourse, they all felt a vasectomy was a good idea. It would be impossible to ground him without drastically restricting his freedom. He took public transportation to work and was one of the few clients who walked places to spend his earnings. The home was a mile away from the nearest grocery, but Roger still took off, regardless of the weather, to buy treats. They decided to add preparation for a vasectomy to his Individual Habilitation Plan (IHP) and drew up these goals: (1) State the pros and cons of parenthood; (2) list factors necessary for good parenting; (3) realistically state his own (lack of) parenting skills; (4) state whether or not he wants to be a father; (5) describe what happens in a vasectomy; (6) list men he knows who have had vasectomies (including a staff member and David); (7) list effects of a vasectomy (some pain with a numbing shot, some pain as the anesthestic wears off, some itching as the incision heals); (8) state his willingness to endure discomfort; (9) list advantages of not impregnating during intercourse. An obligatory routine was to share all IHP revisions with clients' relatives and Mary, the Director of Residential Options. After Greg sent out the revised IHP, he received enthusiastic approval from David and disapproval from Mary. Greg had never had an IHP or a revision rejected, so he had already gone ahead with the program. Roger was an eager, if not efficient, learner. He liked the extra attention.

Greg argued the importance of training and David's support. Mary was persistent in her claim: "This is not training, it's brainwashing. You are getting him to accept his brother's decision, and he already said he does not want the vasectomy." Greg had gotten into morality battles with Mary before. He felt she was too conservative about sex; that she really would prefer clients not be allowed sexual rights in group homes. When MR women had sexual relations, she often said they were "being taken advantage of" or "raped." Although in charge of the male home, Greg felt that the women were more interested in sex than the men. He knew Mary was in the Right to Life movement and had heard her say that sterilization "interfered with the gift of life." Yet Mary was an efficient administrator. He joked with colleagues that Mary often hired people who did not agree with her.

Because Mary and Greg could not agree, they turned to Marv, who was head of all ARC services. Mary did not mention objection to sterilization, but stuck with the brainwashing argument. Greg countered that training was "essentially brainwashing. They don't want to brush their teeth, clean their rooms, or exercise but we get them to see the advantage of these things or just make them do them. How is this different?" Marv was predisposed to side with Greg. He had a vasectomy over 15 years ago and was sold on it. Also, David called Marv about Mary's opposition. He and the Petersons had been good friends, and he admired David's concern about Roger. Many clients had been abandoned by family. On the other hand, Mary was a jewel of an employee, and he could see how fired up she was. Typically compromising, she was not about to change her mind this time. Marv asked for the IHP revision, remarking that he "would need time to think this over." He was glad to get the two tense people out of his office.

The next day Marv started his conversation by stating the importance of working cooperatively with family and respecting their morality systems; then, he informed Mary that they should go along with the training since David wanted it. This was the wrong approach. One of Mary's strengths was working well with families, and she was insulted at Marv's opening speech. She grunted at his announcement, but continued to stew. Marv's siding with Greg undermined her authority. She had hired Greg two years earlier and had backed his promotion to manager. In this case, she felt if David wanted the training for Roger, he should do it himself. She respected a family's positions even when they conflicted with her beliefs, but this situation was unsettling. She felt Roger was too childish to be sexually involved and everybody was giving him the go-ahead. She had known Mrs. Peterson well and thought "she would not like to see this happening." After two days of fretting, Mary called Marv, got his answering machine, and notified him that this was a decision for the Human Rights Commission (HRC), a five-member board set up by the ARC agency to review practices to make sure clients' rights were not violated. Members of the Human Rights Commission reviewed IHPs annually, but rarely saw midyear revisions. Marv had mixed feelings about the message: relief that the decision was to be passed on to another authority and worry that the "whole thing might blow up on us," especially considering the intensity of Mary's feelings and her involvement with several community groups. Mary was middle-aged and single, and he secretly thought of her as "the nun," as much for her prudishness as her dedicated service.

David was not happy about the delay. Once he decided that a vasectomy for Roger was urgent, he was ready to get on with it. He wrote to the HRC stating the reasons for Roger to have a vasectomy. David argued that it was the only male contraception other than a condom and that, in spite of training, Roger had not used a condom properly. He mentioned the times Roger had been known to have sexual relations and went on to state that Roger clearly enjoyed and sought out these interactions. David also said that Roger enjoyed the freedom of going places in the community on foot and by public transit. At 24, Roger had the mental age of a four- to 5-year-old and a prognosis of not maturing significantly in years to come. He argued that Roger was not capable of providing for himself or children either financially or emotionally. He described Roger's immature role in his own family and stated that Roger had never given any indication of wanting to be a parent. Finally, he told of his worry about his own financial liability if Roger were to father a child. David added that group home staff were willing to do the training detailed in the IHP revision.

Perhaps it was no coincidence that Mary was a representative on the HRC. The other staff member was Marcia, an aide in the sheltered workshop. Mrs. Knight, parent of a preschooler, was chair, and Ms. Dunn, the parent of a daughter who attended adult day care, was a member. The last member was Dr. Dewey, a special education faculty member at the university. Mary admitted that she opposed the training on the grounds that it was not informing Roger of his options, but was brainwashing him to accept his brother's preference. She said she worried that the message conveyed to Roger was that it was okay to be sexually active—promiscuous, really, and that it did not matter if he had multiple partners. She also said that the vasectomy would not protect Roger from sexually transmitted diseases and so it was only a partial solution to potential problems from the kind of sexual behavior in which Roger was engaging. She felt the elder Petersons would have liked Roger to have more emphasis on the morality of his acts rather than just letting him do anything he wanted. She then excused herself from the meeting, saying that it was up to the other four to make the decision. Dr. Dewey asked her to respond to David's points before leaving. She agreed Roger was substantially retarded, that he would not make a good parent because of his immaturity, and that he probably was a willing partner in sexual intercourse, but disagreed about his inability to use a condom. She stated her belief that he needed more supervision and less freedom in the community. Then she said: "You know he could meet somebody higher functioning and she might want children. She might be perfectly capable of taking care of a baby. You never know. I have seen very normal people marry our clients and they do okay."

After Mary left the meeting, Ms. Dunn said she appreciated the validity of Mary's arguments, but felt that the brother's point of view, as the only living relative in the immediate family, should be respected. Mrs. Knight disagreed that the relative's request was the most important issue for them to consider, stating: "After all, if our mission is simply to endorse the parent's position, there is no reason for us to exist." She went on to say: "I guess I agree with both David and Mary—Roger should have the vasectomy, but he should continue to be taught the importance of using a condom, and his movement in the community might need more monitoring. He already attends church. Friends of his parents pick him up every Sunday for church. I don't know what else staff can do about morality." Marcia told the group that Roger had very successfully used public transportation for work, shopping, and getting to the YMCA and that it would be hard to monitor him and still let him develop skills for independent living—a goal for all clients. Marcia also reminded them that "three of the four occasions in which he had been caught having sex were right under their noses" in the sheltered workshop. Once he had been found in a nook behind the soda machines, another time in a supply closet, and the third time in a classroom that was empty except for Roger and his partner. With some uneasiness, the four voted unanimously to allow the training as specified in the IHP. They recommended that he continue to be trained to use the condom and be educated about the importance of restricting partners. Mary was not happy, but told a friend, "I did what I could, I have a clear conscience about this."

Three months later, David scheduled an appointment with a urologist in the town where Roger's group home was located. Before the appointment, David sent the doctor a copy of his letter to the HRC, as well as their reply to him. The doctor asked Roger the same questions asked by the last doctor. Roger replied that he knew a vasectomy would "keep me from being a dad" and that he did "not want babies." He dealt with the information about surgery by expressing some apprehension about the pain, but later proudly told David: "I was brave. I was a big boy." He got the banana split he had been offered for cooperation.

At 27, Roger married Marilla, a 35-year-old mildly MR woman he met at work. They had gone steady for about two years and had talked about marriage from the start. Marilla said she wanted children, but did not seem very bothered by their infertility. She literally took care of Roger, who was pleased with the arrangement. The main difficulty in their marriage was that, as Marilla said, "He likes to be on the go and I like to stay put. Sometimes I don't trust him with the women." David had found better employment in a city about 600 miles away, and his brother's marriage lessened his guilt about deserting him. Roger and Marilla visited his family at Christmas, and David spent a few days taking them to an amusement park or camping in the summer. There appeared to be no regrets about the vasectomy.

TRISH

Trish arrived at the Residential Program for Adolescents with Autism (RPAA) two months after her fifteenth birthday. Aside from attending classes for multiply handicapped youth in her rural school district, Trish had spent all her waking hours at home with her parents, her 14-year-old brother, Tom, and her 5-year-old brother, Marcus. Because of her loudness, violence, and unpredictable darting-away behavior, for 10 of the past 15 years the McNeils had almost never taken her out of their home. Trish's behaviors had restricted the whole family's activities. Only recently had Mr. and Mrs. McNeil gone out alone, leaving the capable Tom in charge of his two siblings.

Dissatisfied with local school programming, the McNeils felt that Trish's behaviors had deteriorated. The teacher let Trish pace on the far side of the classroom for hours and admitted that she and her aide were intimidated by Trish's aggressions. This bothered Mrs. McNeil, but she understood. Trish had often hurt members of her family when frustrated or agitated. Both parents were hopeful that Trish would adjust and make progress at the RPAA, but were skeptical because they knew that Trish did not like changes. They worried that staff would not tolerate her moaning or her pinching and scratching. Mrs. McNeil had checked that Trish was toilet trained, but recently she had had accidents once or twice a day. She thought RPAA staff might think that she had lied about toilet training so Trish would be admitted to the program.

Trish was one of eight adolescents attending school and living at the RPAA. She was the most severely retarded and was violent to anyone who moved into her space or tried to get her to do something she did not want to do. Trish had no oral or sign language communication and understood only simple two- to three-word commands. Perhaps due to her mother's patient training, Trish's strong areas were self-care and housecleaning. She could wash and dry dishes and put them on cabinet shelves in an orderly manner. She washed counters and dusted. Trish could dress herself, wash her hands, shower independently, and brush her teeth. And, supposedly, she was toilet trained.

Much to the McNeil's relief, Trish adjusted surprisingly well to life at the RPAA. The McNeils' house was small, and the RPAA had spacious classrooms and living quarters. Trish was a pacer and appreciated space. She had her own room, but shared the three-bedroom group home with another female and a male—the three "lowest functioning" students. Because these three had the most erratic sleep patterns and were the least social and most antisocial, it was decided that they should have private rooms. The other five lived in an identical home across the courtyard.

All eight adolescents attended school in the same two-classroom unit that was attached to, but not administratively part of, a local public elementary and junior high school. The school unit was about two blocks from the group homes. Trish clearly enjoyed the walk—for her, the run—from the group home to the classroom, which the students did four times a day. Although Trish was 5 feet 4 inches and weighed 130 pounds, she loved the sturdy playground swings and a double-sided wooden glider in the courtyard. There were few exits to the courtyard, so Trish could run freely there, a treat she had never been allowed in their yard at home. Trish was a "runner," and Mrs. McNeil had worried that she would run off. With the exception of Tom, Trish was the fastest member of the family. She was also a good climber, so they had to watch her around trees and fences.

Trish's favorite thing about being at the RPAA was going to the Y three times a week. She liked riding in cars, and the five-mile van trip was culminated by running the indoor track, swimming, and showering in an open round shower. In spite of her sour temperament, she lightened up at the Y. It was one setting in which Trish made physical contact with others; while in the swimming pool, Trish wrapped her legs around the male recreation assistant and laughed raucously on three occasions. (Trish had straddled males twice: once in the classroom when a teacher was slouching back in a chair and once in the group home when an assistant was lying on his back on the floor.)

It was when Trish was showering after swimming at the Y that a recreation coordinator noticed her protruding abdomen and enlarged breasts. Trish weighed 130 pounds when she arrived at RPAA; now, two months later, she weighed 142 pounds. They put Trish on a low-calorie diet when she weighed 138, but she seemed frantic about food, often snatching it off people's plates. When they got back to the RPAA, the recreation coordinator promptly called the program director, Ann Harms, to share her observation that Trish might be pregnant. A home pregnancy test administered the next morning turned out to be positive. A nurse practitioner at Planned Parenthood did a pelvic exam on Trish in the afternoon and confirmed the pregnancy, estimating Trish was between 16 and 20 weeks along. The nurse also said that Trish's genitalia resembled those of someone with considerable sexual experience, which indicated that the pregnancy probably did not result from a one-time sexual intercourse experience. Ann Harms was left with the difficult task of informing the McNeils. Because Trish was a minor and could not verbally consent to sexual intercourse, Harms also called Child Protective Services to report the case.

A telephone call to the McNeils got silence, then "Are you sure?" The McNeils' home was in the northern part of the state about 200 miles from the RPAA, but they arrived within three and a half hours of the call. They packed Trish's belongings and headed for home, but not before Harms informed them that she had reported the pregnancy to Child Protective Services, who would be contacting their counterparts in the McNeils' hometown. She watched Mr. McNeil when she made this announcement, but his face remained impassive. Because of Trish's negative reaction to strangers and her need for constant supervision, the director assumed the pregnancy had resulted from incest. The McNeils said they "never left Trish alone," had never hired a babysitter. In Harms' opinion, the most likely perpetrator was Mr. McNeil. Tom was shorter and thinner than his sister— younger-looking than his 14 years, so Harms dismissed him as a suspect.

A few days later, Harms got a request from Mrs. McNeil that Trish return to the RPAA. The director assumed that Trish had had an abortion. Second-trimester abortions are illegal in the state, but not in two neighboring states. They had given this information to the McNeils. On questioning, Harms learned that the family doctor had told the McNeils that second-trimester abortions are very dangerous. Harms expressed concern about the RPAA providing safe and appropriate programming for Trish. Mrs. McNeil's response was: "Do you mean you are going to deny her an education because she is pregnant?" Harms had not expected this, but said that she would speak to the program's attorney.

Harms shared her concerns about risks with the attorney. First, Trish had pica, which meant that she frequently ate such inedibles as nuts and bolts, plastic toys, cleaning fluids, and soap, which, Harms feared, could have disastrous effects on the developing fetus. Trish liked to run and appreciated the open spaces of the RPAA. Sure-footed and well coordinated, Trish had never been observed to fall, but Harms worried that the pregnancy would interfere with her balance and she might injure herself and/or the baby. The RPAA group homes had sturdy tile-covered cement stairs and tiled bathroom facilities—both slippery and hard. It would be easy for Trish to slip.

Although Trish was the most aggressive of the clients, a couple of others pushed and attacked when provoked or stressed. Finally, Trish was nonverbal and would not be able to communicate when she was in labor. Harms did not want her college-aged staff to have to deliver Trish's baby. On the other hand, as Mrs. McNeil had so aptly put it, they did not want to deny Trish an educaton because she was pregnant. Even if she had not been a feminist, the director would have seen the logic of that argument.

The attorney agreed that they could not deny Trish an education, but cautioned that the RPAA needed to protect itself in case an accident occurred. Staff identified risks for the McNeils to consider, and then the attorney drew up a waiver-of-responsibility paper for them to sign. They informed the McNeils that they would keep Trish only through the eighth month of her pregnancy. It was hoped that this timeline would avoid Trish going into labor at the RPAA. Within the week, Trish was back at the RPAA, and it was gratifying to staff that she seemed pleased to be there and even hugged the residential assistants.

They gave Trish the ground-floor bedroom and declared the upstairs off limits. A staff member accompanied her around the clock. They no longer took her on community excursions because the pregnancy was obvious and would raise too many questions among onlookers. Instead of going to the Y, they took Trish to a private home pool that belonged to an acquaintance of a staff member. They felt swimming—or, in Trish's case, thrashing around in the pool—was the safest form of exercise for her. Additionally, water had a calming influence on the frenetic girl. The next three months passed relatively uneventfully; however, Trish pounded her abdomen and bellyflopped onto beds, couches, and even the floor. Everyone assumed she did this to get rid of what to her must have been a mysterious and bothersome bump.

In the meantime, Mrs. McNeil called "15 obstetricians" before she found one willing to deliver Trish's baby. Dr. Thomas almost changed his mind and refused when he learned that Mrs. McNeil wanted Trish to have a tubal ligation. Dr. Thomas had seen Trish during her week at home when she was about five months' pregnant. Mrs. McNeil had warned Dr. Thomas about Trish, but he was still shocked to hear a loud racket in his office. A quick surveillance of his waiting room revealed Trish being physically restrained by her mother and grandmother, although she still was able to pound her head on the wall and wail. His other patients appeared to be in a state of shock and readily agreed that Trish could be examined before them. Thomas made arrangements for a colleague in the town where the RPAA was located to do the remaining prenatal examinations, and a part-time nurse at the RPAA checked Trish's blood pressure and urine on a biweekly basis. Dr. Thomas scheduled a date four months in the future for Trish to have a Caesarean section in a local public hospital. The Catholic hospital where he usually delivered babies would not allow the tubal ligation. Dr. Thomas informed the McNeils that he would not do the sterilization unless they received court permission, which, it turned out, meant that he would have to spend half a day in court giving evidence about the rationale for sterilization.

The McNeils got their lawyer to petition the circuit court judge for permission for the sterilization, but the judge insisted on a "full blown hearing" and assigned a guardian ad litem to the case. Evidence was gathered about the severity and permanency of Trish's mental retardation and autism. These conditions were documented not only by videotapes of Trish at the RPAA, but also by Trish's presence in court on the day. After 10 minutes of listening to Trish roar and bang into the benches, the peaked-looking judge dismissed her from the courtroom.

Dr. Thomas gave evidence that temporary forms of birth control were not feasible. Trish was already on a number of medications, so the birth control pill was not recommended. She was not capable of using temporary barrier methods, and because of lawsuits, no one was taking chances on any of the previously effective intrauterine devices. Although Dr. Thomas had no information about Trish's chances of having a normal baby, he did express the belief that she had no sense of protecting her fetus. He described how Trish had flailed around on his examining table and had flopped off, in spite of the attempts of her mother and grandmother to hold her down. They had eventually given up and done the pelvic examination on the floor. Dr. Thomas stated that because this pregnancy was probably the result of incest, he suspected that the baby would not be normal. The judge granted permission for the tubal ligation and said he would make sure law enforcement officers pursued the sexual abuse charges.

Staff at the RPAA were relieved when Trish left for maternity leave. Many volunteered their time to go to her home and the hospital to help before and after the birth of her baby. Trish had a seven-pound baby boy, diagnosed at birth as microcephalic and likely to be severely MR. Trish showed no maternal instinct; in fact, she ignored her son. Blood tests drawn from the baby and the three males (father, brother, uncle) who had access to her at the time of conception revealed that Trish's 14-year-old brother, Tom, had fathered her baby. Because he was a juvenile, the "rape" was not prosecuted, but Tom, and other family members, had to undergo a year of counseling at the Mental Health Center.

The McNeils raised the baby for the first few years. As predicted, his developmental delays were significant. His temperament, however, was the opposite of Trish's—he was calm and complacent to the point of being lethargic. Trish returned for three more years of education at the RPAA. Unfortunately, her education there was not sufficient to prepare her for existing group-home living and community or sheltered employment. After spending a year at home, because of other family problems, she was placed in a state hospital for MR persons. At about the same time, Trish's son went to a group home for severely MR children.

PENNY

On Penny Carter's eleventh birthday, she had been at the Residential Diagnostic Center for Children with Autism for just over a year. The Center was designed for students to stay no more than six months, but in seven years of operation the average stay was a little over a year and a half. Staff observed students 24 hours a day, kept detailed notes of behaviors, experimented with interventions, designed personalized programs for students, and returned to the home community with them to teach care providers effective techniques. Philosophically aligned with the deinstitutionalization movement, staff were continually frustrated by the lack of appropriate services in communities. School districts clustered students in special classes with these labels: mild, moderate, and severe. Penny, like others with autism, did not fall neatly into one of these categories. Penny had first been placed in a primary class for moderate MR children. The teacher felt Penny was more emotionally disturbed than retarded, so in fourth grade she was transferred to a class for children with serious emotional handicaps. Although Penny had a number of phobias and neurotic behaviors, she did not fit with her peers. She was the only girl in the class, and, perhaps partly because of her bizarre mannerisms and strange behaviors, she was shunned and teased. With the exception of a youngster diagnosed as a "voluntary mute," the other five had been placed in the class because of hostile acting-out behaviors. Their loud and feisty demeanors intimidated and agitated Penny. Penny began to throw tantrums when the special education school bus came to pick her up. The Carters were convinced the present placement was not suitable and were determined to find a calm environment in which Penny could trust those around her and settle down. At the suggestion of the special education director, the Carters had Penny tested at the Diagnostic Center and, shortly thereafter, enrolled her in the program even though they were reluctant to have Penny live so far away from them. As a result of the continuing dearth of appropriate local services, Penny was already into her second year in the program.

Penny's IQ composite score was slightly less than 50, which put her at the high end of the moderate MR range. Although her sentence structure was immature—she typically spoke in two- to three-word sentences—she had a fairly large vocabulary. Penny could usually make her needs and wants known to others. Her receptive language was also fairly good in everyday situations, although she got anxious when she did not understand something. Penny's score on the adaptive behavior inventory was one of the highest of the 27 students who had ever been at the Center. She was efficient in life skills and was usually responsive in social situations. Penny consistently recognized words and symbols connected with everyday living. She used adaptive systems with money and could match amount cards with coins or dollar bills, so she could laboriously figure out the cost of an item.

Penny was a favorite at the center. Although she tended to be stiff and emotionless, she was cooperative and willing to interact with adults. She knew the people who worked with her and talked about them coming using their names ("Joan coming?"). When someone arrived, she did not greet them immediately, but walked away and paced on the opposite side of the room. Within a minute she was back by their side, smiling to herself. When she was particularly fond of someone, she would huddle against them and stroke their arm or back.

In many ways, Penny was more flexible than her peers at the Center. She did not mind going to new places or trying new things as long as she was accompanied by someone she knew and trusted. She conformed to routines in the group home, but was not unduly rigid about them. She made her bed, cleaned the tub after she bathed, helped prepare meals, set the table, and cleaned up after meals. She was a helpful participant on Saturday cleanup day. She could do laundry—even sort light and dark colors—and loved to dust and wash floors. The one thing she did not like to do is run the vacuum cleaner. That was not a problem as one of her three group home companions loved to vacuum. Staff were also fond of Penny's parents. Although they lived 80 miles away, Tom and Patsy Carter visited Penny as often as they could. They were affectionate with Penny and patient in teaching her. Staff felt their diligence resulted in Penny's high adaptive performance and her numerous social skills. The Carters felt Penny had progressed and were reluctant to have the training come to a close.

Staff's goal for all clients was "successful adjustment," which was defined as "the ability to lead an independent, but socially integrated, life in the community." In spite of many accomplishments, Penny continued to have problems that would interfere with successful adjustment. She became distressed at loud sounds, including almost any volume of motor sounds.

She liked doing laundry, but did not like the sound of the washer and drier, so she would quickly put clothes in or take them out and then scoot away with her hands over her ears, saying "get out of here." She would not work if an electric heater to warm the classroom on cold winter days was turned on. She would fret until someone turned it off. Even the whir of computers bothered her. She would not use them herself and insisted on sitting in a distant part of the classroom when someone else used one. Then she mumbled about them to herself until the computers were turned off. Penny never liked to hear the toilet flush. At home she did not flush the toilet, but had learned to do so at the Center. Again, though, she pushed the flush handle and quickly ran away. Although she liked to go places in vehicles, she periodically covered her ears and commented that it was "too noisy." Penny did not like to listen to the radio or television. Although she tolerated them, she was much calmer when they were off.

It was not only the electronic sounds that got to Penny. She did not like people with loud voices; in fact, she refused to look at them or say their names. Her biggest problem was a fear of babies. She hated the sound of a baby crying. If she saw a baby in the distance, she would say "get out of here" and hightail it off in the opposite direction. Although she was usually careful about crossing streets or staying with staff, under such circumstances she would sprint away without looking where she was going. If a baby cried close to her, she would go berserk. Sometimes she would leave the area screaming "bad Penny," but on a few occasions she had fiercely grabbed the offending child and pinched it with her whole fist with all her might, all the while yelling "bad Penny." She knew it was wrong, but could not stop herself. Staff was very careful in scouting out babies to avoid this disaster. At least five times a day Penny would talk about "hurting baby." This phrase would pop up in contexts in which she was seemingly engaged in what she was doing and in which there were no signs of a baby's presence.

Penny's other debilitating problem was a blood phobia. She panicked and became wildly uncontrollable at the sight of blood—"freaked out" or went "bananas or haywire," as staff would say. If another student was hurt, she would yell and throw herself to the floor or would frantically run to find something with which to hurt herself. She might run to a window and thrust herself at it or to a cupboard to find a glass object to smash. The windows at the Center were reinforced glass, but she had gone through windows at home and had scars on her face and hands to prove it. Two times at the Center, she grabbed a hurt peer and pinched, as she had with the babies. Thus, staff devised a system to signal for reinforcement if they were alone with the clients and someone had an accident. Rather than tending to the injured person, the first requirement was to restrain Penny.

It probably is not surprising that Penny was fascinated with scars and wounds. She would perseverate on a staff member or peer with a bandage or scab. Sometimes she would hover around them, saying "bad Penny," "hurt Penny," or "Penny's crying." In spite of reassurances that Penny had no responsibility for the wound, she was so distracted by such signs of physical damage and pain that she could not concentrate on anything else. Attempts to extinguish this reaction had been unsuccessful. Staff carefully assigned a woundfree person to work with Penny.

Once a group home manager took a handkerchief with blood spots on it out of his pocket. She immediately reared back and started to scream "Penny's hurt." He quickly said, "See, Penny, I can wash it out." He promptly went to the sink, washed it, and brought the wet, stain-free hanky back to show her. She seemed intrigued at the disappearance of the marks and quit screaming, but kept going back to scrutinize the wet handkerchief hanging on the towel rack.

Penny also had an excited reaction to glass objects, particularly when they were not in locations where glass objects were usually found. She washed and dried dishes with no problem. She was very careful when she did these tasks and never broke dishes. Once a peer dropped a glass while setting the table. In an instant, she had run to the glass shards and had inflicted several wounds on her fingers and had to be taken to the emergency room for stitches. Penny inevitably noticed and reacted to jars and glasses when they were outside the kitchen area. Nothing could be stored in glass containers in the classroom. Clients had plastic cups in their bathrooms. Once, however, when Penny was visiting in a staff member's apartment, she had gone into the bathroom in a calm mood, but spotting a glass, she had instantaneously swiped it off the shelf. It flew across the room, shattering on the tile. Meanwhile, the staff member grabbed Penny in a half nelson, while Penny flailed around screaming "cut Penny" until she was escorted quite a distance from the area.

The combination of Penny's intense dislike of noises, her blood phobia, and her panic at the sight of glass made it difficult to integrate her into community programs. Because these behaviors meant that she was dangerous to herself and others, she would have to be in carefully controlled settings as long as she had such reactions. This was frustrating because otherwise Penny was a candidate for independent work and living arrangements.

Penny was thin and physically immature when she arrived at the Center, but staff knew puberty would soon arrive, and they wondered how she would react to the blood of her periods. Most projected that she would be "out of hand" with her first period and would probably panic each month or at least perseverate on her condition as long as the blood flowed. The Carters also worried about how Penny would deal with menstruation, and this concern was a central topic at informal and formal conferences that took place that year. Patsy Carter finally said: "I know this sounds cruel and extreme but we have been talking about the possibility of a hysterectomy." The Center director hesitantly replied: "That might be necessary, but I hate to think of how she would react to the operation." Tom Carter said: "I know, but at least it would be a one-time problem. With her periods she might have the trauma every month." Center personnel assured the Carters that if they pursued getting a hysterectomy for Penny, staff at the Diagnostic Center could provide evidence of her extreme reaction to blood. The director warned the Carters that he suspected it would be difficult to get a hysterectomy done—a prophecy that turned out to be very true.

The Carters discussed their worry about menstruation with their family doctor, Ruth Dunlap. Dr. Dunlap was well aware of Penny's blood phobia. Whenever Penny was to receive an injection or blood was to be drawn, both parents accompanied her. They found that the most successful method of drawing blood or doing injections was to blindfold Penny and warn her about the "little sting." Dunlap made sure she put the bandaid on Penny before she could see the punctured spot. Penny still held the arm stiffly and talked continuously about the "little sting" until it was healed enough to remove the bandage. Dr. Dunlap had already thought "hysterectomy," but became anxious when Patsy actually broached the subject. She had known the Carters since before Penny was born and had delivered Penny—a long labor and a difficult birth. Penny was blue from oxygen deprivation, but quickly recovered and seemed normal during the first few months. Dr. Dunlap wondered if this difficult birth had anything to do with Penny's condition and was relieved to read that autism was probably due to genetic or early prenatal problems.

Dr. Dunlap respected the Carters and had often remarked that Penny had been fortunate to be Tom and Patsy's child. Dunlap was proud that she had "done her part" in providing medical care for Penny in spite of the inconvenience, maybe risks, that such care posed. She knew that other doctors simply referred difficult children to Children's Hospital in the city, but it was over 30 miles away, so Dunlap conscientiously provided the routine medical functions needed by Penny. Nevertheless, the idea of becoming involved with the hysterectomy of a minor made her uneasy. After the conversation with the Carters, Dunlap's first step was to call her close friend Ralph Hansen, director of the area hospital. For a minute, she thought they had been disconnected. Then Hansen said: "Oh boy. Everything was going well today until now. Did you have to bring this up?" The hospital was small, serving a few suburbs and surrounding rural counties. Tough cases were rerouted to large city hospitals. Medically this was not a tough case—hysterectomies were common. It was tough because of the characteristics of the patient—both her personal behaviors and the fact that she was a minor with mental disabilities.

Hansen was acquainted with Tom Carter from Rotary Club. He had never met Penny, but had heard about her from two sources. His youngest daughter had been in elementary school with Penny and often had questioned her parents about certain of Penny's behaviors that upset her. He was glad she was exposed to "real life" so that she could see that things were not always easy for everybody. Hansen also heard about Penny from emergency room staff who had treated her for self-inflicted cuts on at least a half dozen occasions. He recalled staff's descriptions of her hysteria—how they had borrowed a straightjacket from the Mental Health Unit to restrain Penny so they could stitch up her wounds.

In reaction to the sensible Ruth Dunlap's announcement of pursuing a hysterectomy for Penny, Hansen said: "Let's see what Bogle [the hospital attorney] thinks." Bogle was aware that the scandal in the *Stump v. Sparkman* case involved the sterilization of an MR minor, but he knew that in that case the diagnosis of mental retardation was debatable. Bogle felt that nobody could dispute Penny's retardation. Bogle knew legislation relating to the sterilization of MR people had been repealed a few years earlier. Although in favor of that decision, he felt the lack of enabling legislation might complicate this case. Bogle first practiced in a rural county where there was a state hospital for MR people. He recalled the lurid stories in the press about the "maiming of little girls" in that place. He had been appalled not only by the wholesale nature of sterilization surgery, but also by the sensationalist report, which did not take into account the advantages of sterilization, and, in his opinion, there were some. In order to convince legislators to overturn the involuntary sterilization law, a lobbying group had collected very personal stories and fed them to the press. Hysterectomies had been performed on preadolescent girls at the institution for hygienic as well as contraceptive purposes. Mildly MR girls usually had tubal ligations, but even that surgery had been done with deceit—they were told they were having appendectomies. Bogle was glad there had been a check on that abuse, but wondered how pregnancy would be prevented in institutions.

A few days later, Bogle, Hansen, Dunlap, and Ashok Radjy, a gynecologist in Dunlap's medical building, met in the hospital cafeteria. After sharing their knowledge of Penny and her blood phobia, all agreed that there seemed to be sufficient evidence that a hysterectomy was in Penny's best interest. Bogle insisted on having a court order for the surgery. Dunlap complained about the expense of the legal route for the Carters, adding that she doubted that the Carters' health insurance would cover the costs of surgery. The others convinced Dunlap that taking a conservative legal route might be cheapest in the long run.

Bogle questioned Circuit Court Judge Louis Price about how to proceed. As Bogle suspected, Judge Price said it would be unwise to do the hysterectomy without having a court hearing and suggested that the Carters hire a lawyer to petition the court for guardianship as well as permission to do the surgery. Price cautioned Bogle that they should avoid reference to any birth control or hygienic reasons for surgery—the federal government had been "down our necks" to avoid sterilization of MR people—and court records should not reflect either of these rationales. Price warned that it was best to confine arguments to Penny's blood phobia and the reaction to menstruation (i.e., the medically indicated reasons) that it was predicted she would have.

Patsy was disappointed about having to go to court, but called their family lawyer, Harold Shock, and urged him to proceed quickly, as Penny was showing signs of puberty. Shock requested that Patsy and Tom make a list of witnesses who could attest to the blood phobia. Patsy compiled a list of 10 without any trouble. A court date was scheduled for the hearing, and the witnesses were sent letters requesting their presence. Shock told all witnesses to focus only on the blood phobia. The court hearing started at 10 a.m. on a rainy spring morning. Penny sat quietly between her parents. Eleven witnesses—two of Penny's previous teachers from her home school district, Dr. Dunlap, two doctors from emergency services, two of the Carters' neighbors, Tom's brother, and three staff from the Autistic Diagnostic Center—were present. Shock called on Dunlap to testify first. She reviewed medical records of the times Penny had been treated for wounds, mainly from broken glass, and showed the judge close-up pictures of Penny's scars. She concluded with her opinion that it was imperative, for health reasons, that menstruation be prevented. The remaining witnesses gave similar reports of Penny's reactions to the sight of blood. One of the Carters' neigbors, a retired social worker, was last to testify. To everyone's consternation, she veered off from the blood phobia to state her opinion that "sterilization was a good idea" because Penny would be "vulnerable to sexual exploitation," adding that as a social worker she had "witnessed firsthand the tragic results of pregnancy for the retarded." Admitting she had been requested not to mention contraception, she argued that it "was a relevant reason" and the judge had "heard enough about the blood phobia." Once the birth control evidence was in the court record, as he had warned, Judge Price would not give approval for the hysterectomy. He told Shock, "You can appeal, but you won't get permission from me. Let someone else take the blame for this one." After conferencing, the Carters decided to appeal.

Bogle called County Superior Court Juvenile Division Judge Sal Notting. Judges had been advised by the Protection and Advocacy Commission that sterilization of minors should not be permitted—the Commission's position was that courts should insist on adequate supervision to prevent sexual intercourse—or "sexual abuse," as they called it. Notting told Bogle he would be appointing a guardian ad litem to represent Penny because of her MR condition and young age.

The Carters were anxious to proceed to prevent the trauma they were sure would occur with her first menses. They asked Dr. Dunlap to document the longevity of Penny's condition. In addition to her own observations, Dr. Dunlap presented reports from two doctors at State Children's Hospital: One had originally diagnosed Penny as retarded and autistic when she was 3 years, 10 months old, and the other had replaced the first doctor and had seen Penny twice during the past four years. Dunlap informed the Carters that she was prepared to assert the opinion that Penny's self-destructive behaviors were life threatening and that menstruation would dangerously aggravate them.

Discussions with Diagnostic Center personnel brought forth four more potential expert witnesses. The psychologist would explain the results of intelligence, adaptive behavior, and language tests that Penny was given prior to coming to the Center. She would administer additional tests to demonstrate Penny's present status. The Center director would give an overview of autism and clarify the nature of Penny's behaviors in the context of that condition. A teacher and a residential supervisor who had spent the most time with Penny since her arrival at the Center planned to talk about her behavior in both home and community settings. Center staff volunteered to bring a videotape that had been running in the classroom and had happened to capture Penny's response to a peer who scraped his leg on a chair. They felt it was a revealing example of her reaction to blood. Bogle requested that they keep their reports to less than five minutes so that the evidence from all parties could be presented within an hour. He warned that they should be thorough, but to the point. The judge would ask questions if he wanted to know more. It was his experience that Judge Notting would cut someone off if he felt the information was irrelevant or redundant. In addition to these parties, the local special education director, who had kept in close touch with the Carters and Center professionals, volunteered to come to the hearing and be a witness, if necessary. She suggested that Penny's preschool teacher accompany her as well. The preschool teacher could attest to the early retardation—since she had first worked with Penny when she was just over two years old.

Judge Notting was impressed with the evidence from all parties as well as the consensus that a hysterectomy was necessary. He had slotted plenty of time in his court schedule for this case and so was able to ask a number of questions after each person shared information. He was impressed with the professionalism of the witnesses and their objective approach to the case. Because of the invasive, irreversible nature of a hysterectomy, Notting wanted to make sure he considered all angles; he said: "I'm going to make certain that no stone is unturned. I don't want my name connected with a shoddy pretense at legality like my friend, Stump." Although he used the term "friend" ironically, he did, in fact, know Stump. Stump was the judge in a juvenile court in a neighboring county.

The guardian ad litem sat in the courtroom throughout the proceedings, silent, but seemingly attentive. A couple sat next to her and, periodically, very discreetly turned and whispered something to her. They were expressionless and did not visibly react to any of the testimony. When Judge Notting asked the guardian if she had anything to say, she said: "Yes. I would like to know if there is evidence that Penny will menstruate?" This question made Judge Notting uneasy. First, it had not occurred to him, and he liked to think that he could come up with all factors relevant to a case during witnesses' testimony. After thinking about it, he believed that there was a good chance that Penny's hormones had been messed up either as part of her condition or due to her perpetual state of stress or her medications. If any one of those factors had interfered with menstruation, the hysterectomy would be unnecessary. Judge Notting was also a little worried about the guardian ad litem's point of view. He had selected her because she was the mother of three children—so he thought she would see the child's and the parents' point of view. In addition, she had recently finished law school, so she would have time. His first impression was that she was an earnest, conscientious person, but it occurred to him that he knew absolutely nothing about her politics.

Notting asked witnesses to address the possibility of suppressed menstruation. Dr. Dunlap made an attempt, but had to admit she could only conjecture because she had no concrete evidence. She did inform Notting that most women, retarded or normal, did eventually menstruate. Nevertheless, Notting asked that Penny be examined by a gynecologist who would attest that she would, indeed, be expected to menstruate. He requested that Dunlap also do a gynecological exam of Penny so that he would have two opinions about the probability of her having periods. A court date one month away was set for reconvening.

Dr. Weinbrenner, a gynecologist at University Medical Center, examined Penny. He was recommended by the Association for Retarded Citizens as being willing to take MR patients as well as someone skilled in working with them. Following the examination, Dr. Weinbrenner wrote to Judge Notting stating his conclusion that there was no biological reason why Penny would not menstruate—that her pelvic organs and reproductive potential appeared normal. He further stated that many women who have Penny's type of brain damage have an irregular and heavy flow during their periods and their excitatory episodes are increased markedly by menstruation, probably due to hormonal abnormalities. He predicted that Penny would be more excitable than ordinary during her premenstrual period as well as during menstruation.

Although Notting recommended that witnesses not refer to the birth control aspects of the case, Dr. Weinbrenner offered the opinion that pregnancy would endanger Penny's life and be devastating to her. He stated his personal knowledge that institutionalized females, especially, are sexually assaulted and the incidence of pregnancies is high. He went on to say that "based on reports and evidence of scars on Penny's body, I believe that her self-destructive actions would be accentuated by menstrual blood, and that a hysterectomy is recommended. It should be done immediately in order to prevent the devastating effects to Penny of experiencing her first menstrual period."

Dr. Dunlap appeared in court for the second time. Her predicted scenario of what might happen with menstruation, in fact, was the testimony that "clinched the case," according to Judge Notting. Dr. Dunlap elaborated:

I have known Penny to draw blood from herself repeatedly by picking at herself and by gouging herself with objects. She appears impervious to pain or, at least, pain does not inhibit or deter her from self-injurious actions. I believe she would become excessively agitated over menstruation and would make an effort to find the source of the blood and attempt to keep it flowing. Due to the pattern that Penny has shown so far, it is very reasonable to expect that she might try to induce bleeding by poking into her vagina or abdomen in an attempt to keep the blood flowing. This, of course, would result in infection or hemorrhaging, and possibly death. The stress of periods would be likely to increase her head banging and other self-destructive activities, which, in turn, would cause further deterioration in her condition.

Following Dr. Dunlap's testimony, Judge Notting turned to the guardian ad litem and asked for comments. Perhaps because she felt outnumbered, she very quietly said: "I object to the surgery. Without her consent, I do not think it should be done." Trying to control his annoyance, Judge Notting promptly replied:

We have heard evidence that Penny cannot now, nor is she ever expected to, make decisions or give consent. I am convinced that the Carters are truly acting in her behalf according to her best interests. It is clear to me that they are conscientious, well-meaning parents, and they have the support of a raft of highly qualified professionals. I humbly take their advice and grant in favor of the hysterectomy. Court adjourned.

A few weeks before the unsuccessful hearing, Tom Carter had been approached by his boss about a promotion. Tom had been head of the appliance department in a national department store chain for 10 years. He had been recommended to run a department at a store that was about to open in an eastern state. Patsy was orginally from that state and was delighted with her husband's offer. As they awaited the appellate court decision, their energy and attention were absorbed by moving. Patsy had scouted schools and liked a program for students with moderate handicaps.

The Carters returned for the appellate court hearing, with many of the same witnesses. This time permission for the hysterectomy was granted, but would only be valid in the state where it was granted. They decided to postpone the surgery until the following summer, when school was out. Before they could reschedule the surgery, Penny had her first menses. Penny was in the bathroom taking a bath. When Patsy went in, she noticed a streak of blood on the underpants that Penny had dropped on the floor, apparently without noticing the blood. Patsy put a sanitary napkin in some clean underpants, and when Penny got out of the bathtub, Patsy calmly informed her, "You have your period, you have to wear this pad to bed tonight." Penny compliantly pulled the underwear on, then her nightie, and went back to the television room. Out of the corner of her eye, Patsy watched Penny pat the pad every few minutes. An hour later, Patsy accompanied Penny to the bathroom, expecting an explosion when Penny noticed blood when she pulled down her pants to urinate. Patsy busied herself cleaning the sink and then looked Penny's direction. Penny was staring at a small circle of blood on the pad. Patsy promptly assured her "that's your period. Don't worry." Penny pulled the pants up and quietly went to bed.

When Tom returned from a meeting, Patsy was delighted to report Penny's calm reaction. He was astounded and remarked: "After all our worries and problems." Then, he added: "Maybe she did not notice it was blood. I bet tomorrow we'll see the reaction we expected." Penny spent most of the next day checking her "period." She calmly and quietly pulled down the pants and looked at the blood. Whenever Patsy suggested that Penny change the pad, she cooperated. She affixed the clean pad to her panties and even wrapped the soiled pad in a newspaper and discarded it properly. When she was not inspecting the pads, however, she was patting them through her clothes. In the afternoon, Patsy informed Penny that they were going grocery shopping, but that Penny could go only if she "didn't touch the pad—that's private." Penny promised to "keep hands away." In relating the shopping trip to Tom later, she laughed that Penny did not touch herself, but kept staring down in that direction.

Having anticipated the worst, Tom and Patsy were very relieved at Penny's reaction. Penny became accustomed to her periods and eventually quit worrying about the pads. Permission for a hysterectomy is in the legal records in the state where she previously lived. It set precedent for permission granted for sterilization based on medical indication of an extreme reaction to blood. Many judges and lawyers in the state are aware of the case, but assume that the hysterectomy was necessary and had been performed.

References

Abbott, J. M., & Ladd, G. M. (1970). Is there any reason why this mentally retarded couple should not be joined together? *Mental Retardation, 8,* 45–48.

Abbott, P., & Sapsford, R. (1990). Health visiting: Policing the family? In P. Abbott & C. Wallace (Eds.), *The sociology of the caring professions* (pp. 120–152). London: Falmer.

Abbott, P., & Wallace, C. (Eds.). (1990). *The sociology of the caring professions.* London: Falmer.

Abelson, R. B., & Johnson, R.C. (1969). Heterosexual and aggressive behaviors among institutionalized retardates. *Mental Retardation, 7,* 28–30.

Abrahams, J. (1958). *Maternal dependency and schizophrenia.* New York: International University Press.

Abramson, P. R., Parker, T., & Weisberg, S.R. (1988). Sexual expression of mentally retarded people: Educational and legal implications. *American Journal on Mental Retardation, 3,* 328–334.

Adams, G. L., Tallon, R. J., & Alcorn, D. A. (1982). Attitudes toward the sexuality of mentally retarded and nonretarded persons. *Education and Training of the Mentally Retarded, 17,* 307–312.

Ainsworth, M. N., Wagner, E. A., & Strauss, A. A. (1945). Children of our children. *American Journal of Mental Deficiency, 49,* 277–289.

Alaszewski, A., & Ong, B. N. (1990). *Normalisation in practice.* London: Tavistock/Routledge.

Alcorn, D. A. (1974). Parental views of sexual development and education of the TMR. *The Journal of Special Education, 8,* 119–130.

Allen, R. C. (1969). Legal rights of the institutionalized retardate: Equal justice for the unequal. *Mental Retardation, 7,* 2–5.

Allport, G. W. (1967). Attitudes. In M. Fishbein (Ed.), *Attitude theory and measurement* (pp. 34–48). New York: Wiley and Sons.

Altman, B. M. (1985). Social structure. In S.E. Browne, D. Connors, & N. Stern (Eds.), *With the power of each breath: A disabled women's anthology* (pp. 69–77). Pittsburgh: Cleis.

Americans with Disabilities Act *(ADA) of 1990, Pub. L. 101–336.* Codified as 42 U.S.C. & 12101 et seq.

Anderson, In re, No. 5–67/1648 (Dane County P. Ct., Wis. 1974).

Andron, L., & Tymchuk, A. (1985). *Marriage and parenting: Effective decision making for the developmentally disabled.* Los Angeles: Stanfield House.

Andron, L., & Tymchuk, A. (1987). Parents who are mentally retarded. In A. Craft (Ed.), *Mental handicap and sexuality: Issues and perspectives* (pp. 238–262). Kent, England: Costello Press.

Arcia, W., Gallagher, J., & Serling, J. (1992). *But what about the other 93 percent?* Chapel Hill: Carolina Policy Studies Program, Frank Porter Graham Child Development Center, University of North Carolina at Chapel Hill.

Argulewicz, E. N. (1983). Effects of ethnic membership, socioeconomic status, and home language on LD, EMR, and EH placements. *Learning Disabilities Quarterly, 6,* 195–200.

Asch, A. (1989). Can aborting imperfect children be immoral? In N. K. Rhoden & J. D. Arras (Eds.), *Ethical issues in modern medicine* (3rd ed.) (pp. 73–89). Palo Alto, CA: Mayfield.

Asrael, W. (1982). An approach to motherhood for disabled women. *Rehabilitation Literature, 43,* 214–218.

B. (A Minor), In re, 2 W.L.R. 1213 (1987).

Bachrach, L. L. (1985). Deinstitutionalization: The meaning of the least restrictive environment. In R. H. Bruininks & K. C. Lakin (Eds.), *Living and learning in the least restrictive environment* (pp. 23–26). Baltimore: Brookes.

Badgley, R. (1984). *Report of the Committee on Sexual Offenses Against Children and Youths.* Ottawa, Ontario: Government of Canada, Ministries of Justice and Attorney General.

Badham, J. N. (1955). The outside employment of hospitalized mentally defective patients as a step toward resocialization. *American Journal of Mental Deficiency, 59,* 666–680.

Bailey, D. B., & Winton, P. J. (1989). Friendship and acquaintance among families in a mainstreamed day care center. *Education and Training in Mental Retardation, 24,* 107–113.

Bakken, J., Miltenberger, R. G., & Schauss, S. (1993). Teaching parents with mental retardation: Knowledge versus skills. *American Journal of Mental Retardation, 97,* 405–417.

Barnes, C. (1991). *Disabled people in Britain and discrimination: A case for anti-discrimination legislation.* London: Hurst.

Bass, M. S. (1963). Marriage, parenthood, and prevention of pregnancy. *American Journal of Mental Deficiency, 68,* 320–325.

Bass, M. S. (1964). Marriage for the mentally deficient. *Mental Retardation, 2,* 198–202.

Bass, M. D. (1978). Surgical contraception: A key to normalization and prevention. *Mental Retardation, 16,* 339–404.

Bearchell, C. (1985, January). Taking advantage of abuse. *The Body Politic, 2,* 17–29.

Beauchamp, T. L., & Childress, J. F. (1989). *Principles of biomedical ethics,* (3rd ed.). New York: Oxford University Press.

Beauchamp, T. L., & Pinkard, T. P. (Eds.). (1983). *Ethics and public policy.* Englewood Cliffs, NJ: Prentice-Hall.

Becker, R. (1976). Job training placement for retarded youth. *Mental Retardation, 14,* 7–11.

Begab, M. J. (1970). Adapting techniques for the mentally retarded. In M. Schreiber (Ed.), *Social work and mental retardation* (pp. 332–345). New York: John Day Co.

Bell, D., Feraios, A. J., & Bryan, T. (1991). Learning disabled adolescents' knowledge and attitudes about AIDS. *Learning Disabilities Research and Practice, 6,* 104–111.

Bell, S. (1992). Birth control. In Boston Women's Health Book Collective, *The new our bodies, ourselves* (pp. 259–307). New York: Simon & Schuster.

Beller, A. H., & Graham, J. W. (1993). *Small change: The economics of child support.* New Haven, CT: Yale University Press.

Bellotti v. Baird, 443 U.S. 622 (1979).

Bennett, B., Vockell, E., & Vockell, K. (1972). Sex education for EMR adolescent girls. *Journal of Special Education of the Mentally Retarded, 9,* 3–7.

Bercovici, S. M. (1983). *Barriers to normalization: The restrictive management of retarded persons.* Baltimore: University Park Press.

Berkowitz, M., & Berkowitz, E. D. (1985). Widening the field: Economics and history in the study of disability. *American Behavioral Scientist, 28,* 405–417.

Bernstein, N. R. (1990). Sexuality in adolescent retardates. In M. Sugar (Ed.), *Atypical adolescents and sexuality* (pp. 44–56). New York: W.W. Norton.

Berry, J., & Shapiro, A. (1975). Married mentally handicapped patients in the community. *Proceedings of the Royal Society of Medicine, 68,* 27.

Bethlehem, D. W. (1990). Attitudes, social attitudes, and widespread beliefs. In C. Fraser & G. Gaskell (Eds.), *The social psychological study of widespread beliefs* (pp. 65–76). Oxford, England: Clarendon Press.

Bijou, S. W. (1983). The prevention of mild and moderate retarded development. In F. J. Menolascino, R. Neman, & J. A. Stark (Eds.), *Curative aspects of mental retardation: Biomedical and behavioral advances* (pp. 223–241). Baltimore: Brookes.

Biklen, D. (1986). Framed: Journalism's treatment of disability. *Social Policy, 16,* 45–51.

Bioethics Committee, Canadian Paediatric Society. (1986). Treatment decisions for infants and children. *Canadian Medical Association Journal, 135,* 447.

Birenbaum, A., & Re, M. A. (1979). Resettling mentally retarded adults in the community—Almost 4 years later. *American Journal of Mental Deficiency, 83,* 323–329.

Blacher, J. (1984). Sequential stages of parental adjustment to the birth of a child with handicaps: Fact or artifact? *Mental Retardation, 22,* 55–68.

Blatt, R.J.R. (1988). *Prenatal tests: What they are, their benefits and risks, and how to decide whether to have them or not.* New York: Vintage.

Bogdan, D. (1993). Order without rules: Wittgenstein and the "communicative ethics controversy." *Sociological Theory, 11,* 55–71.

Bogdan, R. (1988). *Freak show: Presenting human oddities for amusement and profit.* Chicago: University of Chicago Press.

Boggs, E. (1978). Who is putting whose head in the sand or in the clouds as the case may be? In A. P. Turnbull & H. R. Turnbull III (Eds.), *Parents speak out* (pp. 31–59). Columbus, OH: Merrill.

Boston Women's Health Book Collective. (1992). *The new our bodies, ourselves: A book by and for women.* New York: Simon & Schuster.

Bowden, J., Spitz, H. H., & Winters, J. J., Jr. (1971). Follow-up of one retarded couple's marriage. *Mental Retardation, 9,* 42–43.

Bowser, B. P. (Ed.). (1991). *Black male adolescents: Parenting and education in community context.* Lanham, MD: University Press of America.

Boylan, E. (Ed.). (1991). *Woman and disability.* London: Zed Books.

Brakel, S., & Rock, R. (1971). *Eugenic sterilization: The mentally disabled and the law.* Chicago: University of Chicago Press.

Brantlinger, E. A. (1983). Measuring variation and change in attitudes of residential care staff toward the sexuality of mentally retarded persons. *Mental Retardation, 21,* 17–22.

Brantlinger, E. A. (1985a). Mildly mentally retarded secondary students' information about and attitudes toward sexuality and sexuality education. *Education and Training of the Mentally Retarded, 20,* 99–108.

Brantlinger, E. A. (1985b). What low-income parents want from schools: A different view of aspirations. *Interchange, 16,* 14–28.

Brantlinger, E. A. (1987a). Influencing staff attitudes about the sexuality of handicapped persons. In A. Craft (Ed.), *Sex education and counseling for mentally handicapped people* (pp. 177–206). Kent, England: Costello Press.

Brantlinger, E. A. (1987b). Making decisions about special education placement: Do low-income parents have the information they need? *Journal of Learning Disabilities, 20,* 95–101.

Brantlinger, E. A. (1988a). Teachers' perceptions of the parenting abilities of their secondary students with mild mental retardation. *Remedial Education and Special Education, 9,* 31–43.

Brantlinger, E. A. (1988b). Teachers' perceptions of the sexuality of their secondary students with mild mental retardation. *Education and Training in Mental Retardation, 23*, 24–37.

Brantlinger, E. A. (1991). The influence of teacher gender on access to knowledge about their sexual and intimate social selves. *Feminist Teacher, 5*, 25–29.

Brantlinger, E. A. (1992a). Sexuality education in the secondary special education curriculum: Teachers' perceptions and concerns. *Teacher Education and Special Education, 15*, 32–40.

Brantlinger, E. A. (1992b). Professionals' attitudes toward the sterilization of people with disabilities. *Journal of the Association for Persons with Severe Handicaps, 17*, 4–18.

Brantlinger, E. A., & Guskin, S. L. (1987). Ethnocultural and social-psychological effects on learning characteristics of handicapped children. In M. C. Wang, M. C. Reynolds, & H. J. Walberg (Eds.), *Handbook of special education: Research and practice* (Vol. 1, pp. 7–34). Oxford, England: Pergamon.

Brantlinger, E. A., Klein, S., & Guskin, S. L. (1994). *Fighting for Darla*. New York: Teachers College Press.

Brantlinger, E. A., Majd-Jabbari, M., & Guskin, S. L. (1993). *Barriers to integrated schools and classrooms: Affluent parents' thinking about their own and other people's children*. Unpublished manuscript.

Bregman, S. (1984). Assertiveness training for mentally retarded adults. *Mental Retardation, 22*, 12–16.

Brennan, T. A. (1991). *Just doctoring: Medical ethics in the liberal state*. Berkeley: University of California Press.

Bristol, M., Gallagher, J., & Schopler, E. (1988). Mothers and fathers of young developmentally disabled and nondisabled boys: Adaptation and spousal support. *Developmental Psychology, 24*, 441–451.

Brody, B. A. (1987). *Bioethics: Readings and cases*. Englewood Cliffs, NJ: Prentice-Hall.

Bromham, D. R. (1992). *Ethics in reproductive medicine*. London: Springer-Verlag.

Bromham, D. R., Dalton, M. E. & Jackson, J. C. (Eds.). (1990). *Philosophical ethics in reproductive medicine*. Manchester, England: Manchester University Press.

Bronfenbrenner, U. & Neville, P. R. (1994). America's children and families. In S. L. Kagan & B. Weissbourd (Eds.), *Putting families first: America's family support movement and the challenge of change* (pp. 3–27). San Francisco: Jossey-Bass.

Brookhouser, P.E. (1987). Medical issues. In J. Garbarino, P. E. Brookhouser, & K. J. Authier (Eds.), *Special children—Special risks: The maltreatment of children with disabilities* (pp. 161–178). New York: Aldine de Gruyter.

Brown, C. (1990). *My left foot*. London: Mandarin.

Brown, H., & Craft, A. (Eds.). (1989). *Thinking the unthinkable: Papers on sexual abuse and people with learning difficulties.* London: FPA Education Unit.

Browne, S. E., Connors, D., & Stern, N. (Eds.). (1985). *With the power of each breath: A disabled women's anthology.* Pittsburgh: Cleis.

Bruess, C.E., & Greenberg, J.S. (1988). *Sexuality education: Theory and practice.* New York: Macmillan.

Buchanan, A. E., & Brock, D. W. (1989). *Deciding for others: The ethics of surrogate decision making.* New York: Cambridge University Press.

Buck v. Bell, 274 U.S. 200 (1927).

Budd, K. S., & Greenspan, S. (1984). Mentally retarded women as parents. In E. Blechman (Ed.), *Behavior modification with women* (pp. 477–506). New York: Guilford Press.

Budd, K., & Greenspan, S. (1985). Parameters of successful and unsuccessful interventions with parents who are mentally retarded. *Mental Retardation, 23,* 269–273.

Burchard, S. N., Hasazi, J. S., Gordon, L. R., & Yoe, J. (1991). An examination of lifestyle and adjustment in three community residential alternatives. *Research in Developmental Disabilities, 12,* 127–142.

Burgdorf, R. L., Jr. (1983). Freedom of choice: Competency and guardianship. In R. L. Burgdorf, Jr., & P. P. Spicer (Eds.), *The legal rights of handicapped persons: Cases, materials, and text* (pp. 209–222). Baltimore: Brookes.

Burgdorf, R. L., & Spicer, P. P. (1983). *The legal rights of handicapped persons: Cases, materials, and text.* Baltimore: Brookes.

Burt, R. (1984). Constitutional law and the teaching of parables. *Yale Law Journal, 93,* 455.

Calnen, T., & Blackman, L. S. (1992). Capital punishment and offenders with mental retardation: Response to the Penry Brief. *American Journal on Mental Retardation, 96,* 557–564.

Campbell, A. (1990). Withholding neonatal care. A pediatrician's view. In D. R. Bromham, M. E. Dalton, & J. C. Jackson (Eds.), *Philosophical ethics in reproductive medicine* (pp. 107–123). Manchester, England: Manchester University Press.

Carrier, J. G. (1986). Sociology and special education: Differentiation and allocation in mass education. *American Journal of Education, 94,* 281–312.

Carruth, D.G. (1973). Human sexuality in a half-way house. In F. de la Cruz & G. DeLaVeck (Eds.), *Human sexuality and the mentally retarded* (pp. 153–156). New York: Bruner/Mazel.

Cate, H., & Gegenheimer, R. A. (1950). The community supervisor looks at parole. *American Journal of Mental Deficiency, 55,* 275–278.

Chamberlain, S., Rauh, J., Passer, A., McGrath, M., & Burket, R. (1984). Issues in fertility control for mentally retarded female adolescents: I. Sexual activity, sexual abuse, and contraception. *Pediatrics, 73,* 445–450.

Christie, R. J., & Hoffmaster, C. B. (1986). *Ethical issues in family medicine.* New York: Oxford University Press.

Cole, S. S. (1991). Facing the challenges of sexual abuse in persons with disabilities. In R. P. Marinelli & A. E. Dell Orto (Eds.), *The psychological and social impact of disability* (pp. 223–235). New York: Springer.

Coleman, J. S. (1993). Comment on Preston and Campbell's "differential fertility and the distribution of traits." *American Journal of Sociology, 98,* 1020–1032.

Colker, R. (1992). *Abortion and dialogue: Pro-choice, pro-life, and American law.* Bloomington: Indiana University Press.

Comegys, A. (1989). Integration strategies for parents of students with handicaps. In R. Gaylord-Ross (Ed.), *Integration strategies for students with handicaps* (pp. 339–350). Baltimore: Brookes.

Committee on Bioethics. (1988). *Ethical concerns in sterilization of persons with mental retardation.* Washington, DC: American College of Obstetricians and Gynecologists.

Committee on Ethics. (1988, September). *Committee opinion* (No. 63). Washington, DC: American College of Obstetricians and Gynecologists.

Comprehensive Services for Independent Living (1978), added to the Rehabilitation Act of 1973 (29 U.S.C. §796).

Conroy, J. W., & Bradley, V. J. (1985). *The Pennhurst longitudinal study: A report of hospital release programs.* Washington, D.C., Children's Bureau Publications No. 210.

Corbett, K. (1989). System thwarts disabled moms. *New Directions for Women, 18*(5), 4–5.

Costello, A. (1988). The psychosocial impact of genetic disease. *Focus on Exceptional Children, 20,* 1–8.

Craft, A. (1987). Mental handicap and sexuality: Issues for individuals with a mental handicap, their parents, and professionals. In A. Craft (Ed.), *Mental handicaps and sexuality: Issues and perspectives* (pp. 13–24). Kent, England: Costello Press.

Craft, A., & Craft, M. (1979). *Handicapped married couples.* London: Routledge and Kegan Paul.

Craft, M., & Craft, A. (Eds.). (1978). *Sex and the mentally handicapped.* London: Routledge and Kegan Paul.

Craft, M., & Craft, A. (Eds.). (1985). *Sex and the mentally handicapped.* 2nd. ed. London: Routledge and Kegan Paul.

Crain, E. J. (1980). Socioeconomic status of educable mentally retarded graduates of special education. *Education and Training of the Mentally Retarded, 15,* 90–94.

Cranefield, P. F. (1966). Historical perspectives. In I. Philips (Ed.), *Prevention and treatment of the mentally retarded* (pp. 3–24). New York: Basic Books.

Crapps, J. M., Langione, J., & Swain, S. (1985). Quantity and quality of participation in community environments by mentally retarded adults. *Education and Training of the Mentally Retarded, 20,* 123–129.

Crnic, K. A., Friedrich, W. N., & Greenberg, M. T. (1983). Adaptations of families with mentally retarded children: A model of stress, coping, and family ecology. *American Journal of Mental Deficiency, 88*, 125–138.

Crocker, A. C., Cohen, H. J., & Kastner, T. A. (Eds.). (1992). *HIV infection and developmental disabilities: A resource for service providers*. Baltimore: Brookes.

Crowe, M. (1992). Some common and uncommon health and medical problems. In Boston Women's Health Book Collective, *The new our bodies, ourselves* (pp. 561–647). New York: Simon & Schuster.

Cusine, D. (1990). The family and contraception. In E. Sutherland & A.M. Smith (Eds.), *Family rights: Family law and medical advance* (pp. 80–99). Edinburgh: Edinburgh University Press.

Dalley, G. (1991). *Disability and social policy*. London: Political Studies Institute.

Dalley, G., & Berthoud, R. (1992). *Challenging discretion: The social fund review procedure*. London: Political Studies Institute.

Darling, R. B. (1979). *Families against society: A study of reactions to children with birth defects*. Beverly Hills, CA: Sage.

Darling, R. B. (1980). Parental entrepreneurship: A consumerist response to professional dominance. In M. Nagler & E. J. Kemp (Eds.), *Perspectives on disability* (pp. 287–298). Palo Alto, CA: Health Markets Research.

Dartington, T., Miller, E., & Gwynne, G. (1981). *A life together: The distribution of attitudes around the disabled*. London: Tavistock.

Darwin, C. (1871). *The descent of man* and *Selection in relation to sex* (2 vols.). London: John Murray.

Darwin, C. (1898). *The origin of species by means of natural selection: Or, the preservation of favored races in the struggle for life*. New York: D. Appleton.

David, H. P., Smith, J., & Friedman, E. (1976). Family planning services for persons handicapped by mental retardation. *American Journal of Public Health, 66*, 1053–1058.

Davis, A. (1981). *Women, class, race*. New York: Random House.

Davis, S. E., Anderson, C., Linkowski, D. C., Berger, K., and Feinstein, C. F. (1991). Developmental tasks and transitions of adolescents with chronic illnesses and disabilities. In R. P. Marinelli & A. E. Dell Orto (Eds.), *The psychological and social impact of disability* (pp. 70–80). New York: Springer.

Deigh, J. (1989). Human rights and population control. In C. Peden & J.P. Sterba (Eds.), *Freedom, equality, and social change* (pp. 42–50). Lewiston, NY: Edwin Mellen Press.

Deisher, R. (1973). Sexual behavior of retarded in institutions. In F. de la Cruz & G. DeLaVeck (Eds.), *Human sexuality and the mentally retarded* (pp. 145–152). New York: Bruner/Mazel.

Derrida, J. (1976). *On grammatology*. Baltimore: Johns Hopkins University Press.

Diamond, G. W., & Cohen, H. J. (1992). Developmental disabilities in children with HIV infection. In A. C. Crocker, H. J. Cohen, & T. A. Kastner (Eds.), *HIV infection and developmental disabilities: A resource for service providers* (pp. 33–42). Baltimore: Brookes.

Diamond, S. (1979). Developmentally disabled persons: Their rights and their needs for services. In R. Wiegerink & J. W. Pelosi (Eds.), *Developmental disabilities: The DD movement* (pp. 15–26). Baltimore: Brookes.

Diamond, S. (1993). Growing up with parents of a child with a disability: An individual account. In J. L. Paul & R. J. Simeonsson (Eds.), *Children with special needs: Family, culture, and society* (pp. 53–76). Fort Worth, TX: Harcourt Brace Jovanovich.

Dinger, J. C. (1961). Post-school adjustment of former educable retarded pupils. *Exceptional Children, 27*, 353–360.

Diskin, V. (1992). Developing an international awareness. In Boston Women's Health Book Collective, *The new our bodies, ourselves* (pp. 713–732). New York: Simon & Schuster.

Ditzion, J., & Golden, J. (1992). Introduction. In Boston Women's Health Book Collective, *The new our bodies, ourselves* (pp. 239–240). New York: Simon & Schuster.

Doise, W. (1990). Social beliefs and intergroup relations: The relevance of some sociological perspectives. In C. Fraser & G. Gaskell (Eds.), *The social psychological study of widespread beliefs* (pp. 143–159). Oxford, England: Clarendon Press.

Doll, E.A. (1941). The essentials of an inclusive concept of mental deficiency. *American Journal of Mental Deficiency, 46*, 214–219.

Dougan, T., Isbell, L., & Vyas, P. (1983). *We have been there: Families share the joys and struggles of living with mental retardation*. Nashville: Abingdon Press.

Drash, P. W. (1992). The failure of prevention or our failure to implement prevention knowledge? *Mental Retardation, 30*, 93–96.

Ducharme, S., & Gill, K. M. (1991). Sexual values, training, and professional roles. In R. P. Marinelli & A. E. Dell Orto (Eds.), *The psychological and social impact of disability* (pp. 201–209). New York: Springer.

Dugdale, R. (1877). *The Jukes: A study of crime, pauperism, disease, and heredity.* New York: Putnam Publishing Group.

Dunst, C. J., Trivette, C. M., & Cross, A. H. (1986). Mediating influences of social support: Personal, family, and child outcomes. *American Journal of Mental Deficiency, 90*, 403–417.

Dupras, A., & Tremblay, R. (1976). Path analysis of parents' conservatism toward sex education of their mentally retarded children. *American Journal of Mental Deficiency, 81*, 162–166.

Dworkin, R. (1993). Feminism and abortion. *The New York Review of Books, 40*, 27–29.

Edelman, M. (1977). The political language of the helping professions. In M. Edelman (Ed.), *Political language: Words that succeed and policies that fail* (pp. 57–75). New York: Academic Press.

Edgerton, R. B. (1967). *The cloak of competence: Stigma in the lives of the mentally retarded*. Berkeley: University of California Press.

Edgerton, R. B. (Ed.). (1984). Lives in process: Mildly retarded adults in a large city. *Monographs of the American Association on Mental Deficiency* (No. 6).

Edgerton, R. B., & Dingman, H. F. (1964). Good reasons for bad supervision: "Dating" in a hospital for the mentally retarded. *The Psychiatric Quarterly Supplement, 38*, 221–233.

Edmonson, B., McCombs, K., & Wish, J. (1979). What retarded adults believe about sex. *American Journal of Mental Deficiency, 84*, 11–18.

Education for All Handicapped Children Act of 1975, Pub. L. 94–142. Codified as 20 U.S.C. Sec. 143.

Eisenstadt v. Baird, 405 U.S. 438 (1972).

Elgar, S. (1985). Sex education and sexual awareness building for autistic children and youth: Some viewpoints and considerations. *Journal of Autism and Developmental Disorders, 15*, 214–216.

Elkins, T. E., & Andersen, H. F. (1992). Sterilization of persons with mental retardation. *Journal of the Association for Persons with Severe Handicaps, 17*, 19–26.

Ellis, J. W., & Luckasson, R. (1985). Mentally retarded defendants. *George Washington Law Review, 53*, 414–493.

Eshilian, L., Haney, M., & Falvey, M. A. (1989). Domestic skills. In M. A. Falvey (Ed.), *Community-based curriculum* (pp. 115–140). Baltimore: Brookes.

Estabrook, A. (1916). *The Jukes in 1915*. Washington, DC: Carnegie Institute.

Ethics Committee of the American Fertility Society. (1986). *Ethical considerations of the new reproductive technologies*. Birmingham, AL: American Fertility Society.

Evans, A. L., & McKinley, I. A. (1988). Sexual maturation in girls with severe mental handicap. *Child Care, Health and Development, 14*, 59–69.

Evans, C., & Eder, D. (1993). "No exit" processes of social isolation in the middle school. *Journal of Contemporary Ethnography, 22*, 139–170.

Eve v. Mrs. E., 2 S.C.R. 388 (1986).

Faden, R., & Beauchamp, T. (1986). *A history and theory of informed consent*. Oxford, England: Oxford University Press.

Fantuzzo, J.W., Wray, L., Hall, R., Goins, C., & Azar, S. (1986). Parent and social skills training for mentally retarded mothers identified as child maltreaters. *American Journal of Mental Deficiency, 91*, 135–140.

Farber, B. (1959). Effects of a severely mentally retarded child on family integration. *Monographs of the Society for Research in Child Development* (Serial No. 71).

Farber, B. (1968). *Mental retardation: Its social context and social consequences.* Boston: Houghton Mifflin.

Farber, B. (1978). Family organization and crises: Maintenance of integration in families with a severely mentally retarded child. *Monographs of the Society for Research in Child Development* (Serial No. 75).

Farber, B. (1986). Historical contexts of research on families with mentally retarded members. In J. J. Gallagher & P. M. Vietze (Eds.), *Families of handicapped persons: Research, programs, and policy issues* (pp. 3–23). Baltimore: Brookes.

Farran, D. C., Metzger, J., & Sparling, J. (1986). Immediate and continuing adaptations in parents of handicapped children: A model and an illustration. In J.J. Gallagher & P.M. Vietze (Eds.), *Families of handicapped persons: Research, programs, and policy issues* (pp. 143–166). Baltimore: Brookes.

Featherstone, H. (1980). *A difference in the family.* New York: Basic Books.

Fedje, C. G., & Holcombe, M. (1986). Testing for child development and parenting knowledge. *Teaching Exceptional Children, 18*, 253–257.

Felce, D., DeKock, V., & Repp, A. C. (1986). An eco-behavioral analysis of small community-based houses and traditional large hospitals for severely and profoundly mentally handicapped adults. *Applied Research in Mental Retardation, 7*, 393–408.

Feldman, M., Case, L., Rincover, A., Towns, F., & Betel, J. (1989). Parent education project III: Increasing affection and responsivity in developmentally handicapped mothers: Component analysis, generalization, and effects on child language. *Journal of Applied Behavior Analysis, 22*, 211–222.

Feldman, M. A., Case, L., Towns, F., & Betel, J. (1985). Parent education project I: Development and nurturance of children of mentally retarded parents. *American Journal of Mental Deficiency, 90*, 253–258.

Feldman, M. A., Towns, F., Betel, J., Case, L., Rincover, A., & Rubino, C. A. (1986). Parent education project II: Increasing stimulating interactions of developmentally handicapped mothers. *Journal of Applied Behavior Analysis, 19*, 23–37.

Ferguson, P. M., & Ferguson, D. L. (1992). Reader response: Sex, sexuality, and disability. *Journal for the Association for Persons with Severe Handicaps, 17*, 27–28.

Ferguson, P. M., Ferguson, D. L., & Taylor, S. J. (1992). *Interpreting disability: A qualitative reader.* New York: Teachers College Press.

Fernald, W. E. (1896). Some methods employed in the care and the training of feeble-minded children of the lower grades. In *Forty-eighth annual report of the trustees of the Massachusetts School for the Feeble-minded at Waltham, Year ending 1895.* Boston: Wright and Potter.

Fewell, R. (1986). A handicapped child in the family. In R.R. Fewell & P. F. Vadasy (Eds.), *Families of handicapped children* (pp. 3–34). Austin, TX: Pro-Ed.

Fidone, G. S. (1987). Homosexuality in institutionalized retardates. *Infection Control, 8*(6), 231.

Finch, J. (1991). Food for thought. In E. Boylan (Ed.), *Woman and disability* (pp. 66–69). London: Zed Books.

Fine, M. (1988). Sexuality, schooling, and adolescent females: The missing discourse of desire. *Harvard Educational Review, 58*, 29–55.

Fine, M., & Asch, A. (Eds.). (1988). *Women with disabilities: Essays in psychology, culture, and politics*. Philadelphia: Temple University Press.

Finger, A. (1990). *Past due: A story of disability, pregnancy, and birth*. Seattle: Seal Press.

Finkelhor, D. (1984). *Child sexual abuse*. New York: Free Press.

Fischer, H. L., & Krajicek, M. J. (1974). Sexual development of the moderately retarded child: Level of information and parental attitudes. *Mental Retardation, 12*, 28–30.

Fleming, M. A. (1979). Teaching sex to institutionalized retarded people: What society says is accepted behavior. *Disabled USA, 3*, 7–10.

Fletcher, J. F. (1979). *Humanhood: Essays in biomedical ethics*. Buffalo, NY: Prometheus.

Floor, L., Baxter, D., Rosen, M., & Zisfein, L. (1975). A survery of marriages among previously institutionalized retardates. *Mental Retardation, 13*, 33–37.

Foucault, M. (1973). *The birth of the clinic*. New York: Vintage.

Foucault, M. (1985). *The history of sexuality: Vol. 2. The use of pleasure*. New York: Pantheon.

Franklin, D. (1989, September 3). What a child is given. *New York Times Magazine*, pp. 36–41, 49.

Fraser, C., & Gaskell, G. (Eds.). (1990). *The social psychological study of widespread beliefs*. Oxford, England: Clarendon Press.

Fraser, F. C. (1974). Genetic counseling. *The American Journal of Human Genetics, 26*, 637.

Fredericks, B. (1992). Reader response: A parent's view of sterilization. *Journal for the Association of Persons with Severe Handicaps, 17*, 29–30.

Fry, S. T. (1992). The role of caring in a theory of nursing ethics. In H. B. Holmes & L. M. Purdy (Eds.), *Feminist perspectives in medical ethics* (pp. 93–106). Bloomington: Indiana University Press.

Frye, M. (1983). *The politics of reality: Essays in feminist theory*. Freedom, CA: Crossing Press.

Gallagher, J. J. (1993). The future of professional/family relations in families with children with disabilities. In J. L. Paul & R. J. Simeonsson (Eds.), *Children with special needs: Family, culture, and society* (pp. 295–310). Fort Worth, TX: Harcourt Brace Jovanovich.

Garbarino, J., Brookhouser, P. E., & Authier, K. J. (Eds.). (1987). *Special Children—Special risks: The maltreatment of children with disabilities.* New York: Aldine de Gruyter.

Garber, H., & Heber, R. (1982). Modification of predicted cognitive development in high-risk children through early intervention. In D. K. Detterman & R. Sternberg (Eds.), *How and how much can intellect be increased?* (pp. 77–86). Norwood, NJ: Ablex.

Gardner, N.E.S. (1986). Sexuality. In J.A. Summers (Ed.), *The right to grow up: An introduction to adults with developmental disabilities.* Baltimore: Brookes.

Gartner, A., & Lipsky, D.K. (1987). Beyond special education: Toward a quality system for all students. *Harvard Educational Review, 57,* 367–395.

Gath, A. (1983). Mentally retarded children in substitute and natural families. *Adoption and Fostering, 7,* 35–40.

Gaylin, W., & Macklin, R. (1982). *Who speaks for the child? The problems of proxy consent.* New York: Plenum.

Gerber, M. M., & Levine-Donnerstein, D. (1989). Educating all children: Ten years later. *Exceptional Children, 56,* 17–27.

Gerry, M. H. (1988). Section 504 of the Rehabilitation Act, HIV and AIDS : Legal implications. *Issues in Law and Medicine, 4*(2), 175–190.

Gerstel, N., & Gallagher, S.K. (1993). Kinkeeping and distress: Gender, recipients of care, and work-family conflict. *Journal of Marriage and Family, 55,* 598–607.

Geskie, M. A., & Salasek, J. L. (1988). Attitudes of health care personnel toward persons with disabilities. In H.E. Yuker (Ed.), *Attitudes toward persons with disabilities* (pp. 187–200). New York: Springer.

Gilhool, T. K., & Gran, J. A. (1985). Legal rights of disabled parents. In S. K. Thurman (Ed.), *Children of handicapped parents: Research and clinical perspectives* (pp. 11–34). Orlando, FL: Academic Press.

Gillick v. West Norfolk and Wisbech Health Authority and Another, All E.R. 402 (1985).

Gilligan, C. (1982). *In a different voice: Psychological theory and women's development.* Cambridge: Harvard University Press.

Glaser, B. G., & Strauss, A. L. (1965). *Awareness of dying: A study of social interaction.* Chicago: Aldine.

Glaser, B. G., & Strauss, A. L. (1967). *The discovery of grounded theory: Strategies for qualitative research.* Chicago: Aldine.

Gleason, J. J. (1989). *Special education in context: An ethnographic study of persons with developmental disabilities.* Cambridge: Cambridge University Press.

Glidden, L. M. (1986). Families who adopt mentally retarded children: Who, why, and what happens? In J. J. Gallagher & P. M. Vietze (Eds.), *Families of handicapped persons: Research, programs, and policy issues* (pp. 129–142). Baltimore: Brookes.

Glidewell, J. (1961). *Parental attitudes and child behavior. Springfield, IL:* Thomas.

Gliedman, J., & Roth, W. (1980). *The unexpected minority: Handicapped children in America.* New York: Harcourt Brace Jovanovich.

Goddard, H. (1912). *The Kallikak family: A study in the heredity of feeblemindedness.* New York: Macmillan.

Goddard, H. H. (1914). *Feeblemindedness, its causes and consequences.* New York: Macmillan.

Goffman, E. (1961). *Asylums.* Garden City, NY: Anchor Books.

Goffman, E. (1963). Stigma: Notes on the management of spoiled identity. Englewood Cliffs, NJ: Prentice Hall.

Goffman, E. (1967). *Interaction ritual: Essays in face to face behaviors.* Chicago: Aldine.

Gold, R.B., & Daley, D. (1991). Public funding of contraceptive, sterilization and abortion services, Fiscal year 1990. *Family Planning Perspectives, 23*(5), 204–211.

Goldstein, J., Freud, A., & Solnit, A.J. (1979). *Beyond the best interests of the child.* New York: Collier Macmillan.

Gollay, E., Freedman, R., Wyngaarden, M. & Kurtz, N. R. (1978). *Coming back: Community experiences of deinstitutionalized mentally retarded people.* Cambridge, MA: Abt Books.

Goodman, L., Budner, S., & Lesh, B. (1979). The parents' role in sex education for the retarded. *Mental Retardation, 9,* 43–45.

Gordon, S. (1976). Morality and sexuality. *Exceptional Parent, 7,* 47–49.

Gould, S. J. (1981). *The mismeasure of man.* New York: Norton.

Grace, E., Emans, S. J., & Woods, E. R. (1989). The impact of AIDS awareness on the adolescent female. *Adolescent and Pediatric Gynecology, 2,* 40–42.

Grady, In re, 85 N.J. 235, 426 A.2d 467 (1981).

Grant, N. J. (1992). *The selling of contraception: The Dalkon Shield case, sexuality, and women's autonomy.* Columbus: Ohio State University Press.

Green, A. H. (1988). Special issues in child sexual abuse. In D.H. Schetky & A.H. Green (Eds.), *Child sexual abuse: A handbook for health care professionals* (pp. 125–135). New York: Bruner/Mazel.

Green, J., & Armstrong, D. (1993). Controlling the "bed state": Negotiating hospital organisation. *Sociology of Health and Illness, 15,* 141–149.

Greenberg, S., & Campbell, P. B. (1992). Sexism, sexuality, and education: Feminist thought then and now. In S.S. Klein (Ed.), *Sex equity and sexuality in education* (pp. 19–34). Albany: State University of New York Press.

Greenfield, J. (1978). *A place for Noah.* New York: Holt, Rinehart & Winston.

Greenspan, S., & Budd, K. S. (1986). Research on mentally retarded parents. In J. J. Gallagher & P. M. Vietze (Eds.), *Families of handicapped persons: Research, programs, and policy issues* (pp. 115–127). Baltimore: Brookes.

Greenspan, S., & Granfield, J.M. (1992). Reconsidering the construct of mental retardation: Implications of a model of social competence. *American Journal on Mental Retardation, 96*, 442–453.

Greenspan, S., Granfield, J.M., & Becker, S. (1991). Toward an outcome-based definition of mental retardation. *American Association of Mental Retardation: Psychology Division Newsletter, 1*, 27–29.

Griffin, S. (1981). *Pornography and silence: Culture's revenge against nature.* New York: Harper & Row.

Griffiths, D. M., Quinsey, V. L., & Hingsburger, D. (1989). *Changing inappropriate sexual behavior: A community-based approach for persons with developmental disabilities.* Baltimore: Brookes.

Grimes, D. A. (1992). The safety of oral contraceptives: Epidemiologic insights from the first 30 years. *American Journal of Obstetrics and Gynecology, 166*, 1950–1954.

Griswold v. Connecticut, 381 U.S. 479 (1965).

Grossman, H. J. (1973). *Manual on terminology and classification in mental retardation* (rev. ed.). Washington, DC: American Association on Mental Deficiency.

Grossman, H. J. (1983). *Classification in mental retardation.* Washington, DC: American Association on Mental Deficiency.

Haavik, S. F., & Menninger, K. A., II. (1981). *Sexuality, law, and the developmentally disabled person: Legal and clinical aspects of marriage, parenthood, and sterilization.* Baltimore: Brookes.

Habermas, J. (1986). Law as medium and law as institution. In G. Teubner (Ed.), *Dilemmas of law in the welfare state* (pp. 203–220). Berlin: de Gruyter.

Hahn, H. (1987). Public policy and disabled infants: A sociopolitical perspective. *Issues in Law and Medicine, 3*(1), 3–27.

Hahn, H. (1991). Theories and values: Ethics and contrasting perspectives on disability. In R.P. Marinelli & A.E. Dell Orto (Eds.), *The psychological and social impact of disability* (pp. 18–22). New York: Springer.

Haight, S. L., & Fachting, D. D. (1986). Materials for teaching sexuality, love, and maturity to high school students with learning disabilities. *Journal of Learning Disabilities, 19*, 344–350.

Haldeman v. Pennhurst, 451 U.S. 1 (1981).

Hammar, S. L., Wright, L. S., & Jensen, D. L. (1967). Sex education for the retarded adolescent: A survey of parental attitudes and methods of management in fifty adolescent retardates. *Journal of Clinical Pediatrics, 6*, 621–627.

Hamre-Nietupski, S., & Ford, A. (1981). Sex education and related skills: A series of programs implemented with severely handicapped students. *Sexuality and Disability, 4*(3), 179–193.

Harding, S. (1987). Introduction: Is there a feminist method? In S. Harding (Ed.), *Feminism and methodology* (pp. 1–14). Bloomington: Indiana University Press.

Harding, S. (1993, October). *The objectivity of knowledge claims: Contributions from feminism* (School of Education Seminar Series). Bloomington: Indiana University Press.

Harris, A., & Wideman, D. (1988). The construction of gender and disability in early attachment. In M. Fine & A. Asch (Eds.), *Women with disabilities: Essays in psychology, culture, and politics* (pp. 115–138). Philadelphia: Temple University Press.

Harris, J. (1988). Wrongful birth. In D.R. Bromham, M.E. Dalton, & J.C. Jackson (Eds.), *Philosophical ethics in reproductive medicine* (pp. 156–170). Manchester, England: Manchester University Press.

Hartmann, B. (1987). *Reproductive rights and wrongs: The global politics of population control and contraceptive choice.* New York: Harper & Row.

Hauerwas, S. (1982). The retarded, society, and the family: The dilemma of care. In S. Hauerwas (Ed.), *Responsibility for devalued persons: Ethical interactions between society, the family, and the retarded* (pp. 42–65). Springfield, IL: Thomas.

Hayes, In re, 93 Wash. 228, 608 P.2d 635 (1980).

Heber, R., & Garber, H. (1975). The Milwaukee Project: A study of the use of family intervention to prevent cultural-familial mental retardation. In F. Friedlander, F. Sterritt, & G. Kirk (Eds.), *Exceptional infant: Assessment and intervention* (Vol. 3, p. 399). New York: Bruner/Mazel.

Heller, T., Bond, M., & Braddock, D. (1988). Family reactions to institutional closure. *American Journal on Mental Retardation, 92*, 336–343.

Henshel, A. M. (1972). *The forgotten ones: A sociological study of Anglo and Chicano retardates.* Austin: University of Texas Press.

Heshusius, L. (1981). *Meaning in life as experienced by persons labeled retarded in a group home: A participant observation study.* Springfield, IL: Thomas.

Hewitt, S. E. (1987). The abuse of deinstitutionalized persons with mental handicaps. *Disability, Handicap and Society, 2*(2), 127–135.

Hill, B. K., Rotegard, L.L., & Bruininks, R. H. (1984). Quality of life of mentally retarded people in residential care. *Social Work, 29*, 275–281.

Hill, I. B. (1950). Sterilizations in Oregon. *American Journal of Mental Deficiency, 54*, 403.

Hill, R. (1949). *Families under stress.* New York: Free Press.

Hingsburger, D. (1988). Clients and curriculum: Preparing for sex education. *Psychiatric Aspects of Mental Retardation Reviews, 7*, 13–17.

Hirayama, H. (1979). Management of the sexuality of the mentally retarded in institutions: Problems and issues. In D. Kunkel (Ed.), *Sexual issues in social work* (pp. 105–130). Honolulu: University of Hawaii, School of Social Work.

H. L. v. Matheson, 450 U.S. 398 (1981).

Hoffmaster, B. (1982). Caring for retarded persons: Ethical ideals and practical choices. In S. Hauerwas (Ed.), *Responsibility for devalued persons:*

Ethical interactions between society, the family, and the retarded (pp. 28–41). Springfield, IL: Thomas.

Holmes, H. B., & Purdy, L. M. (Eds.) (1992). *Feminist perspectives in medical ethics*. Bloomington: Indiana University Press.

Hudson, F., & Ineichen, B. (1991). *Taking it lying down: Sexuality and teenage motherhood*. London: Macmillan.

Humm-Delgado, D. (1979). Opinions of community residence staff about their work and responsibilities. *Mental Retardation, 17*, 250–251.

Illich, I. (1977). *Disabling professions*. London: M. Boyars.

Individuals with Disabilities Education Act of 1990, Pub. L. 101–476, 20 U.S.C. Codified as 20 U.S.C. Sec. 1400 et seq.

Irvine, A. C. (1988). Balancing the right of the mentally retarded to obtain a therapeutic sterilization against the potential for abuse. *Law and Psychology Review, 12*, 95–122.

Jackson, J. (1988). Withholding neonatal care 2. A philosopher's view. In D. R. Bromham, M. E. Dalton, & J. C. Jackson (Eds.), *Philosophical ethics in reproductive medicine* (pp. 124–139). Manchester, England: Manchester University Press.

Janko, S. (1994). *Vulnerable children, vulnerable families: The social construction of child abuse*. New York: Teachers College Press.

Jaspars, J., & Hewstone, M. (1990). Social categorization, collective beliefs, and causal attribution. In C. Fraser & G. Gaskell (Eds.), *The social psychological study of widespread beliefs* (pp. 121–141). Oxford, England: Clarendon Press.

Jasso, G. (1991). Distributive justice and social welfare institutions. In H. Steensma & R. Vermunt (Eds.), *Social justice in human relations: vol. 2. Societal and psychological consequences of justice and injustice* (pp. 155–192). New York: Plenum Press.

Jendrek, M. P. (1993). Grandparents who parent their grandchildren: Effects on lifestyle. *Journal of Marriage and the Family, 55*, 609–621.

Jensen, A. R. (1969). How much can we boost IQ and scholastic achievement? *Harvard Educational Review, 39*, 1–123.

Joffe, C. (1986). *The regulation of sexuality: Experiences of family planning workers*. Philadelphia: Temple University Press.

Johnson, B. S. (1946). A study of cases discharged from Laconia State School from July 1, 1924 to July 1, 1934. *American Journal of Mental Deficiency, 50*, 437–445.

Jordan, L. (1987). Parents, power, and the politics of special education in a London borough. In T. Booth & W.P. Swann (Eds.), *Including pupils with disabilities* (pp. 218–223). London: Open University Press.

Kaeser, F., & O'Neill, J. (1987). Task analyzed masturbation instruction for a profoundly mentally retarded adult male: A data based case study. *Sexuality and Disability, 8*, 17–24.

Kasachkoff, T. (1989). Paternalistic solicitude and paternalistic behavior: Appropriate contexts and moral justifications. In C. Pedem & J. P. Sterba (Eds.), *Freedom, equality, and social change* (pp. 79–93). Lewiston, NY: Edwin Mellen Press.

Kastner, T. A., DeLotto, P., Scagnelli, B., & Testa, W. R. (1990). Proposed guidelines for agencies serving persons with developmental disabilities and HIV infection. *Mental Retardation, 28*(3), 139–145.

Katz, I., Hass, R. G., & Bailey, J. (1988). Attitudinal ambivalence and behavior toward people with disabilities. In H.E. Yuker (Ed.), *Attitudes toward persons with disabilities* (pp. 47–57). New York: Springer.

Kaufert, P. (1992). Genes, embryos, and public policy. *Women and Therapy, 12*, 83–91.

Kaufman, S. (1984). Friendship, coping systems, and community adjustment of mildly retarded adults. In R.B. Edgerton (Ed.), Lives in process: Mentally retarded adults in a large city (pp. 73–92). *Monographs of the American Association of Mental Deficiency* (No. 6).

Keddie, N. (1973). *The myth of cultural deprivation*. Harmondsworth, England: Penguin.

Kempton, W. (1977). The sexual adolescent who is mentally retarded. *Journal of Pediatric Psychology, 2*, 104–107.

Kempton, W. (1988). *Sex education for persons with disabilities that hinder learning: A teacher's guide*. Chicago, IL: Stoelting Co.

Kempton, W., & Gochros, J.S. (1986). The developmentally disabled. In H.L. Gochros, J.S. Gochros, & J. Fischer (Eds.), *Helping the sexually oppressed* (pp. 224–237). Englewood Cliffs, NJ: Prentice-Hall.

Kennedy, C. H., Horner, R. H., & Newton, J. S. (1990). The social networks and activity patterns with severe disabilities: A correlational analysis. *Journal of the Association for Persons with Severe Handicaps, 14*, 190–196.

Kevles, D. J. (1987). *In the name of eugenics: Genetics and the uses of human heredity*. New York: Knopf.

Kingdom, E. (1989). Birthrights: Equal or special? In R. Lee & D. Morgan (Eds.), *Birthrights: Law and ethics at the beginnings of life* (pp. 17–36). New York: Routledge.

Klein, S. S. (Ed.). (1992). *Sex equity and sexuality in education*. Albany: State University of New York Press.

Kleinfeld, A., & Young, R. (1989). Risk of pregnancy and dropping out of school among special education adolescents. *Journal of Social Health, 59*(8), 359–361.

Koegel, P., & Edgerton, R. B. (1982). Labeling and the perception of handicap among black mildly mentally retarded adults. *American Journal of Mental Deficiency, 87*, 266–276.

Kohlberg, L. (1969). Stage and sequence: The cognitive-development approach to socialization. In D.A. Goslin (Ed.), *Handbook of socialization theory and research*. Chicago: Rand McNally.

Kohlberg, L. (1981). *The philosophy of moral development.* San Francisco: Harper & Row.

Koller, H., Richardson, S. A., & Katz, M. (1988). Marriage in a young adult mentally retarded population. *Journal of Mental Deficiency Research, 32,* 93–102.

Kolodny, R. C. (1979). *Textbook of sexual medicine.* Boston: Little, Brown.

Konstantareas, M. M., & Homatidis, S. (1992). Mothers' and fathers' self-report of involvement with autistic, mentally delayed, and normal children. *Journal of Marriage and the Family, 54,* 153–164.

Koop, C. E. (1989). Life and death and the handicapped newborn. *Issues in Law and Medicine, 5*(1), 101–113.

Kratter, R. E., & Thorne, G.D. (1957). Sex education for retarded children. *American Journal of Mental Deficiency, 62,* 44–48.

Krauss, M. W. (1986). Patterns and trends in public services to families with a mentally retarded member. In J. J. Gallagher & P.M. Vietze (Eds.), *Families of handicapped persons: Research, programs, and policy issues* (pp. 237–248). Baltimore: Brookes.

Kubler-Ross, E. (1969). *On death and dying.* New York: Macmillan.

Lakin, K. C., Prouty, R. W., White, C. C., Bruininks, R. N., & Hill, B. K. (1990). *Intermediate care facilities for persons with mental retardation (ICFs-MR): Program utilization and resident characteristics* (Report No. 31). Minneapolis: University of Minnesota, Center for Residential and Community Services.

Lambert, C. (1974, September). *Profiles of adults living in the community.* Paper presented at the Oxford Symposium on the Adult Retarded in Ontario: Today and Tomorrow, Woodstock, Ontario.

Lancaster, J., & Hamburg, B. (Eds.). (1986). *School age pregnancy and parenthood: Biosocial dimensions.* New York: Aldine de Gruyter.

Lareau, A. (1987). Social class differences in family-school relationships: The importance of cultural capital. *Sociology of Education, 60,* 73–85.

Larry P. v. Riles, 495 F. Supp. 926 (N.D. Cal. 1979).

Lee, R. (1989). To be or not to be: Is that the question? The claim of wrongful life. In R. Lee & D. Morgan (Eds.), *Birthrights: Law and ethics at the beginnings of life* (pp. 172–194). New York: Routledge.

Lee, R., & Morgan, D. (1989a). A lesser sacrifice? Sterilization and mentally handicapped women. In R. Lee & D. Morgan (Eds.), *Birthrights: Law and ethics at the beginnings of life* (pp. 132–154). New York: Routledge.

Lee, R., & Morgan, D. (1989b). Is birth important? In R. Lee & D. Morgan (Eds.), *Birthrights: Law and ethics at the beginnings of life* (pp. 1–16). New York: Routledge.

Lee, S. (1988). Whose consent? In D. R. Bromham, M. E. Dalton, & J. C. Jackson (Eds.), *Philosophical ethics in reproductive medicine* (pp. 236–260). Manchester, England: Manchester University Press.

LeMaistre, J. (1985). Parenting. In S.E. Browne, D. Connors, & N. Stern (Eds.), *With the power of each breath: A disabled women's anthology* (pp. 284–291). Pittsburgh: Cleis.

Levine, C. & Veatch, R. M. (Eds.) (1984). Cases in bioethics from the Hastings Center Report. Hastings-on-Hudson, NY: Hastings Center.

Levy, J. M., Levy, P. H., & Samowitz, P. (1988). *AIDS: Teaching persons with disabilities to better protect themselves.* New York: Young Adult Institute.

Lilford, R. (1988). What is informed consent? In D. R. Bromham, M. E. Dalton, & J. C. Jackson (Eds.), *Philosophical ethics in reproductive medicine* (pp. 211–235). Manchester, England: Manchester University Press.

Livneh, H. (1988). A dimensional perspective on the origin of negative attitudes toward persons with disabilities. In H.E. Yuker (Ed.), *Attitudes toward persons with disabilities* (pp. 35–46). New York: Springer.

Livneh, H. (1991). On the origins of negative attitudes toward people with disabilities. In R. P. Marinelli & A. E. Dell Orto (Eds.), *The psychological and social impact of disability* (pp. 181–196). New York: Springer.

Llewellyn, M. H., & McLaughlin, T. F. (1986). An evaluation of a self-protection skills program for the mildly handicapped. *Child and Family Behaviour Therapy, 8*(4), 29–37.

Luster, T., & Dubow, E. (1992). Home environment and maternal intelligence as predictors of verbal intelligence: A comparison of preschool and school-age children. *Merrill-Palmer Quarterly, 38*, 151–175.

Lusthaus, E. W. (1985). Involuntary euthanasia and current attempts to define persons with mental retardation as less than human. *Mental Retardation, 23*(3), 148–154.

Madsen, M. K. (1979). Parenting classes for the mentally retarded. *Mental Retardation, 17*, 195–196.

Mappes, T. A., & Zembaty, J. S. (1986). Appendix: Case studies. In T. A. Mappes & J.S. Zembaty (Eds.), *Biomedical ethics* (pp. 638–657). New York: McGraw-Hill.

Marchetti, A., Nathanson, R., Kastner, T., & Owens, R. (1990). AIDS and state developmental disability agencies: A national survey. *American Journal of Public Health, 80*, 54–56.

Martin, D. A. (1988). Children and adolescents with traumatic brain injury: Impact on the family. *Journal of Learning Disabilities, 21*, 464–470.

Mason, J. K. (1990). *Medico-legal aspects of reproduction and parenthood.* Aldershot, England: Dartmouth.

Mattinson, J. (1971). *Marriage and mental handicap.* Pittsburgh: University of Pittsburgh Press.

Mayer, D. O. (1979). Legal advocacy for developmentally disabled people. In R. Wiegerink & J.W. Pelosi (Eds.), *Developmental disabilities: The DD movement* (pp. 67–75). Baltimore: Brookes.

Mazumdar, P.M.H. (1992). *Eugenics, human genetics, and human failings: The Eugenics Society, its sources and its critics in Britain.* London: Routledge.

McAfee, J. K., & Gural, M. (1988). Individuals with mental retardation and the criminal justice system: The view from states' attorneys general. *Mental Retardation, 25,* 5–12.

McCarver, R. B., & Craig, E. M. (1974). Placement of the retarded in the community: Prognosis and outcome. In N. R. Ellis (Ed.), *International review of research in mental retardation* (Vol. 7, pp. 145–199). New York: Academic Press.

McClennen, S. (1988). Sexuality and students with mental retardation. *Teaching Exceptional Children, 20,* 59–61.

McCubbin, H., & Patterson, J. (1983). Family transitional adaptations to stress. In H. McCubbin & C. Figley (Eds.), *Stress and the family* (Vol. 1, pp. 5–25). New York: Bruner-Mazel.

McCullough, L. B., Coverdale, J., Bayer, T., & Chervenak, F. A. (1992). Ethically justified guidelines for family planning interventions to prevent pregnancy in female patients with chronic mental illness. *American Journal of Obstetrics and Gynecology, 167*(1), 19–25.

Mercer, J. R. (1973). *Labeling the mentally retarded.* Berkeley: University of California Press.

Meyer, D., Vadasy, P., & Fewell, R. R. (1985). *Living with a brother or sister with special needs.* Seattle: University of Washington Press.

Mickelson, P. (1947). The feebleminded parent: A study of 90 family cases. *American Journal of Mental Deficiency, 51,* 644–653.

Mills, N. (1977). Our daughter's happiness depends on her being sterile. *The Exceptional Parent, 7,* 2–4.

Minuchin, S. (1974). *Families and family therapy.* Cambridge, MA: Harvard University Press.

Mitchell, L., Doctor, R. M. & Butler, D. C. (1978). Attitudes of caretakers toward the sexual behavior of mentally retarded persons. *American Journal of Mental Deficiency, 83,* 289–296.

Mitchell-Kernan, C., & Tucker, M. B. (1984). The social structures of mildly mentally retarded Afro-Americans: Gender comparisons. In R. B. Edgerton (Ed.), Lives in process: Mentally retarded adults in a large city (pp. 173–192). *Monographs of the American Association of Mental Deficiency* (No. 6).

Morgan, R. (Ed.). (1984). *Sisterhood is global: The international women's movement anthology.* Middlesex, England: Penguin Books.

Morgan, S. (1982). Sex after hysterectomy—What your doctor never told you. *MS, 10,* 82–85.

Morris, J. (1991). *Pride against prejudice: Transforming attitudes to disability.* Philadelphia: New Society Publishers.

Morris, P. (1969). *Put away.* London: Routledge and Kegan Paul.

Muccigrosso, L., Scavarda, M., Simpson-Brown, R., & Thalacker, B.E. (1991). *Double jeopardy: Pregnant and parenting youth in special education.*

Washington, DC: ERIC Clearinghouse on Handicapped and Gifted Children.

Mulhern, T. (1975). Survey of reported sexual behaviors and policies characterizing residential facilities for retarded citizens. *American Journal of Mental Deficiency, 79,* 670–673.

Murphy, J. S. (1992). Is pregnancy necessary: Feminist concerns about ectogenesis. In H. B. Holmes & L. M. Purdy (Eds.), *Feminist perspectives in medical ethics* (pp. 181–197). Bloomington: Indiana University Press.

Murray-Seegert, C. (1989). *Nasty girls, thugs, and humans like us: Social relations between severely disabled and nondisabled students in high school.* Baltimore: Brookes.

Myrdal, A. (1945). *Nation and family.* London: Kegan Paul, Trench, Tubner.

Nathanson, C. A. (1991). *Dangerous passage: The social control of sexuality in women's adolescence.* Philadelphia: Temple University Press.

National Down Syndrome Society. (1984). Fact sheet on Down syndrome. *The Exceptional Parent, 14,* 47–49.

Nelson, C. A. (1988). Animals, handicapped children and the tragedy of marginal cases. *Journal of Medical Ethics, 14,* 191.

Neufeld, G. R. (1979). Deinstitutionalization procedures. In R. Wiegerink & J. W. Pelosi (Eds.), *Developmental disabilities: The DD movement* (pp. 115–126). Baltimore: Brookes.

Neville, R. (1981). Sterilizing the mildly retarded without their consent. In. R. Macklin & W. Gaylin (Eds.), *Mental Retardation and Sterilization* (pp. 61–73). New York: Plenum.

Nietro, In re Conservatorship of Valerie, 40 Cal. 3d 143, 707 P.2d 760, 219 Cal. Rptr. 386 (1985).

Nigro, G. (1977). Sexuality and the handicapped. In J. Stubbins (Ed.), *Social and psychological aspects of disability* (pp. 131–136). Baltimore: University Park Press.

Noddings, N. (1993). Caring: A feminist perspective. In K. A. Strike & P. L. Ternasky (Eds.), *Ethics for professionals in education: Perspectives for preparation and practice (pp. 43–53). New York: Teachers College Press.*

North Carolina Association for Retarded Children v. State of North Carolina, 420 F. Supp. 451 (M.D.N.C. 1976).

Oakley, A. (1984). *Captured womb.* Oxford, England: Blackwell.

Oakley, A. (1985). *Subject women.* London: Fontana.

Olshansky, S. (1962). Chronic sorrow: A response to having a mentally retarded child. *Social Casework, 43,* 190–193.

Omenn, G. S. (1978). Prenatal diagnosis of genetic disorders. *Science, 200,* 952–958.

O'Neil, J., Brown, M., Gordon, W., Schonhorn, R., & Green, E. (1981). Activity patterns of mentally retarded adults in institutions and communities—A longitudinal study. *Applied Research in Mental Retardation, 2,* 367–379.

O'Neill, A. M. (1985). Normal and bright children of mentally retarded parents: The Huck Finn syndrome. *Child Psychiatry and Human Development, 15*, 255–268.

O'Toole, C. J., & Bregante, J. L. (1992). Disabled women: The myth of the asexual female. In S. S. Klein (Ed.), *Sex equity and sexuality in education* (pp. 273–301). Albany: State University of New York Press.

Painsky, A., Katz, S., & Kravetz, S. (1986). Sexual behavior patterns of institutionalized mentally handicapped persons. *International Journal of Rehabilitation Research, 9*(3), 276–279.

Park, C. (1982). *The siege: The first eight years of an autistic child.* Boston: Atlantic–Little, Brown.

Pascoe, P. (1990). *Relations of rescue: The search for female moral authority in the American West, 1874–1939.* New York: Oxford University Press.

Patton, M. Q. (1980). *Qualitative evaluation methods.* Beverly Hills, CA: Sage.

Paul, J. L., Porter, P. B., & Falk, G. D. (1993). In J. L. Paul & R. J. Simeonsson (Eds.), *Children with special needs: Family, culture, and society* (pp. 3–24). Fort Worth, TX: Harcourt Brace Jovanovich.

Paul, J. L., & Simeonsson, R. J. (Eds.). (1993). *Children with special needs: Family, culture, and society.* Fort Worth, TX: Harcourt Brace Jovanovich.

Payne, A. T. (1978). The law and the problem parent: Custody and parental rights of homosexual, mentally retarded, mentally ill and incarcerated parents. *Journal of Family Law, 16*(4), 797–818.

Payne, J. E. (1976). The deinstitutional backlash. *Mental Retardation, 14*, 43–45.

Peck, J. R., & Stephens, W. B. (1965). Marriage of young adult male retardates. *American Journal of Mental Deficiency, 69*, 818–827.

Pennsylvania Association for Retarded Citizens v. Commonwealth of Pennsylvania (1972).

Penrose, L. S. (1950). Propagation of the unfit. *Lancet, 259*, 425–427.

Penry, In re, 832 F.2d 915 (5th Cir. 1987).

Petchesky, R. P. (1979). Reproduction, ethics and public policy: The federal sterilization regulations. *Hastings Center Reports, 9*, 29–41.

Petchesky, R. P. (1990). *Abortion and woman's choice: The state, sexuality, and reproductive freedom.* Evanston, IL: Northeastern University Press.

Peterson, S., Robinson, E., & Littman, I. (1983). Parent-child interaction training for parents with a history of mental retardation. *Applied Research in Mental Retardation, 4*, 329–342.

Pincus, J., & Swenson, N. (1992). Pregnancy. In Boston Women's Health Book Collective, *The new our bodies, ourselves* (pp. 401–434). New York: Simon & Schuster.

Pincus, S., Schoenbaum, E., & Webber, M. (1990). A seroprevalence survey for human immunodeficiency virus antibody in mentally retarded adults. *New York State Journal of Medicine, 90*, 139–142.

Planned Parenthood v. Casey, 112 U.S. S.Ct. 2791, 2807 (1992).

Planned Parenthood of the State of Missouri v. Danforth, 428 U.S. 52 (1976).

Pledgie, T. K., & Schumacher, S. H. (1993). Determining the prevalence of human immunodeficiency virus (HIV) within a residential facility for persons with mental retardation. *American Journal on Mental Retardation, 97*(5), 585–588.

Preston, S. H., & Campbell, C. (1993). Differential fertility and the distribution of traits: The case of IQ. *American Journal of Sociology, 98*, 997–1019.

Pueschel, S. M., & Scola, P. S. (1988). Parents' perception of social and sexual functions in adolescents with Down syndrome. *Journal of Mental Deficiency Research, 32*, 215–220.

Quinlan, In re, 355 A. 2d 664 (N.J. 1979).

Ramey, C., & Campbell, F. (1984). Preventive education for high-risk children: Cognitive consequences of the Carolina Abecedrian Project. *American Journal of Mental Deficiency, 88*, 515–523.

Ramsey, E., & Hill, M. W. (1988). Family management correlates of antisocial behavior among middle school boys. *Behavioral Disorders, 13*, 187–201.

Rawls, J. (1971). *A theory of justice*. Cambridge: Harvard University Press.

Reed, E. W., & Reed, S. C. (1965). *Mental retardation: A family study*. Philadelphia: Saunders.

Reed, S. C. (1955). *Counseling in medical genetics*. Philadelphia: Saunders.

Reed, S. C., & Anderson, V.E. (1973). Effects of changing sexuality on the gene pool. In F. de la Cruz & G. DeLaVeck (Eds.), *Human sexuality and the mentally retarded* (pp. 111–125). New York: Bruner/Mazel.

Reed, S. C., Reed, E. W., & Palm, J. D. (1954). Fertility and intelligence among families of the mentally deficient. *Eugenics Quarterly, 1*, 44–52.

Rehabilitation Act of 1973, Pub. L. 93–112, 29 U.S.C. 701 et seq.

Reilly, P. R. (1991). *The surgical solution: A history of involuntary sterilization in the United States*. Baltimore: Johns Hopkins University Press.

Reinert, H. R., & Huang, A. (1987). *Children in conflict: Educational strategies for the emotionally disturbed and behaviorally disordered*. Columbus, OH: Merrill.

Reiss, I. (1970). How and why America's sex standards are changing. In J. H. Gagnon & W. Simon (Eds.), *The Sexual Scene*. New York: Transaction Books.

Relf v. Weinberger, 372 F. Supp. 1196 (D.D.C. 1974).

Richards, D. (1986). Sterilization: Can parents decide. *The Exceptional Parent, 16*(2), 40–41.

Richards, M., & Light, P. (1986). *Children of social worlds: Development in a social context*. Cambridge: Harvard University Press.

Richman, G., & Trohanis, P. (1979). Public awareness as a developmental disability. In R. Wiegerink & J.W. Pelosi (Eds.), *Developmental disabilities: The DD movement* (pp. 85–90). Baltimore: Brookes.

Rienzo, B. A. (1981). The status of sex education: An overview and recommendations. *Phi Delta Kappan, 63*, 192–193.

Rindfleisch, N., & Bean, G. J. (1988). Willingness to report abuse and neglect in residential facilities. *Child Abuse and Neglect, 12*, 509–520.

Robinson, L. H. (1978). Parental attitudes of retarded young mothers. *Child Psychiatry and Human Development, 8*, 131–144.

Roe v. Wade, 410 U.S. 113 (1973).

Rosen, M. (1970). Conditioning appropriate heterosexual behavior in mentally and socially handicapped populations. *Training School Bulletin, 66*, 172–177.

Rosen, M., Clark, G. R., & Kivitz, M. S. (1977). *Habilitation of the handicapped: New dimensions in programs for the developmentally disabled.* Baltimore: University Park Press.

Rosenberg, S. A., & McTate, G. A. (1982). Intellectually handicapped mothers: Problems and prospects. *Children Today, 11*, 24–28.

Rosenholtz, S. J., & Simpson, C. (1984). The formation of ability conceptions: Developmental trend or social construction? *Review of Educational Research, 54*, 31–63.

Rosser, S. V. (1992). Re-visioning clinical research: Gender and the ethics of experimental design. In H. B. Holmes & L. M. Purdy (Eds.), *Feminist perspective in medical ethics* (pp. 127–139). Bloomington: Indiana University Press.

Rousso, H. (1982). Special consideration in counseling clients with cerebral palsy. *Sexuality and Disability, 5*(2), 78–88.

Rousso, H. (1986). Positive female images at last! *The Exceptional Parent, 16*(2), 10–12, 14.

Rousso, H. (1988). Daughters with disabilities: Defective women or minority women? In M. Fine & A. Asch (Eds.), *Women with disabilities: Essays in psychology, culture, and politics* (pp. 139–171). Philadelphia: Temple University Press.

Rowitz, L. (Ed.). (1989). Developmental disabilities and HIV infection: A symposium on issues and public policy. *Mental Retardation, 27*, 197–262.

Russo, N. F., & Jansen, M. A. (1988). Women, work, and disability: Opportunities and challenges. In M. Fine & A. Asch (Eds.), *Women with disabilities: Essays in psychology, culture, and politics* (pp. 229–244). Philadelphia: Temple University Press.

Rutter, M. (1982). Prevention of children's psychosocial disorders: Myths and substance. *Pediatrics, 70*, 883–894.

Sabagh, G., & Edgerton, R.B. (1962). Sterilized mental defectives look at eugenic sterilization. *Eugenics Quarterly, 9*, 213–222.

Saenger, G. (1957). *The adjustment of severely retarded adults in the community* (A Report to the New York State Interdepartmental Health Resources Board). Albany, NY: Graduate School of Public Administration and Social Service Research Center.

Sameroff, A. J., & Chandler, M. J. (1975). Prenatal risk and the continuum of caretaking causality. In F. Horowitz, M. Hetherington, S. Scarr-Salaopatek, & G. Siegel (Eds.), *Review of child development research* (Vol. 4, pp. 187–244). Chicago: University of Chicago Press.

Sameroff, A. J., & Friese, B. (1990). Transaction, regulation, and early intervention. In S. Meisels & J. Shonkoff (Eds.), *Handboook of early childhood intervention* (pp. 119–149). New York: Cambridge University Press.

Sandmaier, M. (1992). Alcohol, mood-altering drugs and smoking. In Boston Women's Health Book Collective, *The new our bodies, ourselves* (pp. 55–64). New York: Simon & Schuster.

Sarrel, L. J., & Sarrel, P. M. (1990). Sexual unfolding in adolescents. In M. Sugar (Ed.), *Atypical adolescents and sexuality* (pp. 18–43). New York: W.W. Norton.

Satterfield, S., & Sugar, M. (1990). Clinical aspects of juvenile prostitution. In M. Sugar (Ed.), *Atypical adolescents and sexuality* (pp. 172–180). New York: W.W. Norton.

Saunders, E. J. (1979). Staff members' attitudes toward the sexual behavior of mentally retarded residents. *American Journal of Mental Deficiency, 84*, 206–208.

Scally, B. G. (1973). Marriage and mental handicap: Some observations in Northern Ireland. In F. de la Cruz & G. DeLaVeck (Eds.), *Human sexuality and the mentally retarded* (pp. 186–194). New York: Bruner/Mazel.

Scarr, S., & Weinberg, R. A. (1978). The influence of family background on intellectual attainment. *American Sociology Review, 43*, 674–692.

Schaefer, E. S. (1991). Goals for parent and future-parent education: Research on parental beliefs and behavior. *The Elementary School Journal, 91*, 239–248.

Scheerenberger, R. C., & Felsenthal, D. (1977). Community settings for mentally retarded persons: Satisfaction and activities. *Mental Retardation, 15*, 3–7.

Schilling, R. F., Schinke, S.P., Blythe, B. J., & Barth, R. P. (1982). Child maltreatment and mentally retarded parents: Is there a relationship? *Mental Retardation, 20*, 201–209.

Schultz, G. L. (1981). Sexual contact between staff and residents. In D.A. Shore & H.L. Gochros (Eds.), *Sexual problems of adolescents in institutions* (pp. 90–103). Springfield, IL: Thomas.

Schweinhart, L. J., & Weikart, D. P. (1981). Perry preschool effects nine years later: What do they mean? In M. J. Begab, H. C. Haywood, & H. L. Garber (Eds.), *Psychosocial influences in retarded performance* (Vol. 2, pp. 113–126). Baltimore: University Park Press.

Scott-Jones, D. (1984). Family influences on cognitive development and school achievement. In E.S. Gordon (Ed.), *Review of research in education* (Vol. 11, pp. 259–304). Washington, DC: American Educational Research Association.

Seginer, R. (1983). Parents' educational expectations and children's academic achievements: A literature review. *Merrill-Palmer Quarterly, 29*, 1–23.

Seligman, M., & Darling, R.B. (1989). *Ordinary families, special children: A systems approach and childhood disability*. New York: Guilford.

Sewell, G. (1981). The microsociology of segregation: Case studies in the exclusion of children with special needs from ordinary schools. In L. Barton & S. Tomlinson (Eds.), *Special education: Policy, practice and social issues* (pp. 17–28). London: Harper & Row.

Sexton, D. (1989, July 26). *Working with parents of handicapped children*. Presentation at the Institute for the Study of Developmental Disabilities, Bloomington, IN.

Shafter, A. J. (1957). Criteria for selecting institutionalized mental defectives for vocational placement. *American Journal of Mental Deficiency, 62*, 599–616.

Shaw, C., & Wright, C. (1960). The married mental defective—A follow-up study. *Lancet, 1*, 273–274.

Shelton, J. D., & Speidel, J.J. (1983). The need for nonsurgical sterilization. In G. I. Zatuchni, J. D. Shelton, A. Goldsmith, & J. J. Sciarra (Eds.), *Female transcervical sterilization* (pp. 1–6). Philadelphia: Harper & Row.

Sherwin, S. (1992a). *No longer patient: Feminist ethics and health care*. Philadelphia: Temple University Press.

Sherwin, S. (1992b). Feminist and medical ethics: Two different approaches to contextual ethics. In H. B. Holmes & L. M. Purdy (Eds.), *Feminist perspectives in medical ethics* (pp. 17–31). Bloomington: Indiana University Press.

Sichel, B.A. (1992). Ethics of caring and the institutional ethics committee. In H. B. Holmes & L. M. Purdy (Eds.), *Feminist perspectives in medical ethics* (pp. 113–126). Bloomington: Indiana University Press.

Silver, L. B. (1989). Frequency of adoption of children and adolescents with learning disabilities. *Journal of Learning Disabilities, 22*, 325–327.

Simpson, In re, 180 N.E. 2d 206 (Ohio P. Ct. 1962).

Siperstein, G. N. (1992). Social competence: An important construct in mental retardation. *American Journal of Mental Deficiency, 96*, iii-vi.

Skeels, H. M., Updegraff, R., Wellman, B., & Williams, H. M. (1938). A study of environmental stimulation: An orphanage preschool project. *Iowa Studies of Child Welfare, 15*(4), 74–80.

Skinner v. Oklahoma, 316 U.S. 535 (1942).

Skodak, M., & Skeels, H. M. (1949). A final follow-up study of one hundred adopted children. *Journal of Genetic Psychology, 75*, 85–125.

Skrtic, T. (1991). *Behind special education: A critical analysis of professional culture and school organization*. Denver: Love.

Sleeter, C. (1986). Learning disabilities: The social construction of a special education category. *Exceptional Children, 53*, 46–64.

Sloan, I. J. (1988). *The law governing abortion, contraception, and sterilization.* London: Oceana Publications.

Smith, A. M. (1990). Is anything left of parental rights? In E. Sutherland & A. M. Smith (Eds.), *Family rights: Family law and medical advance* (pp. 4–20). Edinburgh: Edinburgh University Press.

Smith, C. (1993). Cultural sensitivity in working with children and families. In J.L. Paul & R.J. Simeonsson (Eds.), *Children with special needs: Family, culture, and society* (pp. 113–121). Fort Worth, TX: Harcourt Brace Jovanovich.

Smith, G. P., II. (1990). The ethics of ethics committees. *The Journal of Contemporary Law and Policy, 6,* 157–170.

Smith, G. P., II. (1988). Limitations on reproductive autonomy for the mentally handicapped. *Journal of Contemporary Health Law and Policy, 4,* 71–89.

Smith, J. D. (1994). The revised AAMR definition of mental retardation: The MRDD position. *Education and training in mental retardation and developmental disabilities, 29,* 179–183.

Smith, J. D. (1989). *The sterilization of Carrie Buck.* Far Hills, NJ: New Horizon Press.

Sobsey, D., Grey, S., Wells, D., Pyper, D., & Reimer-Heck, B. (1991). *Disability, sexuality, and abuse: An annotated bibliography.* Baltimore: Brookes.

Soskin, R. (1977). Voluntary sterilization—Safeguarding freedom of choice. *AMICUS, 3,* 40–44.

Sovner, R., & Hurley, A. D. (1989). Ten diagnostic principles for recognizing psychiatric disorders in mentally retarded persons. *Psychiatric Aspects of Mental Retardation Reviews, 8*(2), 9–16.

Spallone, P. (1989). *Beyond conception.* Granby, MA: Bergin & Garvey.

Spicker, P. (1984). *Stigma and social welfare.* London: Croom Helm.

Spitz, R. A. (1946). Hospitalism: A follow-up report on investigation described in Volume 1, 1945. *The Psychoanalytic Study of the Child, 2,* 113–117.

Stepan, N. L. (1991). *"The hour of eugenics": Race, gender, and nation in Latin America.* Ithaca, NY: Cornell University Press.

Stone, D. A. (1985). *The disabled state.* London: Macmillan.

Strauss, A. L. & Corbin, J. M. (1990). Basics of qualitative research: Grounded theory procedures. Newberry Park, CA: Sage.

Stubbins, J. (1991). The interdisciplinary status of rehabilitation psychology. In R. P. Marinelli & A. E. Dell Orto (Eds.), *The psychological and social impact of disability* (pp. 9–17). New York: Springer.

Stubbins, J. (1988). The politics of disability. In H. E. Yoker (Ed.), *Attitudes toward persons with disabilities* (pp. 22–32). New York: Springer.

Stump v. Sparkman, 435 U.S. 349 (1978).

Sugar, M. (Ed.). (1990). *Atypical adolescents and sexuality.* New York: W. W. Norton.

Sullivan, T. (1992). *Sexual abuse and the rights of children: Reforming Canadian law*. Toronto: University of Toronto Press.

Sutherland, E. (1990). Regulating pregnancy: Should we and can we? In E. Sutherland & A.M. Smith (Eds.), *Family rights: Family law and medical advance* (pp. 100–119). Edinburgh: Edinburgh University Press.

Szasz, T. (1991). Psychiatry and social control. *The Humanist, 51*, 24–27.

Taylor, M. O. (1989). Teaching parents about their impaired adolescent's sexuality. *American Journal of Maternal Child Nursing, 14*(2), 109–112.

Taylor, S. J., & Bogdan, R. (1991). On accepting relationships between people with mental retardation and nondisabled people: Towards an understanding of acceptance. In R.P. Marinelli & A. E. Dell Orto (Eds.), *The psychological and social impact of disability* (pp. 165–180). New York: Springer.

Thoene, J., Higgins, J., Krieger, R., Schnickel, R., & Weiss, L. (1981). Genetic screening for mental retardation in Michigan. *American Journal of Mental Deficiency, 85*, 335–340.

Thomas, D. D. (1993). Minorities in North America: African-American families. In J. L. Paul & R. J. Simeonsson (Eds.), *Children with special needs: Family, culture, and society* (pp. 122–138). Fort Worth, TX: Harcourt Brace Jovanovich.

Thurer, S. L. (1991). Woman and rehabilitation. In R. P. Marinelli & A. E. Dell Orto (Eds.), *The psychological and social impact of disability* (pp. 32–38). New York: Springer.

Thurman, S. K. (Ed.). (1985a). *Children of handicapped parents*. New York: Academic Press.

Thurman, S. K. (1985b). Ecological congruence in the study of families with handicapped parents. In S. K. Thurman (Ed.), *Children of handicapped parents* (pp. 35–45). New York: Academic Press.

Tobias, J. (1970). Vocational adjustment of young retarded adults. *Mental Retardation, 8*, 13–16.

Tredgold, A. F. (1903). Amentia (idiocy and imbecility). *Archives of Neurology from the Pathology Laboratory of the London County Asylums, 2*, 363–391.

Tredgold, A. F. (1937). *A textbook of mental deficiency* (6th ed.). Baltimore: Wood.

Trombley, S. (1988). *The right to reproduce: A history of coercive sterilization*. London: Weidenfeld & Nicolson.

Turchin, G. (1974). Sex attitudes of mothers of retarded children. *Journal of School Health, 44*, 490–492.

Turnbull, A. P. (1988). The challenge of providing comprehensive support to families. *Education and Training of the Mentally Retarded, 23*, 261–272.

Turnbull, A., Summers, J., & Brotherson, M. (1986). Family life cycle: Theoretical and empirical implications and future directions for families with mentally retarded members. In J. Gallagher & P. Vietze (Eds.), *Families with handicapped children* (pp. 45–66). Baltimore: Brookes.

Turnbull, A. P., & Turnbull, H. R. (Eds.). (1979). *Parents speak out: Growing with a handicapped child.* Columbus, OH: Merrill.

Turnbull, A. P., & Turnbull, H., III. (1985). Developing independence. *Journal of Adolescent Health Care, 6,* 108–119.

Turnbull, H. R., III, & Turnbull, A. P. (1979). Examining consumers' assumptions. In R. Wiegerink & J. W. Pelosi (Eds.), Developmental disabilities: The developmental disabilities movement (pp. 61–65). Baltimore: Brookes.

Turnbull, H. R., & Turnbull, A. P. (1975). Deinstitution and the law. *Mental Retardation, 13,* 14–20.

Tyor, P. L., & Bell, L. V. (1984). *Caring for the retarded in America.* Westport, CT: Greenwood Press.

Ursprung, A. W. (1990). Family crisis related to the deinstitutionalization of a mentally retarded child. In M. Nagler & J. Kemp (Eds.), *Perspectives on disability* (pp. 302–308). Palo Alto, CA: Health Markets Research.

Varela, R. A. (1979). Self-advocacy and changing attitudes. In R. Wiegerink & J. W. Pelosi (Eds.), *Developmental disabilities: The DD movement* (pp. 77–82). Baltimore: Brookes.

Veatch, R. M. (1987). *The patient as partner: A theory of human-experimentation ethics.* Bloomington: Indiana University Press.

Vitello, S. J. (1978). Involuntary sterilization: Recent developments. *Journal of Mental Retardation, 7,* 31–36.

Voysey, M. (1975). *A constant burden: The reconstitution of family life.* London: Routledge & Kegan Paul.

Walker, P. (1979). *Between labour and capital.* Boston: South End Press.

Warren, K. J. (1989). Reconceiving feminism. In C. Peden & J.P. Sterba (Eds.), *Freedom, equality, and social change* (pp. 135–146). Lewiston, NY: Edwin Mellen Press.

Warren, V. L. (1992). Feminist directions in medical ethics. In H. B. Holmes & L. M. Purdy (Eds.), *Feminist perspectives in medical ethics* (pp. 32–45). Bloomington: Indiana University Press.

Washington, V., & Gallagher, J. J. (1986). Family roles, preschool handicapped children, and social policy. In J. J. Gallagher & P. M. Vietze (Eds.), *Families of handicapped persons: Research, programs, and policy issues* (pp. 261–272). Baltimore: Brookes.

Wasserman, R. (1983). Identifying the counseling needs of the siblings of mentally retarded children. *Personnel Guidance Journal, 61,* 622–627.

Wayment, H. A., & Zetlin, A. G. (1989). Coping responses of adolescents with and without mild learning handicaps. *Mental Retardation, 27,* 311–316.

Webb-Mitchell, B. (1993). Hope in despair: The importance of religious stories for families with children with disabilities. In J. L. Paul & R. J. Simeonsson (Eds.), *Children with special needs: Family, culture, and society* (pp. 97–110). Fort Worth, TX: Harcourt Brace Jovanovich.

Weinberg, J. K. (1988). Autonomy as a different voice: Women, disabilities, and decisions. In M. Fine & A. Asch (Eds.), *Women with disabilities: Essays in psychology, culture, and politics* (pp. 269–296). Philadelphia: Temple University Press.

Weir, R. F. (1984). *Selective non-treatment of handicapped newborns.* London: Oxford University Press.

Weisz, J. R. (1990). Cultural-familial mental retardation: A developmental perspective on cognitive performance and "helpless" behavior. In R. M. Hodapp, J. A. Burack, & E. Zigler (Eds.), *Issues in the developmental approach to mental retardation* (pp. 137–168). Cambridge: Cambridge University Press.

Wells, C. (1989). "Otherwise kill me": Marginal children and ethics at the edges of existence. In R. Lee & D. Morgan (Eds.), *Birthrights: Law and ethics at the beginnings of life* (pp. 195–217). New York: Routledge.

Wendell, S. (1989). Toward a feminist theory of disability. *Hypatia, 4*, 104–124.

Wendell, S. (1992). Feminist theory of disability. In H. B. Holmes & L. M. Purdy (Eds.), *Feminist perspectives in medical ethics* (pp. 63–81). Bloomington: Indiana University Press.

West, R. (1990). Taking freedom seriously. *Harvard Law Review, 104*, 84–85.

Whatley, M. (1992). Goals for sex-equitable sexuality education. In S. S. Klein (Ed.), *Sex equity and sexuality in education* (pp. 83–96). Albany: State University of New York Press.

Wheeless, C. (1975). Abdominal hysterectomy for surgical sterilization in the mentally retarded: A review of parental opinion. *American Journal of Obstetrics and Gynecology, 122*, 872–875.

Whitcraft, C. J., & Jones, J. P. (1974). A survey of attitudes about sterilization of retardates. *Mental Retardation, 12*, 30.

Wikler, L. (1981). Chronic stresses of families of mentally retarded children. *Family Relations, 30*, 281–288.

Winton, P. J., & Bailey, D. B. (1993). In J. L. Paul & R. J. Simeonsson (Eds.), *Children with special needs: Family, culture, and society* (pp. 210–230). Fort Worth, TX: Harcourt Brace Jovanovich.

Wiseman, L. (1979). Beyond the sixty-second solution. In R. Wiegerink & J. W. Pelosi (Eds.), *Developmental disabilities: The DD movement* (pp. 91–96). Baltimore: Brookes.

Wolf, L., & Zarfas, D.E. (1982). Parents' attitudes toward sterilization of their mentally retarded children. *American Journal of Mental Deficiency, 87*, 122–129.

Wolfe, A. (1989). *Whose keeper: Social science and moral obligation.* Berkeley: University of California Press.

Wolfensberger, W. (1974). *The principle of normalization in human services.* Toronto: National Institute on Mental Retardation.

Wolfensberger, W. (1992). *A guideline on protecting the health and lives of patients in hospitals, especially if the patient is a member of a societally devalued class.* New York: Syracuse University Training Institute.

Wolfson, I. N. (1956). Follow-up studies of 92 males and 131 female patients who were discharged from the Newark State School in 1946. In M. Rosen, G. R. Clark, & M. S. Kivitz (Eds.), *The history of mental retardation: Collected papers* (Vol. 2, pp. 277–298). Baltimore: University Park Press.

Wolhandler, J., & Weber, R. (1992). Abortion. In Boston Women's Health Book Collective, *The new our bodies, ourselves* (pp. 353–385). New York: Simon & Schuster.

Wood, S. (1988). Parents: Whose partners? In L. Barton (Ed.), *The politics of special education needs* (pp. 190–207). London: Falmer.

Wright, B. A. (Ed.). (1959). *Psychology and rehabilitation.* Washington, DC: Psychological Association.

Wright, B. A. (1988). Attitudes and the fundamental negative bias: Conditions and corrections. In H. E. Yuker (Ed.), *Attitudes toward persons with disabilities* (pp. 3–21). New York: Springer.

Wyatt v. Stickney, 344 F. Supp. 373, 344 F. Supp. 387 (M. D. Ala. 1972).

Yalnizyan, A. (1988). Economic recovery and labour market adjustment in Canada. *Perception, 12,* 14–18.

Yuker, H. E. (Ed.). (1988). *Attitudes toward persons with disabilities.* New York: Springer.

Yura, M. T., & Zuckerman, L. (1979). *Raising the exceptional child.* New York: Hawthorn.

Zarit, S. H., & Pearlin, L. I. (1993). Family caregiving: Integrating informal and formal systems for care. In S.H. Zarit, L. I. Pearlin, & K. W. Schaie (Eds.), *Caregiving systems: Formal and informal helpers* (pp. 303–316). Hillsdale, NJ: Lawrence Erlbaum.

Zetlin, A. G., & Hosseini, A. (1989). Six postschool case studies of mildly learning handicapped young adults. *Exceptional Children, 55,* 405–411.

Zetlin, A. G., & Turner, J. L. (1985). Transition from adolescence to adulthood: Perspectives of mentally retarded individuals and their families. *American Journal of Mental Deficiency, 89,* 570–579.

Zetlin, A. G., Turner, J. L., & Winick, L. (1988). Socialization effects on the adult adaptation of mildly retarded persons living in the community. In S. Landesman-Dwyer & P.M. Vietze (Eds.), *Impact of residential settings on behavior* (pp. 93–120). Baltimore: University Park Press.

Zetlin, A. G., Weisner, T. S., & Gallimore, R. (1985). Diversity, shared functioning and the role of parenting by retarded persons. In S.K. Thurman (Ed.), *Children of handicapped parents* (pp. 69–95). New York: Academic Press.

Zill, N. & Schoenborn, C. A. (1990). Developmental, learning, and emotional problems: Health of our nation's children. *Advance Data, 190*, 1–20.

Zussman, L., Zussman, S., Sunley, R., & Bjornson, E. (1981). Sexual response after hysterectomy-oophorectomy: Recent studies and reconsideration of psychogenesis. *American Journal of Obstetrics and Gynecology, 140*, 725–728.

Index

Abbott, P., 3, 6, 12
ABCX Family Crisis Model, 71, 72. *See also* Hill, R.
Abortion, 13, 37, 58, 77, 100, 110, 166, 197; among minors, 26, 76–77; of defective fetuses, 43; forced, 13, 44; opposition to, 45, 59; restrictions of, 58, 197; therapeutic, 42
Abuse: charges, 123; child, 10–11, 62, 155; by people with mental disabilities, 19, 45, 92–94, 96, 135, 151, 155; of people with mental disabilities, 19, 60–61
Abusive parents, 44–45, 92–94, 135
Acquired Immune Deficiency Syndrome, 49, 51, 57–58; incidence among mentally disabled, 57
Adaptive behavior, xix, 200; scales, xix, 200
Adjustment. *See* Community adjustment
Adoption: of children of people with mental disabilities, 93, 110, 150–151, 154–156, 179; of disabled children, 11, 75, 82, 100
Adult Protective Services, 120, 126, 133, 135

Advance directive, 35
Advocacy, 60, 139; campaigns, xxi, 20–21; positions, 19, 60
Affect, 111, 143–144, 168–169; importance of, 30, 111, 161, 163–167
Agency: determination of, xxv; personnel, 85; policy, xxiii-xxiv, 33, 94; unwritten, xxv
Agency for International Development, 54
Aid to Families with Dependent Children, 152
American Association on Mental Retardation, xix
Americans with Disabilities Act, 20, 58
Amniocentesis, 42
Andersen, H.F., xvii, xxv, 32–35
Anderson, In re, 25
Andron, L., 9, 12, 79, 90, 92, 95
Asch, A., 39, 43, 74–75, 81–82
Attitudes: of care providers, xxiii-xxv, 7, 12, 63, 78, 85, 114, 128, 139; change, xxiv; toward homosexuals, xxiv; inventories, xxiv; toward impoverished people 12, 15; toward minorities, 28; of parents, 67, 72, 186; toward people with

About the Author

ELLEN BRANTLINGER is Associate Professor in the School of Education, Indiana University. She has published widely on the topics in this book.

ISBN 0-86569-225-4